The Ethic of Care: A Moral Compass for Canadian Nursing Practice (Revised Edition)

Authored by

Kathleen Stephany

Faculty of Health Sciences, Douglas College, BC, Canada

The Ethic of Care: A Moral Compass for Canadian Nursing Practice

Author: Kathleen Stephany

ISBN (Online): 978-981-14-3963-6

ISBN (Print): 978-981-14-3961-2

need for a court order if at any point you breach any terms of this License Agreement. In no event will any delay or failure by Bentham Science Publishers in enforcing your compliance with this License Agreement constitute a waiver of any of its rights.

3. You acknowledge that you have read this License Agreement, and agree to be bound by its terms and conditions. To the extent that any other terms and conditions presented on any website of Bentham Science Publishers conflict with, or are inconsistent with, the terms and conditions set out in this License Agreement, you acknowledge that the terms and conditions set out in this License Agreement shall prevail.

Bentham Science Publishers Pte. Ltd.
80 Robinson Road #02-00
Singapore 068898
Singapore
Email: subscriptions@benthamscience.net

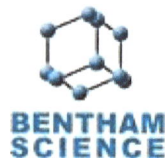

CONTENTS

FOREWORD

"Nurses support oppression when they actively participate in oppression; deny or ignore oppression; or recognize oppression but take no action. Noticing or witnessing oppression, and taking the moral stance that it is none of our business, or that it is someone else's responsibility to speak up, is the same as not doing anything in the face of need – silence is assent."[1]

Ethics, as a discipline and as an intellectual pursuit, has existed for thousands of years and has sought to resolve questions on human morality. Health care professionals are faced with uniquely complex ethical questions every day on continuously evolving topics such as the withdrawal of treatment, medical assistance in dying, resource allocation, the use of substances, and reproductive rights and technologies. Being equipped with an understanding of ethics is crucial in providing nurses with the needed skills to speak up when they encounter ethical situations, and to work collaboratively toward a resolution with the client and their family at the center of the health care team.

Nurses work in wide variety of areas beyond acute care settings, including in the community, long term care, assisted living facilities, forensic systems, and postsecondary institutions. A study of nursing of ethics is not only critical in equipping nurses to understand their own perspectives, but also in respecting and understanding the perspectives of others who may differ from their own. Working collaboratively requires a team that can clearly communicate and articulate their roles and viewpoints. This, in turn, enhances the quality of care provided, helps to improve client outcomes, and increases job satisfaction for health care providers (Weiss, Tilin, & Morgan, 2018).

I have been fortunate to work in a number of clinical areas both within Canada and overseas. Before embarking on a graduate degree in nursing, I distinctly remember the early years I spent practicing as a nurse in various clinical areas, and the moral questions that would keep me awake at night. A few years ago, I slowly began to realize the impacts of trauma and violence on physical, mental and emotional health and how these health effects can be compounded by poverty, oppression, stigma, racism, substance use, as well as pervasive systemic violence. As a nurse, I found myself becoming more and more uneasy by the labeling and stigmatization of patients, and particularly of women seeking pain treatment who were dismissed as "drug-seekers." It was my frustration and confusion with this very term, and my gradual awareness of the harmful discourses that are deeply embedded and normalized within health care practice environments (Doane & Varcoe, 2015) that became the catalysts in my pursuit of graduate studies. I completed my MSN degree exploring women's pain experiences in relation to pressing health concerns and the need for creating culturally safe environments for clients, families and health care providers alike. In my graduating project, I made several recommendations for nursing education, health care, and research that asked nurses to engage with other key stakeholders in addressing the ethics of adequate pain treatment and assessment while exploring the unique circumstances and experiences of Indigenous women as a case in point (Heino, 2018). Nurses have both the opportunity and an ethical responsibility to provide the best quality of care possible and to ensure all individuals feel safe and respected, especially when they are at their most vulnerable.

To become a nurse is to embark on a lifelong learning journey requiring openness, humility and the ability to embrace the inherent complexity of the health care system and of relationships. Health care providers are shaped by their knowledge, experiences, and their interactions with clients and with members of the health care team. Given the emerging societal awareness of the necessity of embracing diversity and inclusion, it is critical that nursing students and nurses to engage in ongoing reflection throughout their education and beyond, so that they continually unpack their own assumptions as they provide care. Bias can be both conscious and unconscious, and it can influence clinical decision making in ways that can have profound impacts on patient outcomes (Pauly & Browne, 2015; Persaud, 2019). It can take great moral courage to have the self-awareness to continually self-evaluate and self-assess as we journey toward understanding and change.

When the author of this book asked me to contribute the foreword, I was delighted and I was greatly encouraged to see how the elements of dignity, trust, and respect are front and center throughout. Her writing resonates with many of my own experiences. Dr. Stephany has a distinguished set of qualifications, knowledge, and experience as a nurse, psychologist, educator, ethicist and author that uniquely qualify her to speak about the practice of applied ethics in nursing. Throughout her book, she provides research and specific examples to help bring the concepts and ideas she explores within its pages to life. While many of us come into nursing knowing about ethics on some level, being given the language with which to understand these ideas is crucial in defining nursing to ourselves and to the people with whom we collaborate. Throughout the chapters, there are boxes and tables that highlight especially useful and salient information such as definitions, narratives and cases in point that assist the reader in integrating the concepts with actual clinical practice. In my experience as an educator, giving students such examples to consider and work through is a powerful learning tool that helps to consolidate learning and prepare students for what they might encounter in their practice.

Technological advancements and shifting societal norms and values are changing the landscape of the health care system. Nurses have a duty and a responsibility to continually reflect on their practice using an ethical model throughout their professional careers (Canadian Nurses Association, 2017). The inevitable ethical situations that arise in everyday nursing practice can have enormous implications for clients and families. Having the skills and tools to navigate the uncertainty of these waters can mean the difference between life, and death, for clients who place their trust in the health care team. A solid footing in ethics can guide nurses in their decision-making and help them to become key contributors, and leaders, in this process. This book will serve the reader well on their journey in developing into a thoughtful, ethical and compassionate practitioner. It is a must-read for students and clinicians alike.

NOTES

[1]McGibbon, Mulaudzi, Didham, Barton & Sochan, 2014, p. 187.

REFERENCES

Canadian Association of Nursing (2017). Code of Ethics for Registered Nurses. https://www.cna-aiic.ca/~/media/cna/page-content/pdf-en/code-of-ethics-2017-edition-secure-interactive

Doane G.H, Varcoe C. , . (2015). How to nurse: Relational inquiry with individuals and families in changing health and health care contexts.. Philadelphia:: Wolters Kluwer, Lippincott Williams & Wilkins;

Heino A. N. (2018, April 30). Toward a better understanding of the chronic pain experiences of Indigenous women who experience violence: Implications for nursing education, practice and research [G]. doi:http://dx.doi.org/10.14288/1.0365526.

McGibbon E, Mulaudzi F.M, Didham P, Barton S, Sochan A. [http://dx.doi.org/10.1111/nin.12042] [PMID: 23837570] (2014). Toward decolonizing nursing: The colonization of nursing and strategies for increasing the counter-narrative. Nursing Inquiry, 21(3), 179-191.

Pauly B.B, McCall J, Browne A.J, Parker J, Mollison A. [http://dx.doi.org/10.1097/ANS.0000000000000070] [PMID: 25932819] (2015) Toward cultural safety: Nurse and patient perceptions of illicit substance use in a hospitalized setting. Advances in Nursing Science, 38(2), 121-133.

Persaud S. [http://dx.doi.org/10.1097/NAQ.0000000000000348] [PMID: 30839450] (2019). Addressing unconscious bias: A nurse leader's role. Nurs Admin Q, 43(2), 130-137.

Weiss D, Tilin F, Morgan M. , . (2018). The interprofessional health care team: Leadership and development, 2nd ed. Burlington, MA: Jones & Bartlett Learning.

Angela Heino
New Westminster,
British Columbia

PREFACE

"We do not live as isolated fragments, completely separate, but as parts of a great, dynamic, mutable whole." Sharon Salzberg, Author of Lovingkindness: The Revolutionary Art of Happiness.

The ethic of care is the moral imperative to act justly. It is built on the premise that we are all interconnected, that humans are inherently good and that our relationships to one another matter. The ethic of care inspires us to honour and respect the lived experiences of others and to do whatever we can to end suffering, discrimination and social injustice. It has been greater than 37 years since the ethic of care began to inform moral decision making in nursing and it continues to be as valid today as it was back then. For example, today's nurses face new ethical challenges due to the way in which health care delivery is implemented. There is an increased use of technology, heavier workloads and advances in the way in which disease processes are managed. Yet, when compared with other health professionals, nurses are still the ones who spend a great deal of time in direct contact with clients. Nurses do much more than give medications and perform treatments. They stay at the bedside, listen to their clients' stories, empathize, give comfort and advocate. The aim of this book is to inspire nurses to be as skillful, and compassionate as they can be so that they will leave every encounter with their clients, better than when they first arrived.

In this book the following topics are covered with clarity and depth: caring notions, moral principles, the CNA Code of Ethics, legal issues, values clarification, professionalism, accountability, advocacy, gender issues, spirituality, challenges created by the advancement of technology and matters pertaining to social justice. Practical tools for ethical decision-making are offered to assist nurses to effectively deal with sorting through actual ethical dilemmas and moral distress. Nurses are encouraged to sincerely and wholeheartedly embrace diversity including the multiplicity of issues that relate to ethnicity, culture and gender. Worthy goals are recommended such as working toward achieving sustainability in the Canadian publicly funded health care system and ending social inequities. At the end of each chapter a Case in Point brings the subject of ethics to life and serves as a means for applying newly acquired ethical knowledge. Within some of the Chapters narratives will also sometimes be utilized to help elucidate specific explanations. Narratives are real situations and encourage an inductive process where a person can examine the notions of morality that are embedded in the story (Keatings & Smith, 2016).[1]

Changes to the Revised Edition

The revised edition of *The Ethic of Care: A Moral Compass for Canadian Nursing Practice* differs from the original textbook in several ways. Many of the quotes and pictures are new and the book is reformatted to be more accessible and easily read on hand-held devices. Outdated information has been corrected, new information added, and some of the material contained in the previous book has been condensed. Learning activities, new narratives, recommended readings and web resources have also been added.

Overview of New Additions to the Chapters

Each Chapter in this revised book includes exciting new content. Chapter One forms the foundation for everything else that follows and has been expanded upon significantly. A section on biomedical ethical theories has been included. The origins of the ethic of care has been more fully developed. Watson's (2008) caritas dimensions for healing are presented followed by dynamic strategies to practice unconditional positive regard. Chapter Two focusses on moral principles and care. The topic of moral courage is intensified which includes identifying its key attributes.

The legal portion of Chapter Three contains a summary of exceptions for the duty to maintain confidentiality. Part I of the newly revised version of the Canadian Nurses Association (CNA) Code of Ethics (2017) is presented with attention to additional content such as, the nurse's role in end of life care and medical assistance in dying (MAID). Chapter Four emphasizes the importance of values clarification and includes strategies to facilitate empathetic listening and to enhance self-care.

Chapter Five introduces tools for moral decision making in nursing in the form of a model and framework. In the first edition of this textbook nurses were presented with one model for ethical decision making, *The Mosaic Model for Ethical Decisions* (Stephany, 2012). This revised edition includes that tool but in a very condensed and easy to use form. *A Framework for Ethical Decision Making* has been added as an additional resource (Oberle & Bouchal, 2009). This framework has been added because it is applicable in many venues and it is highly recommended by the CNA Code of Ethics (2017).

Chapter Six combines professionalism and accountability to inspire nurses to act responsibly. Redundant information has been removed and the bulk of the content is focused on the ethical responsibilities expected of nurses. Chapter Seven promotes advocacy as the heart of nursing. The focus includes ethical endeavours that protect public access to health care and actions that promote social justice. Chapter Eight explores how constantly changing technological advances can enhance healthcare delivery but create new moral situations for nurses that keep changing. Chapter Nine encourages nurses to whole-heartedly embrace diversity and to practice trauma-informed care to combat systemic racism and improve the health outcomes for Indigenous peoples [2] (Allan & Smylie, 2015; First Nations Health Authority (FNHA), 2016). A new Code of Conduct for inclusion is also proposed for nursing.

Chapter Ten deals with the somewhat sensitive subject matter of ethics, gender and sexual orientation. The goal is to encourage nurses to move beyond tolerance and to accept and respect life choices that differ from their own. The discussion highlights the fact that persons who identify as lesbian, gay, bisexual, transgender, queer or questioning their sexual identity, and 2 spirit (LGBTQ2S), are often victims of both acute and chronic trauma. Members of this population are also not very well understood or treated well by health professionals. Additional education and training are key to changing some of these factors.

Chapter Eleven covers the topic of spirituality in nursing and very little has been changed in this edition. Chapter Twelve is completely new and introduces the topic of ethical nursing leadership where nurses are inspired to take on the challenge of being agents for change.

NOTES

[1]Note: The details of all the Cases in Point, stories and narratives in this textbook have been altered sufficiently to ensure confidentiality.

[2]Note: In this textbook "Indigenous" is used as an inclusive and international term to describe individuals and collectives who consider themselves as being related to and/or having historical continuity with "First Peoples," whose civilizations in what is now known as Canada, the United States, the Americas, the Pacific Islands, New Zealand, Australia, Asia, and Africa predate those of subsequent invading or colonizing populations (Allan & Smylie, 2015, p. 3).

REFERENCES

Allan B, Smylie J. (2015). *First Peoples, second class treatment: The role of racism in the health and well-being of Indigenous peoples in Canada.* Toronto: OntarioThe Wellesley Institute. http://www.wellesl eyinstitute.com/wp-content/uploads/2015/02/Summary-First-Peoples- Second-Clas--Treatment-Final.pdf

Canadian Nurses Association (CNA. (2017). *CNA Code of Ethics for Registered Nurses* (Revised Edition). Ottawa: Author

First Nations Health Authority (FNHA) (2017). *Creating a climate for change: Cultural safety and humility in health services delivery for First Nations and Aboriginal Peoples in British Columbia (BC).* BC: Author http://www.fnha.ca/Documents/ FNHA-Creating-a-Climate-For-Change-Cultural-H-mility-Resource-Booklet.pdf

Keatings M, Smith O.B. (2016). *Ethical & legal issues in Canadian nursing* (Kindle ed.). Canada: Saunders

Oberle K, Bouchal S.R. (2009). *Ethics in Canadian nursing practice.* Toronto: Pearson

Watson J. (2008). *Nursing: The philosophy of caring (Revised edition).* Boulder, Colorado University Press of Colorado

Kathleen Stephany
Full Time Nurse Educator in the Faculty of Health Sciences,
Douglas College,
BC,
Canada

ACKNOWLEDGEMENTS

I want to extend heartfelt gratitude to all my former nursing students. You forever inspire me to be my best and to role model what it means to practice the ethic of care. I am grateful to my beloved husband, Harold for always encouraging me to write about the topics that I care most about. To my children, Connie, Kent, Kim and Nathan and my daughter-in-law, Renee, thank-you for your love and loyalty. To my darling grand-daughters, Kaileia and Kamiah, I dedicate this book to you. Thank-you Bentham Science Publishing for publishing this new edition.

CONFLICT OF INTEREST

The author confirms that the contents of this ebook have no conflict of interest.

Kathleen Stephany
Full Time Nurse Educator in the Faculty of Health Sciences,
Douglas College,
BC,
Canada

ABOUT THE AUTHOR

Dr. Kathleen Stephany PhD, is a Registered Nurse (RN) and Psychologist. She is a nurse educator, author, ethicist, ethic of care theorist, suicidologist and motivational speaker. Kathleen has a PhD in Counselling Psychology. She also obtained a MA in Counselling Psychology from Simon Fraser University (SFU), a BA in Psychology from SFU, a BSN from the University of Victoria and a Diploma in Nursing from the British Columbia Institute of Technology (BCIT). Kathleen is a practicing RN with the BC College of Nursing Professionals (BCCNP) and a Certified Counsellor with the Canadian Counselling & Psychotherapy Association (CCPA). Kathleen is also a member of many other professional associations: the Xia Eta Chapter of Sigma Theta Tau International, Honor Society of Nursing; the Western Northern Region of Canadian Association of Schools of Nursing; the International Association for Suicide Prevention (IASP); the Canadian Association for Suicide Prevention (CASP); and the Canadian Mental Health Association (CMH). Kathleen has a diverse employment history. She previously worked as a critical care nurse, Coroner, psychiatric nurse clinician, psychotherapist and researcher. Kathleen is currently employed as a Full-time Faculty Member in Health Sciences at Douglas College in BC, where she teaches nursing students courses in applied nursing ethics, mental health and addictions. She is also a motivational speaker. When she is not teaching, writing or doing public speaking, she enjoys reading, gardening, cooking and spending time with family.

DEDICATION

To my beloved grand-daughters, Kaileia and Kamiah, may you always remember to be caring and compassionate toward everyone.

CHAPTER 1

The Ethic of Care: Our Moral Compass

Abstract: Chapter One forms the foundation for everything that follows. The ethic of care, or the moral imperative to act justly, is presented as a moral compass to guide nurses when making ethical choices. Nurses are inspired to adopt the ethic of care into their practice and into their everyday lives as a lived virtue. Ethics is defined. A brief overview of the philosophical ethical theories of utilitarianism and deontology are presented followed by an explanation of the origins of the ethic of care. A connection is drawn between the ethic of care and the theoretical premises of feminism, humanism and phenomenology because they all pay attention to the contextual features of people's lives. The ethic of justice is compared with the ethic of care. A supported argument is made that the ethic of care is still valid for today's nurses. Watson's caritas dimensions of healing practice are presented. It was revealed that Florence Nightingale was a strong proponent of virtue ethics, which laid the foundation for the ethic of care. Special attention is given to specific multifaceted concepts associated with care as demonstrated by three theorists: Mayerhoff, Perlman & Stephany. The Chapter ends with a Case in Point where a student nurse is assigned the challenging task of caring for a client diagnosed with a catatonic type of schizophrenia.

Keywords: Acceptance, Act utilitarianism, Applied nursing ethics, Act deontology, Autonomy, Alternating rhythms, Beneficence, Caritas, Categorical imperatives, Consequentialism, Caring, Courage, Caring-concern, Compassion, Distributive justice, Deontology, Esthetics, Ethic of care, Ethic of justice, Ethics, Empathy, Feminism, Florence Nightingale, Genuineness, Generosity, Hypothetical imperatives, Honesty, Humanism, Humility, Hope, Justice, Kantianism, Knowledge, Logic, Maxim, Morals, Metaphysics, Morality, Nightingale, Narratives, Non-maleficence, Presencing, Politics, Philosophy, Principlism, Phenomenology, Patience, Rule utilitarianism, Rule deontology, Trustworthy, Unconditional Positive Regard, Utilitarianism, Virtue ethics, Warmth.

LEARNING GUIDE

After Completing this Chapter, the Reader Should be Able to

* Define ethics.

Kathleen Stephany
All rights reserved-© 2020 Bentham Science Publishers

* Gain a brief understanding of the philosophical ethical theories of utilitarianism & deontology along with their key premises and differing emphasis.

* Describe what distributive justice consists of.

* Explain the focus of applied nursing ethics.

* Define the ethic of care.

* Understand the historical underpinning of the ethic of care.

* Draw a connection between the ethic of care, feminist philosophy, humanism and phenomenology.

* Be able to compare the ethic of justice and the ethic of care.

* Explain why the ethic of care is still valid for today's nurses.

* Identify each of Watson's caritas dimensions of healing practice that cultivate caring.

* Understand the connection between Florence Nightingale, virtue ethics and the ethic of care.

* Illustrate each of the multifaceted concepts that are associated with care as presented by Mayerhoff (1971), Perlman (1979) & Stephany (2007).

* Be able to give examples of how each of the multifaceted concepts of care are demonstrated in nursing practice.

* Apply the ethic of care to the Case in Point: Presencing & Care.

INTRODUCTION

"Conscience is a man's compass." Vincent Van Gogh, famous Post Impressionist painter

Chapter one offers a brief introduction to ethics, traditional philosophical ethical theories and applied nursing ethics. The ethic of care is presented from a historical perspective and compared with the ethic of justice, followed by a discussion of multi-faceted aspects of care and how they are played out in the actions of nurses.

What exactly is a compass? (Fig. **1.1**). A compass is a device that was used by ancient sailors as well as modern seafarers alike, to assist in navigating the correct course, especially when lost at sea. The compass points to the North Star and once you know where this star is located you can find your way home. A moral compass acts in a similar fashion. It helps us to plot a course of right action when we do not know how to proceed. Nurses, not unlike sailors, sometimes need assistance in knowing how to navigate their way, not through waterways, but through the many ethical issues that arise in practice. The **ethic of care**, which is the moral imperative to act justly, acts as a moral guide for nurses. The ethic of care takes into consideration contextual factors, the subjectivity of human experience, the need for human connection and emphasizes the importance of relationships (Watson, 2008; Wood, 2011). The ethic of care also prioritizes the nurse's ability to respond to their clients' needs (Watson, 2008).

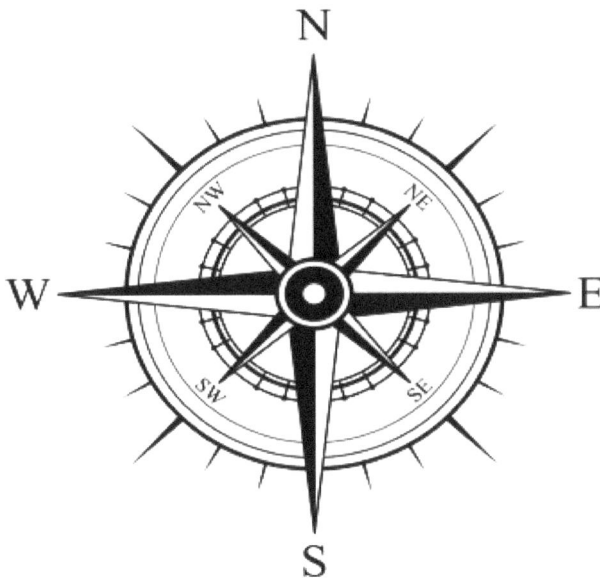

Fig. (1.1). Compass. Source: www.pixabay.com.

This book is unique and different from other ethics textbooks in several ways. Traditionally, ethics in health care has been approached through a rule orientated focus. However, this ethical approach has been criticized as not being very well suited to the unique role that nurses play (Gilligan, 1982). Nurses are in a somewhat unique position when compared to other health professionals. They are the ones who spend the most time with their clients in the hospital setting and even in the community. Therefore, the subject matter of this book is less concerned with philosophical underpinnings associated with traditional ethical theories and places greater emphasis on the actual practice of applied nursing ethics. In this revised edition, just like in the original version, nurses are encouraged to embody the ethic of care as a lived virtue.

Ethics

Ethics falls under the discipline of **Philosophy,** which studies the fundamental nature of knowledge and is dedicated to the pursuit of truth (Durant, 1961). Philosophy critically evaluates human beliefs and assumptions about the world and life, and philosophers ask questions, such as, *"Why are we here?"* According to Durant (1961) philosophy includes five areas of inquiry: logic, esthetics, politics, metaphysics and ethics. **Logic** is involved with research while **esthetics** studies beauty. **Politics** is concerned with social organization and the dynamics of power. **Metaphysics** focuses on perception and knowledge and the surreal or the ultimate reality of all things (Durant, 1961). **Ethics** is the study of moral conduct or the right and noble action of groups and how we all should ideally act (Bjarnason & LaSala, 2011). For example, ethics focusses on issues related to social values that include the importance of respecting life and protecting freedom (Burkhardt, Nathaniel & Walton, 2015). Words like, *ought, should, right, wrong, good, and bad*, are often associated with ethics (Burkhardt *et al.*, 2015).

Since ethics is concerned with right conduct it is also closely aligned with terms referred to as morals or morality. There is however, a notable distinction between these terms. **Morals** and **Morality** have been more readily associated with the good or bad thoughts and actions of individuals and have been traditionally aligned with religious views (Smith, 2017). **Ethics** is more concerned with moral values and the humanitarian duty as it pertains to a group or society, and is not affiliated with religion (Smith, 2017). However, in this current book the terms ethics, morals and morality will be used interchangeably.

PHILOSOPHICAL ETHICAL THEORIES: A BASIC OVERVIEW

It is beyond the scope of this textbook to delve into ethical theories that differ from the ethic of care in depth. However, due to their historical significance, it is important for nurses to have at least a basic understanding of some traditional philosophical ethical theories. Therefore, the following two competing ethical theories will be briefly discussed: utilitarianism and deontology.

UTILITARIANISM

Utilitarianism is a moral theory that is concerned with outcomes and an action is considered good or bad in relation to the result of that activity. This theory is not in any way concerned with the morality of the person who is performing the act. Utilitarianism dates back as far as 200 – 300 B.C.E. but it gained notoriety among the eighteenth and nineteenth century philosophers (Burkhardt *et al.*, 2015). Jeremy Bentham (1748 – 1832) was a popular political philosopher and considered to be the parent of modern-day utilitarianism. Bentham declared that any action is judged as good if it gives us pleasure, happiness or decreases misery. Alternatively, any act is considered bad if it causes us suffering or pain (Bosek & Savage, 2007; Burkhardt *et al.*, 2015). What is considered morally right is simply what is regarded most highly in value by human beings (Ford, 2006). Since utilitarianism focuses on the end result or consequences of an action, this theory is also often referred to as **Consequentialism** (Xu & Ma, 2016).

Many of the notions derived from utilitarianism also directly or indirectly influence decision making concerning individuals in medical venues (Bosek & Savage, 2007; Ford, 2006). For example, some of the ethical dilemmas encountered in the medical setting can be associated with people's happiness. Quality of life is determined by an individual's conception of what is worthwhile and what is intolerable. However, one's perception of what consists of quality of life often changes when health challenges occur. Similarly, issues of withdrawing or withholding treatment can be viewed as a way to end suffering (Bosek & Savage, 2007).

Act Utilitarianism *versus* Rule Utilitarianism

There is more than one utilitarian viewpoint in how to best address moral issues. **Act Utilitarianism** applies the pleasure criteria where an individual judges the moral status of each action by its consequences (Ford, 2006). An act utilitarian believes that tenets should not be rigidly followed and should only be used as guidelines. They do not believe in the application of strict rules for decision-making (Burkhardt *et al.*, 2013). An act utilitarian will allow diverse and even somewhat opposing actions in different situations (Burkhardt *et al.*, 2015). For example, although they believe that telling the truth is best, they realize that there are certain circumstances when telling the truth may cause harm. This type of incidence can occur when a family member conveys that if the client is informed that they have cancer, they will give up, refuse all treatment and die. In this sort of situation an act utilitarianist would agree that it would be better for everyone concerned, the client and the family, if the guideline of truth telling is not followed.

However, in rule utilitarianism withholding the truth is not acceptable. In **rule utilitarianism** the moral status of general rules of conduct are evaluated by judging the possible consequences if everyone is expected to behave according to the same moral rules (Ford, 2006). People are expected to act according to specific rules in order to maximize happiness and decrease unhappiness (Burkhardt *et al.*, 2015). However, a rule utilitarian insists that people tell the truth, keep their promises, refrain from killing and follow other similar rules, in every circumstance. There are no exceptions to these rules because the overall good is believed to be maximized by consistently following these moral rules (Burkhardt *et al.*, 2015). Let's examine the previous example of not telling the truth to a cancer client because it will cause them harm. The rule utilitarian would argue that lying is wrong. Even though a certain client's situation may benefit through the act of deception, overall pervasive use of lying will inevitably cause more harm than good and that good can only be maximized if rules of truth telling are consistently followed (Burkhardt *et al.*, 2015).

Utilitarianism, Distributive Justice & Health Care Service

The political philosopher, Bentham also promoted a sort of social justice where action that is taken should ultimately increase the happiness of the community as a whole (Burkhardt *et al.*, 2015; Ford, 2006). Bentham's argument was that the greatest happiness is determined by the greatest good for the greatest number of people (Bosek & Savage, 2007). This notion is utilized in the health care setting with the distributions of medical resources (*e.g.*, the greatest number of people should get the most benefit from what medical resources arc on hand) (Ford, 2006). This method of decision making is associated with distributive justice (Burkhardt *et al.*, 2015). **Distributive justice** is concerned with the notion of fairness and requires that resources be distributed proportionately and equally, (Bosek & Savage, 2007). In the delivery of health care service, this is not always that easy to do. What health care services are considered necessary? What sort of services are expendable? How much revenue will be allocated to specific health services? What is considered to be a reasonable wait time for elective surgery? These are just a few questions that come to mind when considering an appropriate level of services that would benefit the majority of people. A utilitarian would use a material rule to decide how resources should best be allocated. Box (**1:1**).

Box 1:1. DISTRIBUTIVE JUSTICE & MATERIAL RULES (as adapted from Burkhardt *et al.*, 2015)
To each person an equal share
To each person according to need
To each person according to merit
To each person according to social contribution
To each according to the person's rights
To each person according to effort
To each person according to ability to pay
To each person according to the greater good to the greatest number

Criticisms of Utilitarianism

This Utilitarianism/Consequential ethical theory is problematic in several ways. It has been criticized as too simple and not equipped to adequately address the complexities of many real situations (Bosek & Savage, 2007). The following discussion outlines some commonly cited weaknesses of this ethical theory. First there is the matter of definitions and their subjective interpretations. It is difficult to define in an objective and concrete manner what is a good consequence. Besides, who gets to decide what is good and desirable, and under what circumstances (Bosek & Savage, 2007)?

Secondly, there is the issue of a lack of respect for the disadvantaged in society. Utilitarianism is not concerned with individuals or minority groups and what harm could occur to them in the name of the overall good for most people (Xu & Ma, 2016). Thirdly, there is the problem of focusing solely on what optimizes pleasure or happiness while excluding other moral values in decision-making (Burkhardt *et al.*, 2015). A fourth problem with this theory lies in the belief that real ethical dilemmas do not exist because in every situation, the only relevant moral consideration is that which will maximize the balance of pleasure over pain (Ford, 2006).

DEONTOLOGY

Deontology is a main challenger to utilitarianism (Bosek & Savage, 2007).

Deontology is an ethical theory that is based on the point of view that the rightness or wrongness of an act is dependent on the very nature of the act and not on its outcome or consequences (Burkhardt *et al.*, 2015). Since this book is focused on the ethic of care theory, we will not cover all deontology theories, but we will briefly touch upon act and rule deontology, Kantianism and principlism. Even though there are many types of deontology, what most forms have in common is the resolve that an action is only morally right if it conforms to a person's moral duties and obligations (Bosek & Savage, 2007; Xu & Ma, 2016). The key way specific deontological theories vary is in their view of what specific moral duties and obligations are paramount (Bosek & Savage, 2007).

How Deontology Differs from Utilitarianism

As an introduction to deontology it is beneficial to do a simple comparison of utilitarianism and deontology. For instance, when we ask the question, what makes an act right, how would a utilitarianist or deontologist answer? The utilitarianist would reply that good consequences, or nonmoral values such as happiness or utility, makes an act right, because the end justifies the means (Pojman, 2017). In contrast, the deontologist would reply to the same question differently. For them, it is not the consequences that determines what is right or wrong, but whether the action satisfies a moral obligation. The end never justifies the means in deontology (Bosek & Savage, 2007). Acting unjustly is wrong even if it will increase or maximize utility. For instance, when a person is acting as a deontologist, telling the truth and keeping promises are right even if they may cause harm (Pojman, 2017).

Act Deontology

Deontological theories can be divided into two types: act deontology and rule deontology. Act deontologists believe that because people have a conscience, they can decide what is right or wrong. In this manner, **act deontology** views each act as unique and separate. The decision to label a situation as right or wrong must be made by consulting our intuition and our choices must be also be made without the application of rules (Pojman, 2017).

One stark criticism of act deontology is that intuitive guidance between individuals many differ (Pojman, 2017). For example, what if one person believes that abortion is morally wrong and another believes that it is morally permissible? Act deontology would require that both individuals reflect deeply into their conscience to find the answer. Reason or theory cannot guide them (Pojman, 2017). It seems obvious how this may prove to be problematic.

Rule Deontology

According to Pojman (2017) most deontologists follow rule deontology. **Rule deontology** embraces the notion of universality in addition to making moral judgments, and argues that moral rules are universal. Some of the accepted collective moral rules in rule deontology would include never telling a lie, always keeping our promises, and never executing an innocent man (Pojman (2017). Although there are many forms of rule deontology the focus of the remaining discussion will be on Kantian rule deontology and principlism.

Kantian Rule Deontology: The Hypothetical Imperative & Categorical Imperative

"Live your life as though your every act were to become a universal law." Immanuel Kant, German Philosopher.

The German Philosopher, Immanuel Kant (1724 – 1804) has been esteemed by many as one of the most important philosophers of all time (Pojman, 2017). Kant is known as a rationalist who rejected the idea of using intuition to assess the morality of an act (Bosek & Savage, 2007). He believed that truth could be revealed solely through the principles of logic and reason and that is why Kant's ethics is readily associated with rule deontology (Ford, 2006; Pojman, 2017).

Kant believed that because every person is a rational human being, they are therefore capable of discerning the universal validity of rational moral principles and in order to evaluate the moral rightness of an action, one must focus on the person's intentions (Smolkin *et al.*, 2010; Ford, 2006).

Kant asserted that people act on one of the following two types of reason, hypothetical imperatives or categorical imperatives, which are readily explained by the word, "ought" (Smolkin *et al.*, 2010). **Hypothetical imperatives** are statements of what a person ought to do given the existence of a certain desire or goal (Smolkin *et al.*, 2010). Hypothetical imperatives are everyday decisions that we make in order to achieve our goals (Smolkin *et al.*, 2010). Consider the following example. If you want to pass your nursing ethics class then you ought to take notes in class and study your readings.

In contrast, **categorical imperatives** are commands that direct what a person ought to do that are associated with morality and moral maxims. According to Kant, a **maxim** is the principle behind an action (Smolkin *et al.*, 2010). A moral maxim is consistently expressed in the form of a universal command, like, *"Thou must not kill"* (Ford, 2006). One of Kant's famous categorical imperative is, *"Always act in a manner that in so doing you can will that your action become a universal principle"* (Rodney, Burgess, Phillips, McPherson & Brown, 2013, p. 60). According to a categorical imperative, a lie is immoral even if the outcome of telling a lie is in some way beneficial (Rodney *et al.*, 2013. Kant's categorical imperative directs that a maxim can be tested to decide whether its abiding principle constitutes a moral law that is in alignment with the laws of reason (Ford, 2006). Kant argued that when people act in harmony with reason, they will consistently treat others in the manner that rational human beings would want to be treated (Ford, 2006).

Criticisms of Kantianism

Kantianism is not without its critics. The question arises, can you really reduce morality to two categorical imperatives (Pojman, 2017)? To many people absolute universality also appears counter intuitive. Pojman (2017) asserts that although the categorical imperative is a way to evaluate moral principles more is needed because it leaves out necessary criteria to test what qualifies. For instance, for a principle to be judged as rational or moral it needs to be universalizable and must be applicable to everyone under similar circumstances (Pojman, 2017).

Principlism

Another form of deontology is called principlism. It is an approach that was proposed by Tom Beauchamp and James Childress (2009) as a means to address issues that arise in the practice of medicine. **Principlism** proposes that clinical decisions in medical practice be evaluated, not by philosophical theory or even moral codes of practice, but by these four moral principles: autonomy, beneficence, non-maleficence and justice (Sorell, 2010). All of these principles will be discussed more fully in Chapter two, but for the sake of their association to principlism they will be briefly defined here. **Autonomy** consists of the recognition that persons are capable of governing themselves and making decisions about their welfare (Ford, 2006). **Beneficence** is the duty to do what will benefit the client, and **non-maleficence** is an aspect of beneficence that consists of the commitment to do no harm (Burkhardt *et al.*, 2015). **Justice** is about ensuring fairness for all human beings (Ford, 2006). One criticism of principlism as proposed by Beauchamp and Childress is that it does not allow for a resolution of conflicting principles. All of the four principles are treated equally (Heinrichs, 2010).

Applied Nursing Ethics & Ways of Knowing

"Nursing encompasses an art, a humanistic orientation, a feeling for the value of the individual, and the intuitive sense of ethics, and of the appropriateness of action taken."

Myrtle Aydetolle, American Nurse, Professor and Hospital Administrator.

Applied nursing ethics is a sub-category of ethics and is more involved with the practice of nursing and less concerned with just applying philosophical rules to deal with the problems that nurses face. The practice of nursing involves at least four ways of obtaining knowledge. The first way is through empirics, or the science of nursing. The art of nursing or aesthetics is a second way. Personal knowledge in nursing is a third means of gaining understanding and ethics is the fourth mode (Collaborative Nursing Program in British Columbia (BC), 2004). Oftentimes, nurses have placed more emphasis on the empirics or science of nursing in the form of evidence-based practice and less weight on the other three ways of learning. All ways of knowing are necessary for obtaining nursing knowledge. Watson (2008) has made a strong case for caring as being all encompassing. She specifically argues that a science of caring embraces all ways of knowing, ethics, intuition, lived experience, research, art and spirituality.

THE ORIGINS OF THE ETHIC OF CARE

"In a different voice of women lies the truth of an ethic of care, the tie between relationship and responsibility, and the origins of aggression in the failure of connection." Carol Gilligan, Psychologist and Seminal Ethic of Care Theorist.

The **Ethic of care** is a special proponent of applied nursing ethics that incorporates caring and meaning making into decisions. The ethic of care emphasizes the interconnectedness of all of life, places significant importance on relationships, context and lived experiences, and values equality (Gilligan, 1982). For example, the ethic of care places the person at the center and what matters to them is important. What matters to their family is also a priority because all personal relationships are to be respected.

Many Philosophers have contributed to the theory of the ethic of care such as Aristotle, Mayerhoff (1971) and Slote (2007) (Woods, 2011). However, it was a Psychologist named Carol Gilligan (1982), who provided the impetus for the development of the ethic of care as it pertains specifically to nursing. Gilligan challenged the status quo on moral thought that had historically excluded the voice of women and their experiences (Held, 2006; Wood, 2011). For example, in her book entitled: *In a different voice: Psychological Theory and Women's Development*, Gilligan (1982) pointed out that women had repeatedly been excluded from "critical theory-building studies of psychological research" (p. 1). Furthermore, a woman's caring ways was traditionally associated with weakness (Gilligan, 1982). Subsequently, Gilligan set out to record different modes of thinking about relationships from both male and female voices by reviewing texts associated with psychology and literature (Gilligan, 1982). Gilligan referred to three studies throughout her book that she reflected upon in depth and that supported her research. The key assumption of her research was that the way in which people talk about their life experiences is of significance, the language they use to describe their experiences is relevant, as are the connections that they make with others (Gilligan, 1982). Gilligan concluded that moral knowledge that is solely derived from the application of rules and abstract principles is insufficient. Being aware of and sensing the needs of others was deemed to be as important as being able to use universalized maxims (Smolkin, Bourgeois & Findler, 2010).

Gilligan (1982) defined the concept of **care** as a web of connection and that being aware of another's need and responding to their need was crucial to caring. Gilligan asserted that care is also concerned with taking responsibility for others, a responsibility that condemns exploitation and the intentional hurting of others.

Other theorists quickly followed Gilligan and built upon her work (Fig. **1.2**). For example, Noddings (1984) in her book, *Caring: A Feminine Approach to Ethics and Moral Education*, encouraged people to act in a caring manner toward all others with genuineness and emotional sensitivity (Slote, 2007). Noddings proposed that when setting out to help another person, we must be engrossed with their experience. We must pay close attention to the other person's perspective, to the way in which they see their world, and become absorbed into their lived experiences (Slote, 2007). Noddings believed that engrossment was more than empathy. **Empathy** is the action of trying to understand what another person is experiencing, whereas, **engrossment** is the process of receiving the other person's experience into oneself (Noddings, 1984).

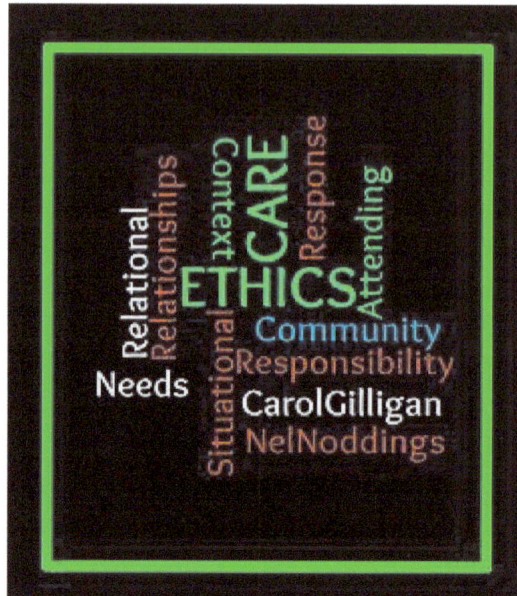

Fig. (1.2). Care Ethics. Source: www.pixabay.com.

However, Noddings (1984) did not believe that anyone could truly care for someone they did not know. Virginia Held (2006) and Michael Slote (2007) disagreed with Nodding's assertion that one could not care for a stranger. Held and Slote asserted that caring altruistically for others who are distant from our personal realm of contact, is possible in a broader form which consists of being involved in humanitarian causes. Watson (2008) also made a strong case that caring for everyone is crucial for the survival of humanity. She carefully articulated that nurses must take on a leadership role in preserving and sustaining universal caring.

During the 1990s, the beginning of the new millennia and beyond, many other theorists contributed to the dynamic dialogue about the ethic of care and its relevance. Wood (2011) pointed out that the ethic of care confirmed the main arguments that were emerging from care-based research into nursing practice. For example, research reveals that nurses value the importance of caring as a moral impetus to act, and view caring as a means to meet the needs of others through the avenue of relationships (Watson, 2008; Woods, 2011). The ethic of care "now has a central, though not exclusive place in feminine moral theorizing, and has drawn increasing interest from moral philosophers of all kinds" (Held, 2006, p. 28). Box (**1:2**).

Box 1:2. CARING AS A MORAL IMPETUS TO ACT (as adapted from Watson, 2008; Woods, 2011; Held, 2006)
Research reveals that nurses value the importance of caring as a moral impetus to act, and view caring as a means to meet the needs of others through the avenue of relationships. Subsequently, the ethic of care now has a central, though not exclusive place in feminine moral theorizing, and has drawn increasing interest from moral philosophers of all kinds.

The Ethic of Care, Feminism, Humanism & Phenomenology

Feminism

The ethic of care aligns well with many other theoretical premises which includes feminism. **Feminism** is concerned with subjectivity and the ways that politics and the establishment shape experience. It entails being involved in causes that aim to end discrimination against women and all other minorities. Since the ethic of care emphasizes relationships, context and condemns prejudicial acts, it aligns well with feminist philosophy (Watson & Marilyn, 1990; Tschudin, 2005). For instance, feminism is involved in causes that aim to end discrimination, not just against women but includes all other minorities. Modern day feminists also strive to increase our understanding of the importance of honouring personal autonomy and insist that we become more sensitive to the background circumstances that affect peoples' lives (Smolkin *et al.*, 2010).

Carl Rogers, the Forefather of Humanism & Phenomenology

"In my early professional years I was asking the question, How can I treat, cure, or change this person? Now I would phrase the question in this way: How can I provide a relationship which this person may use for his own personal growth? Carl Rogers, famous 20th Century Psychologist & forefather of Humanism & Phenomenology.

At the time that the ethic of care was introduced into nursing practice, nursing as a profession began to also personify key aspects from psychological theories such as humanism and phenomenology. Both psychological theories fit nicely into the notion of the importance of relationships and context in the realm of the ethic of caring.

Carl Rogers was a famous 20th Century American Psychologist and the forefather of both humanism and phenomenology. **Humanism** emphasizes the human capacity for goodness and places the emphasis on the whole human being with special attention being given to the personal, interpersonal and context (Monte, 1995; Schneider & Langle, 2012). It was Roger's (1951) belief that people are essentially good and that every human being has an innate tendency to grow into something better.

Phenomenology is closely tied to humanism. It is the psychological study of structures of consciousness as experienced by the person. Rogers (1951) argued that every person is at the center of their own experiences amid living in a world that is constantly changing. In this manner, phenomenology accentuates each person's uniqueness and focuses on lived experiences (Nietzel, Bernstein & Milich, 1998). Monte (1995) when describing the essence of phenomenology proposed that experience speaks for itself, and that the individual's experiences be taken as is and unfettered by research analyses and kept free from theoretical predictions.

Why are the lived experiences of clients important? Nurses need to be able to emphasize with what someone has been through. This action is the basis of building trust and rapport. In fact, Bishop and Scudder (1996) point out that the caring presence of the nurse contributes the most to achieving the therapeutic connectedness between the nurse and client.

So how does feminism, humanism and phenomenology in nursing practice bond with the ethic of care? Feminists focus closely on issues involving gender, power and social justice. Humanism accentuates the human capacity for good and for growth, and phenomenology stresses each person's uniqueness and honours lived experience. All these notions align well with the premises associated with the ethic of care because they draw attention to the important contextual features of people's lives (Fig. **1.3**).

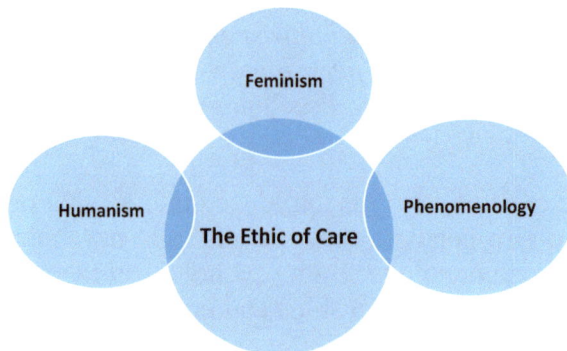

Fig. (1.3). The Ethic of Care, Feminism, Humanism & Phenomenology. Source: K. Stephany.

THE ETHIC OF CARE & THE ETHIC OF JUSTICE

The ethic of care is not without its critics. Some argue that the ethic of care is a polar opposite to the ethic of justice. I will demonstrate that the ethic of care and the ethic of justice can actually be complimentary when practiced together. The **ethic of justice** is related to distributive justice. It proposes that ethical decisions should be made by making use of universal principles and rules and that decision-making be impartial (Rawls, 1999). Furthermore, the fair and equitable treatment of everyone should be ensured (Rawls, 1999; Botes, 2000). The **ethic of care** proposes that context and subjectivity matter and prioritizes the following three processes: responding to other's needs, fostering connection and ensuring that no one gets hurt (Burkhardt *et al.*, 2015). Botes (2000) proposed that both the ethic of justice and the ethic of care are needed because if health professionals only use one of these perspectives when making ethical decisions in practice, some ethical dilemmas would be unresolved. Botes further stressed that, although rules and principles (ethic of justice), are needed to guide decisions, if the needs of clients or their voice is excluded (ethic of care), then harm may occur. Gilligan (1982) also clearly argued that the ethic of justice and the ethic of care go well together Box (**1:3**).

Box 1:3. THE ETHIC OF JUSTICE & THE ETHIC OF CARE (Gilligan, 1982, p. 174)
While an ethic of justice proceeds from the premise of equality – that everyone be treated the same – an ethic of care rests on the premise of nonviolence – that no one should be hurt.

The Case for the Ethic of Care

Critics of the ethic of care argue that not all relationships require attending to. They assert that morality ought to be concerned with more than just relationships and that principles are necessary when dealing with conflicting relationships (Smolkin *et al.*, 2010). Others contend that one should apply principles to help decide which relationship should take priority, or which one needs to be attended to first and so forth (Smolkin *et al.*, 2010). To argue that the ethic of care is somewhat inadequate to deal with moral issues in nursing, and that it does not apply moral principles to deal with conflicting relationships, leaves the impression that one may not fully grasp the rich scope and magnitude of this dynamic applied theory. The ethic of care not only acts as a guiding moral compass, but it takes into consideration many other factors within the milieu of relationships. What will be made evident in this book is that multifaceted components of care, sound moral principles and the values and ethical responsibilities as laid out by the CNA Code of Ethics for Registered Nurses (2017) are drawn upon to inform decision-making. It is within this juxtaposed framework that the ethic of care is utilized to assist nurses with the many moral challenges that they face in the clinical setting.

Is the Ethic of Care Still Valid for Today's Nursing Practice?

"It is entirely possible to claim that the use of the ethic of care is not only desirable within nursing practice but also that, overall, it continues to guide both the moral ideals and ethically focused practice of competent and committed nurses." Martin Woods, Nurse Educator & Ethicist

Is the ethic of care still valid in today's nursing practice? (Fig. **1.4**). I believe that the answer to that question is a resounding, *"Yes."* **Ontology** is defined as the study of the basic nature of human beings (Stephany, 2007). Jean Watson (2008) proposed that a caring science perspective rests upon a foundation of relational ontology of being, relationship and a world view of unity and connectedness. Watson also strongly believed that caring is the essence of nursing. To be a nurse is to care and for many of us, the reason we became a nurse is to care for others. As Woods (2011) so poignantly points out, in the practice of nursing, an ethic of care is an all-embracing moral response that is as much an integral part of nursing as any other aspect of the profession. For example, although important, conventional science in and of itself, is insufficient to inform nurses on how to best deal with being confronted with the suffering and loss faced by their clients. More is needed and that something more is our capacity to care.

Care as a Foundation for Nursing

Care, as a core foundation for the profession of nursing, also informs our practice in many ways (Watson, 2008). For example, our ability to care for others as a nurse includes science but also resides in an environment that honours our humanity and all that being human encompasses (Watson, 2008). Furthermore, the ethic of care enhances a nurse's ability to genuinely respond to clients' vulnerabilities (Woods, 2011). In this manner, responding to the specific needs of clients and being sensitive to their experiences is a key aspect of exceptional nursing practice (Woods, 2011).

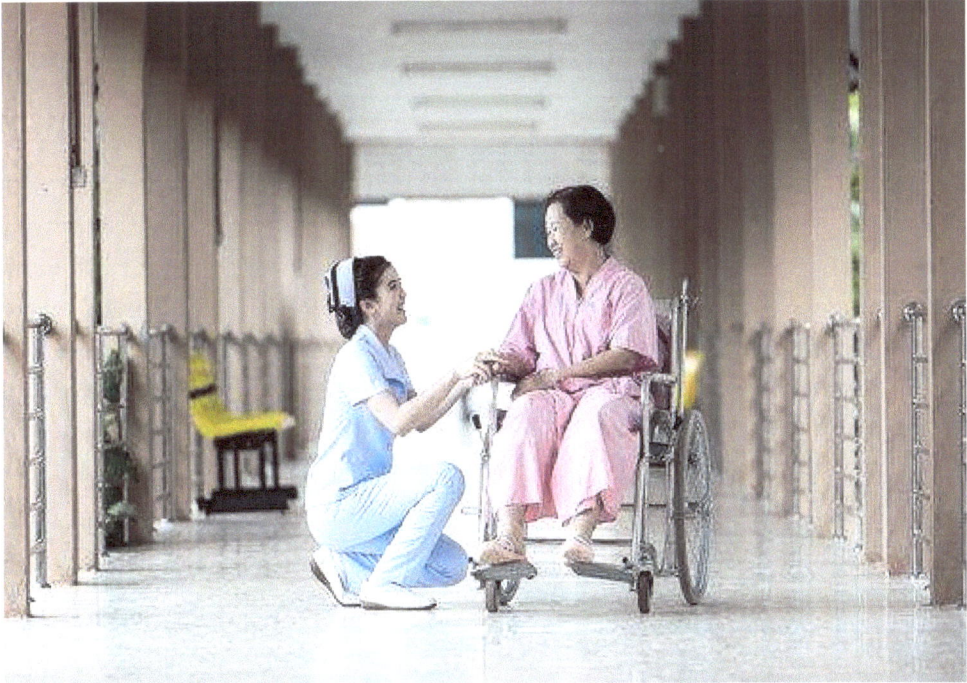

Fig. (1.4). Nursing & Care. Source: www.pixabay.com.

It is also worthy to note that caring practice in nursing is also associated with positive outcomes for both clients and nurses. For instance, research has demonstrated that offering care to our clients in the form of empathy and understanding, can enhance the quality of the client's experience and also contributes to a nurse's overall work satisfaction (Palese, Tomietto & Suhonen, 2011).

The question is often posed, "*In today's climate of enhanced work-loads and so many additional technological demands on nurses, how do we still keep caring in our practice?*" We keep caring in our practice by making a conscious choice to do so. If caring becomes an integral part of our way of being, it will not necessarily take time away from nursing tasks. We can get the job done in a timely manner, but it is "*how*" we do the job that also matters. Watson (2008) has proposed caritas dimensions and healing practices for nurses to employ that will help them to cultivate caring. **Caritas** refers to the belief that caring and devotion are the most important forces in all of life (Watson, 2008). I highly recommend them. Refer to Box (**1:4**).

Box 1:4. WATSON'S CARITAS DIMENSIONS & HEALING PRACTICES (as adapted from Watson, 2008, pp. 25 – 26)
* Cultivate a caring consciousness as a starting point.
* Centre yourself before entering a client's room or be still.
* Be present - *Be* as well as *Do* for the other.
* Accurately identify and address the person by name.
* Maintain eye contact as appropriate for cultural sensitivity.
* Accurately detect what the other person is feeling.
* Encourage the client to tell you their story and authentically listen.
* Hold the other person within an attitude of unconditional loving-kindness.
* Be silent and wait for the other to respond, allowing their inner thoughts to emerge.

The Ethic of Care as a Lived Virtue

"Just as treasures are uncovered from the earth, so virtue appears from good deeds, and wisdom appears from a pure and peaceful mind. To walk safely through the maze of human life, one needs the light of wisdom and the guidance of virtue."

Buddha, Spiritual leader and founder of the Buddhist Religion

I believe that the desire to make a positive difference in the lives of others is at the heart of nursing. Therefore, it is with sincerity and fervor that I set out to inspire nurses to adopt virtue and ethic of care into their practice and everyday lives. **Virtue** is concerned with the character of the human being and the pursuit of moral excellence. The ethic of care has strong ties to virtue ethics and virtue ethics represents a unique approach (Woods, 2011). Instead of placing the focus on right or wrong action, or justified or unjustified principles, **virtue ethics** places the emphasis on the moral character of the person (Smolkin *et al.,* 2010). It was the Greek philosopher, Aristotle who promoted virtues as good habits that we make a part of our way of being. Western theorists who study the subject of virtue advocate that we should avoid undesirable character traits, and MacIntyre (2007) encourages us to have ethics do its job through how we conduct our lives. Virtue ethics also places more emphasis on *being* and less on *doing* which is totally in sync with the ethic of care (Benner, 1997). Morality is seen as stemming from the disposition of the person rather than through the conduct of the individual. Furthermore, note that, characteristics of nursing that appear to be highly esteemed are courage, trustworthiness and practical wisdom. These attributes also align well with key attributes of the ethic of care (Benner 1997; Sellman, 2007; Woods, 2011). Refer to Box (**1:5**). As Allmark (1998) proposed, even if caring is not a virtue, being virtuous entails caring about what is the right and noble way to act.

Box 1:5. VIRTUE ETHICS & THE ETHIC OF CARE (as adapted from Benner 1997; Sellman, 2007)
Virtue ethics and the ethic of care both focus more on *being* and less on *doing*. Furthermore, characteristics of nursing, such as courage, trustworthiness and practical wisdom, align well with the main attributes of an ethic of care.

Florence Nightingale, Virtue Ethics & Nursing as a Calling

"Let whoever is in charge keep this simple question in her head, not how can I always do this right thing myself, but how can I provide for this right thing to be always done?"

Florence Nightingale, (1820 – 1910) Nurse, Social Reformer & Statistician.

Virtue and virtuous acts have been highlighted as foundational within the history of nursing (Ray, 2016). Florence Nightingale was one of the most re-known nurses and she was a strong proponent of virtue as central to nursing practice (Burkhardt *et al.*, 2015). Florence Nightingale was born in 1820 in England at a time when it was very rare that a woman was awarded the opportunity to obtain a first-class education. However, Florence Nightingale did become well educated because she was one of two sisters born into a wealthy family with no sons. Her father decided to give his two daughters an exceptional education which at the time, was almost unheard of for women (Zinner, 2014). Florence studied history, geography, math, science, French, Greek and Latin. She was also an avid reader of Plato and Homer (Zinner, 2014).

Florence was a nurse leader. She was instrumental in elevating the leadership role of nurses by ensuring that they were a part of the administration of health care delivery (Zinner, 2014). However, her greatest leadership achievement occurred during the Crimean war. The Crimean war was fought between the British, Russians, French and Turks between October 1853 and February 1856 (Strachey, 2013). Through the introduction of increased cleanliness in the hospital setting, enhanced nutrition and wound sanitation, Florence Nightingale and her fellow nurses saved many lives (Strachey, 2013). Florence Nightingale was also known for recording accurate client data in the form of statistics which proved to be instrumental in improving medical care and saving lives (Zinner, 2014).

Florence Nightingale believed that nurses should possess virtuous characteristics and she encouraged virtue in her nursing students. For instance, in her recruitment of nurses she chose women who were upstanding in character, honest and trustworthy. Florence strove to further add punctuality, quiet fortitude and tidiness to these virtuous character traits (Skretkowicz, 2010; Zinner, 2014).

Florence Nightingale also perceived the profession of nursing as a calling. A **calling** can be described as a way in which our work allows us to demonstrate passion, dignity, integrity and greater service to the greater good for all (Miller-Tiedeman (1999). Florence believed that nurses, while caring for the sick and injured could experience the divine by restoring clients' health and helping them to achieve a higher purpose for their life (Zinner, 2014).

Miller-Tiedeman (1999) also emphasizes the importance of viewing our work as a mission. She proposes that a job should not merely be about just earning a living. Society would be better served if we felt passion for the work we did and if our means of employment was concerned with using our gifts and abilities to serve others (Miller-Tiedeman, 1999).

The Multifaceted Aspects of Care

The ethic of care is about the practice of caring. In the health professions, **caring** has been interpreted as being engrossed in, and acting to promote another's wellbeing (Bishop & Scudder, 1996). Caring is a process that is multifaceted and sometimes difficult to articulate in precise, concrete terms, but that does not mean that the distinct aspects of care should not be delineated into practice (Stephany, 2007). Specific components of care as put forward by theorists such as Milton Mayerhoff, Helen Perlman and me, Kathleen Stephany, will now be introduced followed by examples of how each caring trait are demonstrated in the practice of the ethic of care. Box (**1:6**).

Milton Mayerhoff (1971), a well-known Philosopher and a strong supporter of the ethic of care, put forward what he referred to as, **Qualities of Care** that consisted of: knowledge & care; alternating rhythms of care; demonstrating patience; being honest & trustworthy; showing humility; having hope and maintaining courage. Helen Perlman (1979) a famous Social worker and care theorist who studied psychology and its implications for clinical work, formed an **Inventory of Caring Traits** such as: warmth, acceptance, caring-concern, genuineness and empathy. I have added a mosaic of caring actions to this already rich list. Specific **Components of the Mosaic of Care** that I focus on consist of compassion, generosity & care, unconditional positive regard and presencing (Stephany, 2007).

The aforementioned list of specific caring features may appear overwhelming at first and seem like too much for a nurse to ascribe to. Many will argue that nurses are merely human and not capable of consistently demonstrating all of these in practice. However, I contend that as nurses, if we desire to exemplify the ethic of care as a lived virtue, we should at least endeavour to incorporate most of these qualities into our relationship with clients. The key here is that different situations require diverse aspects of care. Whatever specific helping motif that is employed depends on the context. The degree to which we can succeed in this task reflects the magnitude to which we are successful as caregivers and will enhance our satisfaction with what we do (Stephany, 2007). Let us take a closer look at some of these specific caring features and how they relate to the practice of the ethic of care.

Box 1:6 Multifaceted Aspects of Care (as adapted from Mayerhoff, 1971; Perlman, 1979; Stephany, 2007)

MAYERHOFF'S QUALITIES of CARE	PERLMAN'S INVENTORY of CARE	STEPHANY'S COMPONENTS of the MOSAIC OF CARE
* Knowing	* Warmth	* Compassion
* Alternating Rhythms of care	* Acceptance	* Generosity & Care
* Demonstrating Patience	* Caring-Concern	* Unconditional Positive Regard
* Being Honest & Trustworthy	* Genuineness	* Presencing
* Showing Humility	* Empathy	
* Having Hope		
* Maintaining Courage		

MAYERHOFF'S QUALITIES OF CARE

Knowledge & Care

The first quality of care as introduced by Mayerhoff (1971) is that of knowledge and care. **Knowledge and care** refer to the proficiency of applying our intelligence and competence to the situation that we are confronted with (Schmidt, 2002). As nurses knowing is about competence and skillfulness. We want the person who is attending to us to be knowledgeable and to be able to apply what they know. When we undergo surgery we are counting on the skillful competence of the surgeon (Stephany, 2007). When we are being assessed by a nurse we are depending on the assumption that the assessment is thorough and that the nurse knows what to do with their findings.

When teaching I inform my nursing students that they are never allowed to pretend that they do not know if they know the answer to a basic health inquiry. For instance, the ethic of care would dictate that nurses cannot completely leave behind what they know just because their shift of work has ended. A nurse's knowledge base becomes a part of who they are (Stephany, 2007). The example that I use to illustrate this point centers on a mother's concern about her child's fever. She phones her nurse friend asking what she should do. As a nurse you must share knowledge with the mother even though you may be off duty because not doing so, would be unethical and uncaring (Stephany, 2007).

Alternating Rhythms of Care

Another quality of care introduced by Mayerhoff (1971) is **alternating rhythms of care** which consists of the notion of flexibility and spontaneity in helping relationships. Often nurses get locked into doing things the same way by habit. In contrast, alternating rhythms requires nurses to choose their responses, interventions and strategies carefully, with a willingness to vary behavior based on the situation at hand (Schmidt, 2002). What is needed is an eagerness on the part of the nurse to be adaptable and sensitive enough to look beyond the obvious and to ascertain what might really be needed (Stephany, 2007). It is about placing the human connectedness component of the ethic of care alongside priority setting and safety, and not just following some set formula as a guide for our actions. An example in the clinical setting where a nurse may be acting without the guidance of alternating rhythms and care occurs when a client is prescribed an anti-hypertensive medication and the nurse neglects to do essential assessment skills. The nurse doesn't check the client's blood pressure to ensure that the medication is being effective, because vital signs have not been ordered by a physician. Yet, it is well within a nurse's scope of practice to check vital signs without a doctor's order.

Another example of a nurse not applying alternating rhythms and care occurs when they do not develop a safety plan with a highly suicidal client before they are leaving the hospital on a day pass. A **safety plan** is a written list of healthy coping strategies and resources and people to call when the person feels like self-harming (Stephany, 2017). The nurse may actually be aware that a safety plan is warranted under the guidance of safe and best practices but they refuse to implement one because it isn't in the ward policy manual. Both aforementioned decisions by a nurse not to act on what they know is best practices, goes against the application of alternating rhythms and care.

Demonstrating Patience

Mayerhoff (1971) points out that **demonstrating patience** contributes to the caring relationship through the process of tolerance and encouraging personal growth. By demonstrating patience with our clients we are permitting them to process sensitive information and to make health decisions on their own time and at their own pace (Stephany, 2007). It is about exhibiting sensitivity to their particular circumstances.

A nurse's deliberate action of patience and care is extremely important when a person is amid a crisis. For instance, finding out that they have a life-threatening disease or being diagnosed with a mental illness may render clients to feel overwhelmed and unable to cope. Customary methods of problem solving can seem elusive or irrelevant. The nurse needs to be able to give their client time to sort through their feelings, but still convey that they are there to assist, support and help guide them through the available options when they are ready.

Being Honest and Trustworthy

Caring entails being **honest and trustworthy** because without honesty and openness there can be no trust (Mayerhoff, 1971). Nurses must be truthful in all of their interactions and keep their promises to their clients. Actions speak louder than words (Stephany, 2007). If we inform a client that we will get them a warm blanket or something to alleviate their physical pain or anxiety, we need to carry through with what we promised in a timely fashion. Alternatively, if a nurse is dishonest or neglects to carry through with their promises, the message that may be inadvertently sent is that they do not care. Being honesty also consists of being sensitive in the way in which we tell the truth. We need to state the facts but not without ensuring that we are compassionate and that we make provisions for what the person is feeling (Stephany, 2007).

Showing Humility

For nurses, demonstrating **humility** consists of being able to admit when you are wrong as well as taking responsibility for when you do not know (Mayerhoff, 1971). As a nursing instructor, sometimes a student will ask me a question that I do not have the answer to. I honestly inform them that I will find the answer and get back to them as soon as possible.

Another nursing characteristic of humbleness is the ability to truly listen. Listening sends the message that you care about what is going on for the person and validates their experience. Schmidt (2002) refers to this trait as the way in which people care with their eyes. The message is, what you are saying is important to me and it matters (Schmidt, 2002). Box (**1:7**) tells the story of how a Catholic priest was able offer humility and care in a very sad time.

Box 1:7. Narrative: Humility in Action (as adapted from Stephany, 2007, pp. 50 – 51)
I recall when my mother was lying on her death bed. She was a practicing Catholic, so I summoned the priest to perform the last rites. I was very sad and despondent at the thought of her impending death and I was overcome with grief. I looked into the priest's eyes and saw them fill with tears, although he was able to contain them. That act was one of compassion and humility. It takes a lot of courage to let your humanness show through when you are trying to act professionally, but sometimes that is exactly what is needed in the moment.

Having Hope

Mayerhoff (1971) believed in the importance of having hope when circumstances are less than desirable. **Hope** is the belief that beneficial outcomes can be realized. It is not blind optimism but consists of unwavering confidence that anything is possible if we only believe (Stephany, 2012). For example, a nurse can instill hope in a person who is suicidal by genuinely sending the message, *"I care about you, even though I don't know you. I care enough about you to help you to choose life"* (Stephany, 2002, p. 7). Perlman (1979) points out that, what happens when this message is sent is that hope is caught from the helper. It buoys the spirit and restores energy. The suicidal person begins to see themselves in the eyes of the caregiver and they begin to think that maybe they are lovable and worth caring about (Stephany, 2002).

Maintaining Courage

Maintaining courage is another important quality of caring action. **Courage** consists of working to improve a situation to enhance the good of other people even in the presence of opposition (Cleary & Horsfall, 2014). Mayerhoff (1971) asserted that maintaining courage when situations become difficult is as crucial as having hope. For example, like hope, courage sometimes needs to be demonstrated by the caregiver on behalf of the client, especially when a person is most vulnerable and afraid. It also may require that a nurse speak up when client care is at risk (Cleary & Horsfall, 2014).

PERLMAN'S INVENTORY OF CARING TRAITS

"I've learned that people will forget what you said, people will forget what you did, but people will never forget how you made them feel." Maya Angelou, American Poet.

Warmth

Warmth is the ability to truly connect with others on a human level. Perlman (1979) described warmth as a positive, lively, outgoing and genuine interest in another person's experience that is physically felt by the person on the receiving end of the experience. Although warmth is sometimes difficult to articulate into words, many of us who have experienced it can describe how it made us feel. Warmth consists of feeling genuinely cared for, just by being in the other person's presence. The opposite of warmth is cold indifference. Most clients will attest that they trust a nurse who is caring and warm and that they instinctively mistrust a nurse who is cold and dismissive.

Acceptance

Perlman (1979) describes **acceptance** as the act of taking people as they are and where they are. It is about understanding that the way that people act is an aspect of their behaviour and that their behaviour is not who they actually are (Perlman, 1979). A person is not inherently bad even if they behave badly (Stephany, 2015). Therefore, being accepting means that we consider someone to be a valuable human being even if they are exhibiting less than desirable traits. For example, someone who is suffering from an addiction may act in ways that seem to lack consideration for others. Even if the nurse does not approve of the person's behaviour, a message must be sent that the nurse still cares for them as a person of worth (Stephany, 2007). Perlman (1979) pointed out that people often come to us when they are in trouble. Sometimes they may even be the cause of many of their problems. Oftentimes they merely lack the means or ability to embark upon a different course. It is the helper's role to assist the person to see that there is a better way, but they will only listen to the advice that is given if they feel accepted and understood (Perlman, 1979).

Caring-Concern

According to Perlman (1979) caring-concern exists within the milieu of helping relationships through the act of demonstrating genuine interest in the complete and full welfare of those we seek to help. This action concerns being interested in the person's present set of health challenges and everything else that is going on in their life. For instance, in addition to health problems, our clients may be experiencing psycho-social and/or economic difficulties. In this manner, caring-concern aligns perfectly with the ethic of care and social justice. **Social justice** is concerned with the comparative position of one social group in relation to other social groups. Social justice draws attention to the disparities in socio-economic status, the root causes of inequalities, and what can be done to eradicate these disparities (CNA, 2009). In fact, Canadian nurses are mandated by the Part II of the CNA Code of Ethics to pursue active ethical endeavours related to broad societal issues associated with enhancing health and wellbeing (CNA, 2017).

Genuineness

Genuineness consists of honesty and being authentic and real in our interactions and communication with others (Stephany, 2015). It is the way that we convey to our clients that we are human just like them and that it is safe for them to be entrusted into our keeping (Perlman, 1979). To be genuine also entails being free of self-importance. It is about portraying wholeness, knowing who we are and what our guiding values consist of (Perlman, 1979). Being genuine consists of being self-aware, self-accepting of one's strengths and weaknesses, and being bold in the face of uncertainty (Perlman, 1979). Genuineness is also closely tied to humility and having the courage to admit when you are wrong.

Empathy

Empathy is the capacity to relate on an emotional level to the experience of another person and includes identifying with all their emotions, both happy and sad (Stephany, 2015). The key to empathy is a clinician's desire to understand the world from the client's perspective. It is the ability to feel with the other person and being able to imagine what it might be like to walk a mile in their shoes (Perlman, 1979). Empathy is an important communication technique because it enhances the connection between the nurse and the client, which is the essence of the ethic of care in action (Noddings, 1984). In other words, empathy as an integral aspect of the ethic of care consists of the action of a motivated sensitivity to the experience of others (Stephany, 2015).

What Deliberate Actions are Associated with Empathy?

The Psychologist, Carl Rogers (1951) who was a proponent of person-centered counselling was a strong supporter of cultivating empathy in order to facilitate trust and rapport with clients. Rogers asserted that there are three deliberate actions associated with empathy: active listening, reflection and non-verbal communication. **Active listening** is intentionally being fully present and listening to what is being said while also giving your full attention to the person who is speaking (Stephany, 2015). Oftentimes active listening may also require that you ask a question to ensure that you understood the intended message. Reflection may also be needed. **Reflection** involves paraphrasing what you think the client may have stated to ensure that you have truly understood their intended message (Stephany, 2015). Paying attention to **nonverbal cues** is crucial because if the client's verbal response differs from what their body language demonstrates, their non-verbal communication is likely more indicative of what is really going on for them (Stephany, 2015). When active listening, reflection and attention to non-verbal cues are employed by the nurse, a client is likely to feel understood (Stephany, 2015).

What Impedes Empathy?

There are four specific activities that nurses should avoid because they impede empathy: giving advice, offering superficial reassurance, explaining your own position or sharing your own feelings (Rosenberg, 2003). Giving advice is a bad idea because it can be condescending and disempowering (Stephany, 2015). Offering superficial reassurance in statements like, *"Everything will be alright,"* undermines the client's experience, especially if they are expressing sadness (Stephany, 2015). If we explain our own position on the issues we undermine the client's ability to choose for themselves. If we resort to sharing our feelings the focus of the interaction becomes more about us and less about them (Stephany, 2015).

So why do health professionals resort to these tactics if they are not helpful? When another person expresses intense emotions we may become uncomfortable and want to do something to fix the situation but trying to fix it doesn't work. What I recommend is that you stay silent and just listen. Say nothing at all if you don't know what to say. Allow the other person to fully experience what they are feeling, just listen and be a safe place for them.

We Can Learn to be More Empathetic

Frequently nursing students want to know how they can improve their empathy skills. I suggest that they consider regular reflective journaling to increase self-awareness and to reflect on how interactions went between them and clients. I also recommend that they seek constructive feedback from others on how their behaviour is interpreted, especially their non-verbal cues. I likewise inform my student nurses to never underestimate how much they have already learned about how to be empathetic from their prior life experiences, such as personal loss and suffering (Stephany, 2015).

STEPHANY'S COMPONENTS OF THE MOSAIC OF CARE

A **mosaic** is a pattern created by small pieces of material that when viewed together form an artful picture that is beautiful to behold. (Fig. **1.5**). I have called my list of caring concepts, **Components of the Mosaic of Care** and they include: compassion, generosity & care, unconditional positive regard and presencing.

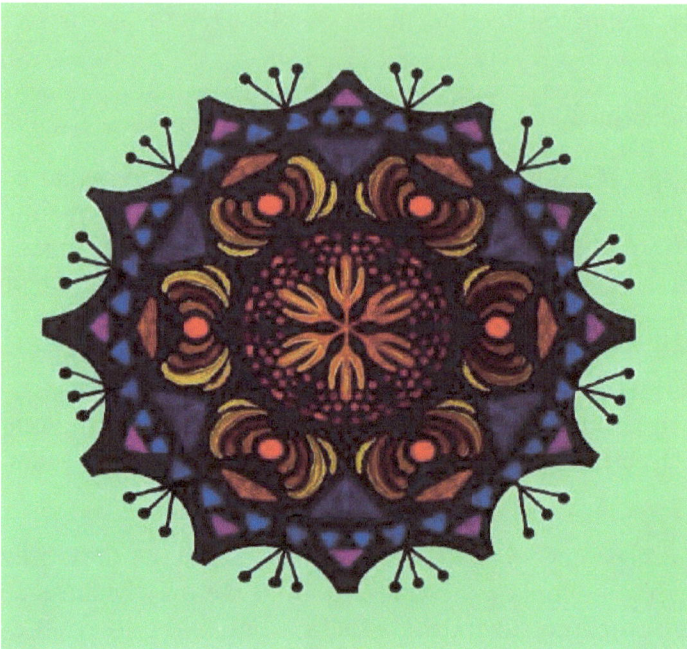

Fig. (1.5). Mosaic. Source: www.pixabay.com.

COMPASSION

"If you want others to be happy, practice compassion, if you want to be happy, practice compassion." His Holiness, the 14th Dalai Lama

Compassion is similar to empathy in that both compassion and empathy involve our willingness to want to understand what another person is experiencing (Stephany, 2015). However, compassion and empathy are also somewhat different. For example, whereas empathy is about identifying with both positive and negative feelings of others, **compassion** is solely concerned with identification with a person's suffering (Stephany, 2015). I believe that when one of us suffers we all suffer and as Chopra (2005) so poignantly explains, "when you feel someone else's suffering, understanding is born" (p. 26).

Compassion in nursing practice identifies with whatever type of anguish the client is facing and suffering does not merely occur in the body. Many of our clients also experience emotional and psychological pain. Therefore, as a nurse we must never focus exclusively on physical wounds without also attending to the matters of the heart. Box (**1:8**) tells the story of how personal suffering can teach us how to be compassionate with others.

Box 1:8. Narrative: The Embodiment of Compassion & Care (Source: K. Stephany)
One of the most compassionate people in my life was my beloved mother. My mother was a woman who suffered numerous losses throughout her life, which included the untimely death of several of her children. Yet there was something of beauty in her character that arose from the pangs of pain. My mother developed tremendous compassion for everyone, especially those whom no one seemed to care about, and she was courageous enough to act on what she believed. In this fashion she embodied compassion and care.

The Importance of Self-Compassion

"It is lack of love for ourselves that inhibits our compassion toward others. If we make friends with ourselves, then there is no obstacle to opening our hearts and minds to others." Anonymous.

Compassion begins with examining and nurturing ourselves first (Brammer & MacDonald, 1999). In fact, we can only genuinely offer compassion to others if we first learn how to be compassionate with ourselves, because if we judge ourselves harshly, we tend to project that same judgment onto others (Rosenberg, 2003). We also need to be willing to attend to our own pain before we can genuinely be concerned with the pain and suffering of others.

Generosity & Care

"Real giving is the art of transmitting ourselves to others and to the conditions and situations that surround us. This is not something for special occasions only, for it should become a habit of growing out of our desire to live life to the fullest. Just as life belongs to the one who lives it, to the one who enjoys it, so the fuller life belongs to the one who scatters every good he has." Ernest Holmes, author of The Science of Mind

Some equate generosity with the giving of money and material goods. However, in the practice of nursing, **generosity** consists of the imparting of non-material substance. It is the giving of care through our actions (Salzberg, 2004). For example, every contact with a client is an opportunity to offer generosity. You can offer the client who is discouraged, encouragement. To someone who is feeling down, hope. To the person who needs to talk, you can listen. For a client who is alone, you can spend some time just being with them. Rosenberg (2003) points out that giving of ourselves and our time generously benefits both the nurse and the client. The person who is doing the giving feels better about themselves because they are helping another person and the person who is on the receiving end feels cared for and cherished (Rosenberg, 2003).

Unconditional Positive Regard

Carl Rogers viewed caring at its best when a helper gives unconditional positive regard to their client (Rogers, 1951). **Unconditional positive regard** is the act of offering an atmosphere that demonstrates that you truly do care for the person and that there are no obstacles or conditions to your capacity to care for them. It is not about caring for the individual if they behave in a certain, acceptable fashion, but caring about them and for them, even if they misbehave (Rogers, 1980). Unconditional positive regard is the action of non-judgment. There are four strategies that I recommend to nursing students to learn how to offer genuine unconditional positive regard (Stephany, 2017). Box (**1:9**).

Box 1:9. HOW TO PRACTICE UNCONDITIONAL POSITIVE REGARD (as adapted from Stephany, 2017)
1.   **Make unconditional positive regard a conscious choice.**
It is not helpful to judge others. You need to make a conscious choice not to judge.
2.   **Imagine that your client is someone in your life that you care about.**
If you imagine that the person you are caring for is someone in your life that you love, you are much more inclined not to judge them so harshly.
3.   **Remind yourself that your client is human just like you.**
This strategy was developed by Chopra (2005). Just like you, your client has people in their life that love them. Just like you they have experienced joy and sorrow. Just like you they will someday die. They deserve your respect.
4.   **Take the time to listen to their story.**
We are quick to judge when we do not understand what has happened to our clients. Many of them have experienced trauma. Listening to their story helps us to relate to them on a more compassionate level.

Presencing & Silence

"Few delights can equal the presence of one whom we trust utterly." George MacDonald, Scottish Author, Poet and Christian Minister.

Presencing involves being a safe, non-judgmental place for someone and in its purest form it occurs in complete silence. Presencing is being fully present and with the person in the moment. The only action that accompanies the silence is for the nurse to send kind caring thoughts to the client. Bishop and Scudder (1996) describe caring presence as fostering wellbeing and when caring presence permeates the room, the whole atmosphere of that room is changed in a positive way. The environment becomes a haven for healing to take place. Being comfortable with silence is often difficult for nurses, yet sometimes it is exactly what is needed. If a client is extremely ill or even dying and they have no family or friends present to support them, then the nurse must offer their presence to the client. I believe that it is an honour to be present when a person is born, but that it is also an honour to be present when someone dies and as Gilligan (1982) so poignantly put it, no one should die alone. It is a privilege to spend time with a dying client and to offer them caring presence because they get to take part in helping the person to leave. It is about offering our clients care and dignity in their final moments.

Box 1:10. CASE IN POINT: PRESENCING & CARE
Susan was a student nurse in a mental health setting and she was assigned to do her clinical practice on a ward for clients diagnosed with serious mental illness. When Susan came onto the ward for her first shift, her instructor assigned her to Mark, a young client diagnosed with schizophrenia, catatonic type. A person suffering from this type of mental illness is extremely ill. This was Mark's first psychotic breakdown and he had lost all contact with reality. He was so sick that he did not speak or maintain any contact with the outside world. He just sat and stared. Mark needed help with every task including being bathed, dressed and fed. The nursing staff asked the instructor to assign a student to care for Mark because they knew that he was badly in need of the attention. Mark was prescribed more than one anti-psychotic medication but he didn't appear to be responding to them yet. Susan had just learned in her communications lab about the importance of caring presence. Her instructor encouraged her to spend as much time as possible just "being with" Mark and sending him caring, healing thoughts and energy. At first Susan found this task difficult but she did her best and spent a couple of hours each clinical day over the course of six weeks, just presencing. Nothing seemed to change in Mark's condition until the last day of clinical, then something amazing happened. Susan went into the common room where Mark was seated and when she approached him and said hello, he looked up at her and smiled. This was Mark's first attempt at any connection with another person since he was admitted. Susan was elated. She informed her instructor, who notified the rest of the staff. A team conference was held and the Psychiatrist asked if Susan would be willing to come and visit Mark as a volunteer. She agreed and her instructor ensured that this arrangement was okay with the nursing school rules. Over the course of the next month Mark only spoke to Susan but in time he also began to speak to other staff members and he was on his way to becoming well.

Questions Pertaining to the Case in Point:

1. What effect do you think presencing and care had on Mark?
2. Did he get well because of the medications were working or was Susan's presencing a part of his journey to healing?
3. Is caring presence something that needs to be taught in the nursing curriculum of all nursing schools? Why or why not?

REFLECTING BACK

Summary of Key Points Covered in Chapter 1

* Ethics is primarily concerned with the study of moral conduct or the right and noble action of groups and how we all should ideally act.

* The philosophical ethical theories of utilitarianism & deontology were presented along with their key premises and different emphasis.

* Utilitarianism, also referred to as consequentialism, is a moral theory that asserts that any action is judged as good or bad relative to the consequences or outcome resulting from that action. What is deemed good is anything that brings us pleasure and/or freedom from pain.

* Distributive justice as an aspect of utilitarianism, is concerned with the notion of fairness and requires that the privileges awarded to people in given situations be distributed proportionately and equally.

* Deontology as an ethical theory asserts that the rightness or wrongness of an act is dependent on the very nature or morality of the act and not on its outcome or consequences.

* Applied nursing ethics was identified as a sub-category of ethics. It is more involved with the practice of nursing and less concerned with just applying philosophical rules to deal with the problems that nurses face.

* The ethic of care is a special proponent of applied nursing ethics.

* The ethic of care emphasizes the interconnectedness of all of life, places significant importance on relationships, context and lived experiences, and incorporates caring and meaning making into decisions.

* In 1982, a Psychologist named Carol Gilligan, provided the impetus for the development of the ethic of care.

* During the 1990s and the beginning of the new millennia and beyond, many other theorists contributed to the dynamic dialogue about the ethic of care and its relevance.

* It was pointed out that the ethic of care aligns well with many other theoretical premises that focus on the contextual features of people's lives such as: feminism, humanism and phenomenology.

* The ethic of justice is related to distributive justice. It proposes that ethical decisions should be made by making use of universal principles and rules and that decision making be impartial.

* The ethic of justice and the ethic of care are complementary but their focus is different. While an ethic of justice proceeds from the premise of equality, that everyone be treated the same, an ethic of care rests on the premise of nonviolence, that no none should be hurt.

* The ethic of care was deemed to still be valid for today's nurses because conventional science in and of itself, is insufficient to inform nurses on how to best deal with being confronted with human suffering.

* Watson's (2008) caritas dimensions and healing practices were recommended to nurses to cultivate caring.

* Virtue is concerned with the pursuit of moral excellence and virtue ethics in nursing can be traced back to Florence Nightingale.

* Virtue ethics has a great deal in common with the ethic of care. For example, both focus more on *being* and less on *doing*. Furthermore, the virtuous characteristics of nursing, such as courage, trustworthiness and practical wisdom, merge relatively seamlessly with similar attributes associated with an ethic of care.

* The ethic of care is about the practice of caring. The following multifaceted aspects of care were carefully delineated, including ways that these caring features play out in nursing practice.

Mayerhoff's (1971) **Qualities of Care**: knowledge & care; alternating rhythms of care; demonstrating patience; being honest & trustworthy; showing humility; having hope and maintaining courage.

Perlman's (1979) **Inventory of Caring Traits**: warmth, acceptance, caring-concern, genuineness and empathy.

Stephany's (2007) **Components of the Mosaic of Care**: compassion, generosity & care, unconditional positive regard and presencing.

* The famous 20th Century Psychologist, Carl Rogers was the founder of humanism and phenomenology. Rogers was also the originator of person-centered counselling that focused on the importance of empathy and unconditional positive regard.

* The following Four Strategies were recommended to learn how to practice unconditional positive regard.

1. Make unconditional positive regard a personal choice.

2. Imagine that your client is someone in your life that you care about.

3. Remind yourself that your client is human just like you.

4. Take the time to listen to their story.

SOMETHING TO PONDER

1. What does the ethic of care mean to you?

2. How do you incorporate aspects of the ethic of care into your nursing practice?

3. Which of the multifaceted components of care resonate most closely with who you are and whom you wish to evolve into?

4. What specific elements of the multifaceted aspects of care still elude you and how will you incorporate some of these into your daily round?

CLASSROOM GROUP EXERCISES

1. For discussion as a large group or smaller groups. Scenario: You are busy changing a client's dressing and they begin to cry. You have lots of other tasks to perform on other clients and you are pressed for time. What do you do? Will you carry on with business as usual or will you tend to what the client may be needing in the moment?

2. Break into groups of two. For each group place two chairs side by side, slightly facing each other. One student will assume the role of the student nurse and the other will act as a mental health client who is suffering from depression. Both actors sit in silence. For five minutes, just sit there. The only action that is required is for the person playing the role of the student nurse, to send kind, caring, healing thoughts to the acting client. After breaking the silence, ask the person who was on the receiving end to tell the group what it felt like. Were they able to feel warmth and care without words? Time permitting, have the two students switch places and do it all over again.

RECOMMENDED READINGS

Gilligan, C. (1982). *In a different voice: Psychological theory and women's development.* Cambridge: MA: Harvard University Press.

Herbland, A., Goldberg, M., Garric, N., & Lesieur, O. (2011). Thank-you letters from clients in an intensive care unit: From expression of gratitude to an applied ethic of care. *Intensive & Critical Care Nursing, 43* (10), 47 – 54.

Rawls, J. (1999). *A theory of justice* (Revised Edition). USA: Harvard University Press.

Sealy, P. (2011). The power of empathy. *Canadian Nurse, 107* (8), 30 – 31.

Stephany, K. (2015). *Cultivating empathy: Inspiring health professionals to communicate more effectively.* United Arab Emirates: Bentham Science Publishing Ltd.

WEB RESOURCE

Web Resource: Unconditional Positive Regard – What it is and Why you Need it https://www.harleytherapy.co.uk/counselling/unconditional-positive-regard-w-at-it-is-and-why-you-need-it.htm

CONSENT FOR PUBLICATION

Not applicable.

CONFLICT OF INTEREST

The authors confirm that this chapter contents have no conflict of interest.

ACKNOWLEDGEMENTS

Declared none.

REFERENCES

Allmark, P (1998) Is caring a virtue? *J Adv Nurs,* 28, 466-72.
[http://dx.doi.org/10.1046/j.1365-2648.1998.00803.x] [PMID: 9756212]

Beauchamp, TL & Childress, JF (2009) *Principles of biomedical ethics*, 6th ed. Oxford University Press, New York.

Benner, P (1997) A dialogue between virtue ethics and care ethics. *Theor Med,* 18, 47-61.
[http://dx.doi.org/10.1023/A:1005797100864] [PMID: 9129392]

Bishop, AH & Scudder, JR (1996) *Nursing ethics: Therapeutic caring presence.* Jones and Bartlett Publishers, London.

Bjarmason, D & LaSala, A (2011) Moral leadership in nursing. *J Radiol Nurs,* 30, 18-24.
[http://dx.doi.org/10.1016/j.jradnu.2011.01.002]

Bosek, MS & Savage, TA (2007) *The ethical component of nursing education: Integrating ethics into clinical experience.*Lippincott Williams & Wilkins, New York.

Botes, A (2000) A comparison between the ethics of justice and the ethics of care. *J Adv Nurs,* 32, 1071-5.

[http://dx.doi.org/10.1046/j.1365-2648.2000.01576.x] [PMID: 11114990]

Brammer, LM & MacDonald, G (1999) *The helping relationship: Process and skills.*Allyn and Bacon, Toronto.

Burkhardt, MA, Nathaniel, AK & Walton, NA (2015) *Ethics and issues in contemporary nursing* Nelson, Toronto, Ontario.

Canadian Nurses Association (CNA) (2009) *Ethics in practice for registered nurses series: Social justice in practice* Retrieved from: https://cna-aiic.ca/sitecore%20modules/web/~/media/cna/page-content/p-f-fr/ethics_in_practice_april_2009_e.pdf

Canadian Nurses Association (CNA) (2017) *CNA Code of Ethics for Registered Nurses.* (Revised Edition). Ottawa: Author.

Chopra, D (2005) *Peace is the way.* Three Rivers Press, USA.

Cleary, M & Horsfall, J (2014) Nursing and enacting the courage of one's convictions. *Issues in Mental Health Nursing,* 35, 724-6.
[http://dx.doi.org/10.3109/01612840.2014.938965]

Collaborative Nursing Program in British Columbia (2004) *Collaborative curriculum* (Revised Edition).

Collis, C & Nolan, M (2005) Sites of benevolence. *J Aust Stud,* 85.

Durant, W (1961) *The story of philosophy.*Simon & Schuster, Toronto.

Ford, GG (2006) *Ethical reasoning for mental health professionals.*Sage, London.

Gilligan, C (1982) *In a different voice: Psychological theory and women's development.*Cambridge: MA: Harvard University Press..

Held, V (2006) *The ethic of care: Personal, political, and global.*Oxford University Press, UK.

Heinricks, B (2010) Single-Principle *versus* multi-principles approaches in biomedical ethics. *J Appl Philos,* 27, 72-84.
[http://dx.doi.org/10.1111/j.1468-5930.2009.00474.x]

Keatings, M & Smith, OB (2016) *Ethical & legal issues in Canadian nursing*

MacIntrye, A (2007) *After virtue: A study of moral theory* Lippincott Williams & Wilkins, New York.

Mayerhoff, M (1971) *On caring.*Harper & Row, New York.

Miller-Tiedeman, A (1999) *Learning, practicing, and living the new careering.*Taylor & Francis Group, USA.

Monte, CF (1995) *Beneath the mask: An introduction to theories of personality.*Harcourt Brace College Publishers, Toronto.

Nietzel, MT, Bernstein, DA & Milich, R (1998) *Introduction to clinical psychology* Prentice Hall, Upper Saddles River, New Jersey.

Noddings, N (1984) *Caring: A feminine approach to ethics and moral education.*University of California Press, Berkeley.

Oberle, K & Bouchal, SR (2009) *Ethics in Canadian nursing practice.*

Palese, A, Tomietto, M, Suhonen, R, Efstathiou, G & Tsangari, H Papastavrou, E. (2011). Surgical client satisfaction as an outcome of nurses' caring behaviors: A descriptive and correlational study in six European countries *Journal of Nursing Scholarship,,* 43, 341., 350.

Perlman, H H (1979) *Relationship: The heart of helping people.*The University of Chicago Press.

Pojman, LP (2017) *Ethics: Discovering right and wrong* Cengage, USA.

Rawls, J (1999) *A theory of justice* Harvard University Press, USA.

Ray, M (2016) *Transcultural caring dynamic in nursing and health care*

Rodney, P, Burgess, M, Phillips, J, McPherson, G & Brown, H (2013) Our theoretical landscape: A brief history of health care ethics.*Toward a moral horizon: Nursing ethics for leadership and practice* 59 – 83.

Rogers, CR (1951) *Client-centered therapy.*Houghton Mifflin, Boston.

Rogers, CR (1980) *A way of being.*Houghton Mifflin Company, New York.

Rosenberg, MB (2003) *Nonviolent communication: A language of life*

Salzberg, S (2004) *Lovingkindness: The revolutionary art of happiness.*

Schmidt, J J (2002) *Intentional helping: A philosophy for proficient caring relationships.*

Schneider, KJ & Längle, A (2012) The renewal of humanism in psychotherapy: a roundtable discussion. *Psychotherapy (Chic),* 49, 427-9.
[http://dx.doi.org/10.1037/a0027111] [PMID: 23205823]

Sellman, D (2007) On being of good character: Nurse education and the assessment of good character *Nurse Education Today,* 27, 762-7.

Skretkowicz, V (2010). *Florence Nightingale's notes on nursing and notes on nursing the laboring classes: Commemorative edition with historical commentary.*

Slote, M (2007) *The ethics of care and empathy.*Routledge, New York.
[http://dx.doi.org/10.4324/9780203945735]

Sorell, T (2011) The limits of principlism and recourse to theory: The example of telecare. *Ethical Theory Moral Pract,* 14, 369-82.
[http://dx.doi.org/10.1007/s10677-011-9292-9]

Smith, M A (2017) The ethics/advocacy connection: What are the ethical leadership qualities of nurses and how do these traits contribute to competent, safe care? *Nursing Management,* 48, 18-23.

Smolkin, D, Bourgeois, W & Findler, P (2010) *Debating health care ethics.*McGraw-Hill Ryerson, Canada.

Stephany, K (2002) Preventing suicide by increasing understanding of the commonalities of suicide risk, learning from past misconceptions and instilling hope *Life Notes,* 6, 6-7.

Stephany, K (2007) *Suicide intervention: The importance of care as a therapeutic imperative*(unpublished doctoral dissertation). Breyer State University, Alabama, USA..

Stephany, K (2012) *The ethic of care: A moral compass for Canadian nursing practice.*United Arab Emirates: Bentham Science Publishing Ltd.
[http://dx.doi.org/10.2174/97816080530491120101]

Stephany, K (2015) *Cultivating empathy: Inspiring health professionals to communicate more effectively.*United Arab Emirates: Bentham Science Publishing Ltd.

Stephany, K (2017) *How to help the suicidal person to choose life: The ethic of care & empathy as an indispensable tool for intervention.*United Arab Emirates: Bentham Science Publishing Ltd.

Strachey, L (2013) *The biography of Florence Nightingale.*Simon & Schuster, London.

Tschudin, V (2005) *Ethics in nursing: The caring relationship.*Elsevier, Philadelphia.

Watson, J & Marilyn, AR (1990) The ethics of care and the ethics of cure: Synthesis in chronicity. *Synthesis*New York: National League of Nursing.

Watson, J (2008) *Nursing: The philosophy of caring (Revised Edition).*

Woods, M (2011) An ethic of care in nursing: Past, present and future considerations *Ethics and Social Welfare,* 5, 267-276.
[http://dx.doi.org/10.1080/17496535.2011.563427]

Xu, ZX & Ma, HK (2016) How can a deontological decision lead to moral behaviour? The moderating role of

moral identity. *J Bus Ethics,* 137, 537-49.
[http://dx.doi.org/10.1007/s10551-015-2576-6]

Zinner, S E (2014) Paragons of virtue: Is Florence Nightingale working in the next cubicle? *Public Integrity,* 16, 411-21.

CHAPTER 2

Integrating Sound Moral Principles into Practice

Abstract: Moral principles are a set of ethical values that are used to guide decision making in practice. In Chapter Two an important connection between the ethic of care, nursing practice and key moral principles is made evident. Integrity consists of integrating honest ways consistently into one's everyday actions and is the moral principle that guarantees all other values. Veracity, which is the duty to tell the truth, and fidelity, which is about being loyal, are both related to integrity. Nurses are expected to view all people as worthy of dignity. They are cautioned to avoid blaming the victim because it holds people burdened by social conditions as accountable for their own situations. Beneficence is the obligation to do what will benefit the client and non-maleficence is the duty to prevent harm. However, sometimes medical interventions with known associated risks are utilized prior to considering less harmful options. Autonomy is having the freedom to make choices and nurses are expected to do their best to ensure that client autonomy is honoured as much as possible. Nurses are encouraged to be morally courageous which consists of performing the ethical right action even in the face of opposition. The seven key attributes of a morally courageous nurse are identified. Although impediments to moral courage do exist, nurses are inspired to develop strategies to overcome them. The Case in Point at the end of the Chapter is particularly challenging. A nurse is expected to practice non-maleficence while taking care of a client who is accused of a brutal crime.

Keywords: Autonomy, Advocacy, Beneficence, Cognitive behavioural therapy (CBT), Electroconvulsive therapy (ECT), Fidelity, Integrity, Moral principles, Moral courage, Mental Health Act, Non-maleficence, Paternalism, Parentalism, Respect for self-worth, Veracity.

LEARNING GUIDE

After Completing this Chapter, the Reader Should be Able to

* Be aware of the important connection between the ethic of care, nursing practice and key moral principles.

* Define each of the following: integrity, veracity, fidelity, respect for self-worth, beneficence, non-maleficence, autonomy and moral courage.

* Describe what victim blaming consists of and explain how it interferes with respect for self-worth.

* Realize that consistently looking for the good in others can sometimes be morally challenging.

* Understand why nurses should avoid practicing paternalism.

* Be able to describe what moral courage entails.

* Be conscious of each of the seven key attributes of a morally courageous nurse.

* Recognize that impediments to acts of moral courage do exist and brain-storm ways to over come them.

* Apply what was learned to the Case in Point: Practicing non-maleficence.

HOW MORAL PRINCIPLES FIT IN WITH THE ETHIC OF CARE

Chapter two begins by drawing attention to the important connection between the ethic of care, nursing practice and key moral principles. This discussion proceeds to explain how victim blaming interferes with respect for self-worth. Nurses are also cautioned to avoid practicing paternalism because it violates a client's right to choose. Acts of moral courage are encouraged which consists of performing the ethical right action in the face of opposition. The seven key attributes of a morally courageous nurse are then identified. Although impediments to moral courage do exist, nurses are inspired to develop strategies to overcome them. The Chapter ends with a Case in Point that is particularly challenging. A nurse is expected to practice non-maleficence while taking care of a client who is accused of a brutal crime.

Moral principles are a set of ethical values that are used to guide decision-making. Fig. (**2.1**) Cooper (1991) argues that nurses can focus on caring and also draw upon moral standards when faced with ethical conflicts. In fact, select ethical principles may sometimes assist nurses in helping their clients to sort through the challenging situations they may find themselves in. In the discussion that ensues an important connection will be made between the ethic of care, nursing practice and the following moral principles: integrity, veracity, fidelity, respect for self-worth, beneficence, non-maleficence, autonomy, and moral courage.

INTEGRITY: The Ethical Value that Guarantees All Other Values

"Live so when your children think of fairness and integrity, they think of you." H. Jackson Brown, American Author.

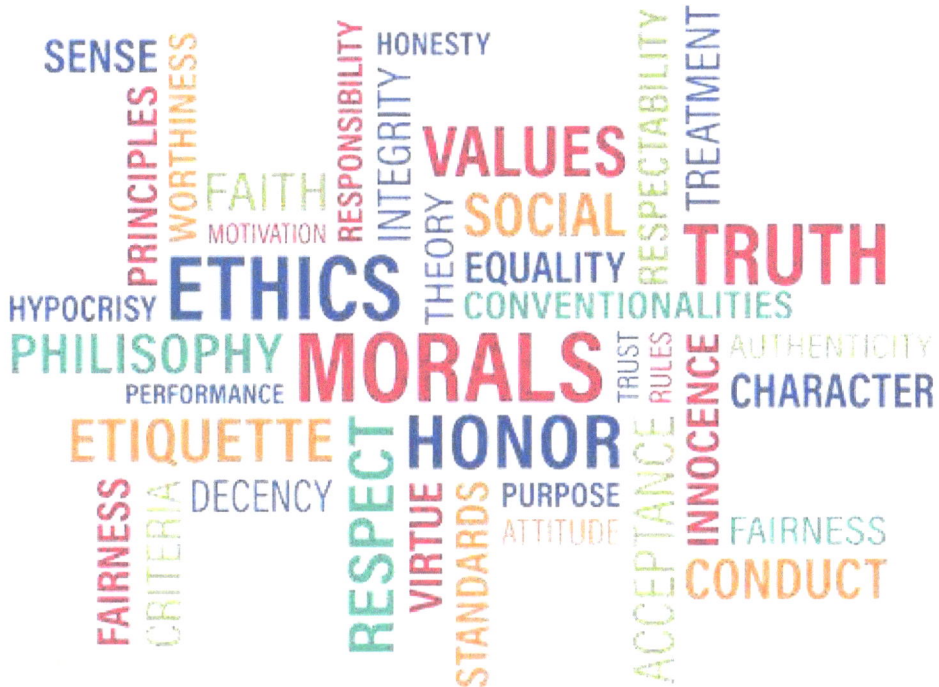

Fig. (2.1). Moral Principles. Source: www.pixabay.com.

Integrity consists of integrating honest ways consistently into one's everyday actions. Integrity has been identified as the moral principle that guarantees all other values, because in the absence of honesty your actions cannot be trusted. Integrity is also referred to as walking the talk or being true to your word and is exemplified by your actions. For example, you are a good nurse to the degree to which you live your life to the highest values that you espouse. Integrity becomes the external manifestation of high standards of expectations that one will be totally honest, will strive for excellence, and live authentically under the guidance of personal responsibility for the decisions one makes (Miller-Tiedeman, 1999). To live authentically is to be true to who you are in the stewardship of self (Hasser-Herrick, 2005).

VERACITY: Only the Truth Will Do

"Proclaim the truth and do not be silent through fear." Catherine of Siena, Scholastic Philosopher & Theologian.

Veracity is the duty to tell the truth and veracity is a likely ally of integrity

(Keatings & Smith, 2016). (Fig. **2.2**) When a client is suffering from an ailment they are vulnerable and fear of the unknown is often paramount. The expectation is that the nurse will be someone who can be trusted to do the right thing and not intentionally deceive the client in any way. However, the nurse's willingness to tell the truth can sometimes be challenged when they are asked to withhold valuable knowledge from the client who is desperately seeking answers. This problem readily occurs when a client is waiting for important test results or a definitive diagnosis that may include bad news. The rule is that it is the physician who does the telling. So where does that leave the nurse? Do they lie to the client? Of course not. Even if the nurse cannot be the one to share the facts about the tests or the diagnosis, they still must be honest about their role. The client needs to be informed that the doctor will discuss the test results and/or diagnosis with them, but the nurse will be there to follow up with additional queries and to offer support. The nurse can do what they can to help the client to sort through some of their emotions and fears after learning the truth, but that task can also be emotionally overwhelming for the nurse. The following story illustrates this point in a touching way. Box (**2.1**).

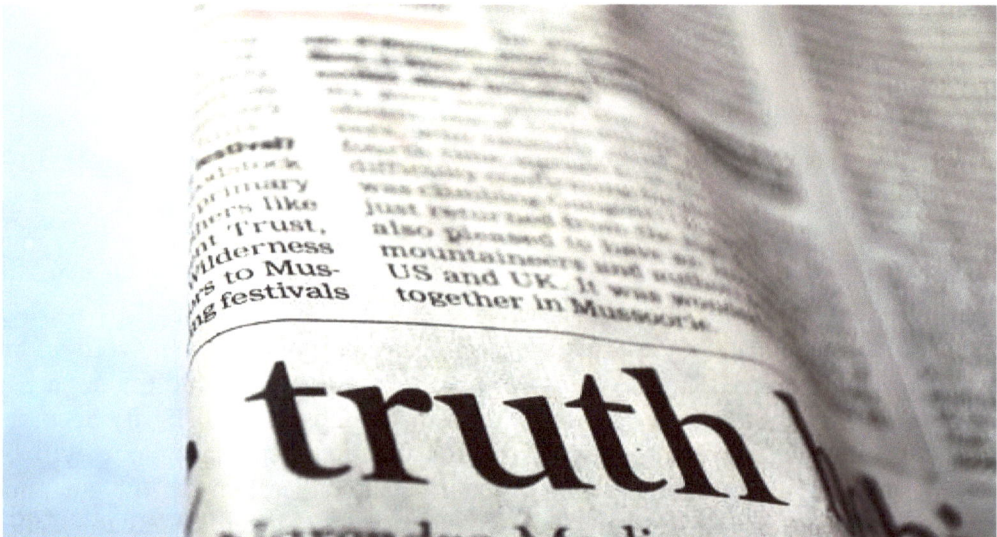

Fig. (2.2). Truth. Source: www.pixabay.com.

FIDELITY

"Keep every promise you make and only make promises you can keep." Anthony Hitt, American Businessman.

Fidelity is the act of keeping promises and being loyal and flows naturally from the lived morals of integrity and veracity. Fidelity is also foundational to the trust relationship between the nurse and the client (Burkhardt, Nathaniel & Walton, 2015; Keatings & Smith, 2016). According to Noland (1991) moral fidelity in nursing must start with the values of the client above loyalty to the physician, hospital or profession. This assertion does not in any way infer that the nurse deliberately disregards the authority and respect associated with other health care provider's wishes, the institutional policies or professional standards. Rather, one ought to strive to keep the client first and at the heart of the care that is provided.

Box 2:1. Narrative: Helping a Client Who has been Given Grave News.

Jane was a 30-year-old woman who had been admitted to hospital with shortness of breath that required oxygen therapy. Jane suffered from an aggressive form of cancer that had metastasized. Her haemoglobin was extremely low even though she had just received a blood transfusion a few days ago. The attending physician compassionately explained to Jane and her spouse, that after speaking with the Oncologist, he felt palliative measures were the only option left. The couple knew what that meant and they were somewhat prepared. However, when the doctor left the room Jane's husband summoned the nurse, Tom, to her bedside. Jane was sobbing quietly. She explained how upset she was that her two girls, who were mere toddlers, would never remember her and that she would not be able to see them grow up. Tom felt so sad for Jane but held his composure. He paused to just listen and be fully present and then he had an idea. Tom informed Jane that he had just read a story where someone was dying and had written letters to her children, sharing who she was and what her hopes and dreams were for them. The woman had instructed her next of kin to keep the letters in a safe place until her children turned 21. Tom asked Jane if that was something that she might want to consider. Jane's eyes lit up, she stopped crying and asked for a pen, paper, and two envelopes. Tom went and gathered the materials and handed them to Jane. Tom then left on his break for some time alone to cry.

The Importance of Keeping Promises

It is the ethical duty of the nurse to never *intentionally* make a pledge that they know they cannot keep. However, what if the nurse, in all fairness is unaware that they cannot carry through with what was promised due to unforeseen circumstances? In this situation the nurse is obliged to be upfront and admit to the person why it is that they could not keep their word. The humility of admitting the truth helps to re-build a foundation of trust. Furthermore, the nurse can endeavour to carry through with an action related to what was originally promised, even if there is a delay.

Respect for Self-Worth: Planting the Seeds of Self-Esteem

"When it comes to human dignity, we cannot make compromises." Angela Merkel, First Woman Chancellor of Germany.

Respect for self-worth views each person as equal and deserving of dignity and has the power to transform when it is applied consistently and from the heart. Respect for self-worth builds quite naturally on some of the previously introduced concepts from Chapter One like: acceptance, compassion, and unconditional positive regard. However, how do you help a person who has a poor self-esteem learn to feel worthy of love and care? Helping others to feel that they matter is not unlike planting seeds of flowers in a garden. You begin with small actions that in time result in something beautiful (Fig. **2.3**). For example, when a nurse believes in a person first through acts of kindness, praise and appreciation what follows is the faint hope that the client will begin to see themselves as a person of value. Once a seed of self-esteem is planted the individual can become more in touch with their deeper needs, feelings and values. In time they will hopefully rely less on other's opinions of their worth (Brammer & MacDonald, 1999). With the development of a healthy self-esteem the journey out of despair appears more hopeful.

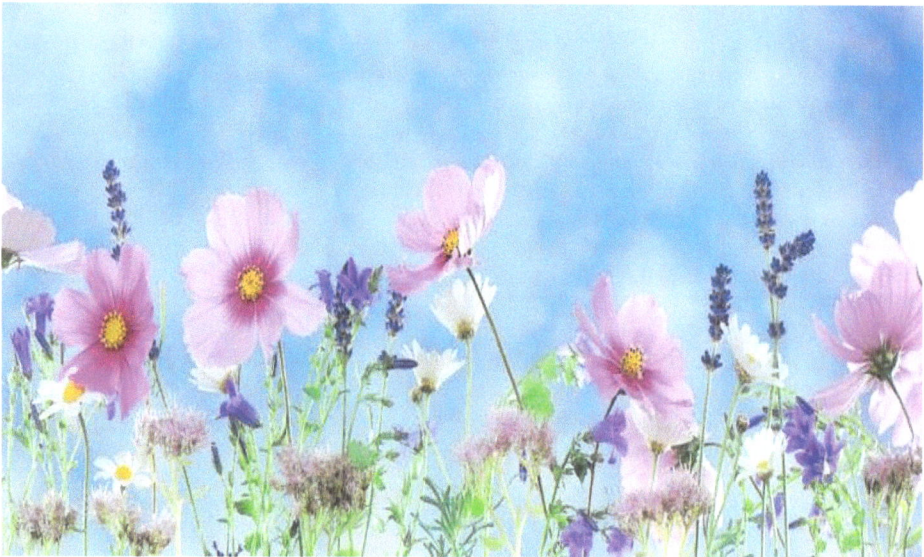

Fig. (2.3). Beautiful Flower Garden. Source: www.pixabay.com.

Blaming the Victim Poses a Barrier to Honouring Self-worth

In an ideal world all people would be viewed as worthy of dignity and respect, yet often finding fault and blame in another person is what has been taught as the norm. Similarly, nurses are sometimes prone to judge some of their clients because of their unscrupulous choices or actions. The perception of personal weakness or inferiority due to less than favourable conduct stems from a social notion of blaming the victim and blaming the victim poses a barrier to honouring a person's self-worth.

What is victim blaming? **Victim blaming** holds the people living under poor social conditions as accountable for their own situations and solely responsible for finding their way out of their impoverished circumstances (Burkhardt *et al.*, 2015). Yet in fact, social injustice is often a primary contributing factor to a person's less fortunate circumstances. I have often heard lay people and even nurses make statements like, *"Homelessness is a choice. People who are homeless are using their money for drugs and alcohol instead of for food and shelter."* Attitudes like this are counterintuitive to what is happening and these assumptions are not necessarily based on fact. The ethic of care admonishes nurses to be cognizant of the background circumstances that affect a person's choices and plight (Smolkin, Bourgeois & Findler, 2010). The truth of the matter is that homelessness is on the rise in many parts of Canada and the Canadian federal government still has not implemented a national housing strategy that addresses this crucial issue (Hulchanski, 2017).

Deliberately Looking for the Good in Others

"Each person matters, no human life is redundant." Basil Hume (1953 – 1999) The Monk Cardinal.

In the practice of the ethic of care nurses need to make it their deliberate intention to look for the good in their clients. Box (**2.2**). However, the act of concentrating on the decency in another person does not suggest that all their actions be condoned. Consequences rightfully follow the act of intentionally harming another (Stephany, 2012). However, the nurse must always strive to relinquish the tendency to condemn or treat a client with neglect or disrespect, regardless of what they have done. Nurses are ethically obligated to offer competent and compassionate care even in the presence of wrong action. This theme is threaded throughout this textbook because it is one of the greatest challenges to the lived moral practice of the nurse. Salzberg (2004) argues that we may be able to find at least one good quality in someone with character flaws, although sometimes we may be reluctant to do so.

Box 2:2. DELIBERATELY LOOKING FOR THE GOOD IN OTHERS: A MORAL CHALLENGE (Source: K. Stephany).
In the practice of the ethic of care nurses need to make it their deliberate intention to look for the good in their clients. For example, nurses are ethically obligated to offer competent and compassionate care even in the presence of wrong action. This theme presents itself throughout this textbook because it is one of the greatest challenges to the lived moral practice of the nurse.

BENEFICENCE

Beneficence closely aligns with the notion of respect for self-worth and consists of the duty to do what will help the client (Oberle & Bouchal, 2009). Beneficence not only requires careful consideration of the best interests of the people under our watch, it also consists of the ability to see issues and circumstances from the perspective of the other person (Burkhardt *et al.*, 2015). Austin & Boyd (2010) describe beneficence in action as occurring when the health care provider uses knowledge of science and draws upon aspects of caring to develop an environment in which individuals achieve maximum health care benefit. The role of the nurse in ensuring beneficence can sometimes be complex. It may require that the nurse integrate knowledge from a scientific, ethical, humanistic, holistic and cultural perspective into the overall plan for client care (Ray, 2016). Furthermore, the action of beneficence compels nurses to intervene when a medical order is harmful (*e.g.* unsafe drug dose). Similarly, a nurse needs to be aware of when their own behaviour or attitude does not benefit the client (Ray, 2016). These actions blend well into our next discussion which concerns the topic of non-maleficence, which is derived from the concept of beneficence.

NON-MALEFICENCE

"If you can, help others; if you cannot do that, at least do no harm." His Holiness the 14th Dalai Lama.

Non-maleficence is the duty to prevent harm whether intentional or unintentional (Burkhardt *et al.*, 2015). Keatings and Smith (2016) point out that some actions by a nurse may cause temporary harm (*e.g.*, intramuscular or subcutaneous injections, intravenous punctures, catheterizations and painful dressing changes). However, in these situations temporary harm is justified as a way of ultimately producing good for the client.

Non-Maleficence & Choosing Less Harmful Treatment Options

Sometimes medical interventions with known associated risks are utilized prior to considering less harmful options. An example is the use of **electroconvulsive therapy (ECT)** for the treatment of a suicidal client in the absence of trying other less invasive treatments first, such as counselling and **cognitive behavioural therapy (CBT)**. ECT is a treatment modality in psychiatry that induces a self-limiting seizure in a controlled fashion under general anesthesia and results in changes in mood. A series of ECT treatments has been demonstrated to be useful in the treatment of someone who is suicidal, but it is not without its risks (Austin & Boyd, 2010; Patel, Patel, Hardy, Benzies & Tare, 2006). CBT is an alternative to ECT as a treatment option for the suicidal client and is a non-invasive counselling strategy. For example, CBT teaches clients to change their negative self-talk and a negative world view into something positive. CBT, when applied consistently is known for its relative success in alleviating suicidal ideation and in improving overall coping and it does not pose any physical risk to the client (Cutcliffe & Stevenson, 2007; Stephany, 2017).

Another example of not following the ethical principle of non-maleficence, although with good intentions, is the practice of locking a suicidal person up in a seclusion room to protect them from acts of self-harm. The staff proceed with this strategy with the rational that at least the client is safe and free from access to a means to hurt themselves. Yet research demonstrates that placing a suicidal person in seclusion can induce increased psychological distress. For example, placing someone who is suicidal in seclusion for long periods of time can actually perpetrate increased suicidal thoughts, and enhance feelings of isolation, worthlessness and hopelessness (Cutcliffe & Stevenson, 2007; Stephany, 2017). Furthermore, neglect or not spending quality time with a suicidal client may be interpreted by them as a lack of care (Stephany, 2017). What is so badly needed in place of seclusion, is human connection and instillation of hope. Ideally seclusion room usage should be kept to a minimum and as soon as feasible, be replaced by close surveillance and interaction with a caring, empathetic helper who can instill hope (Cutcliffe & Stevenson, 2007; Stephany, 2017).

RESPECTING CLIENT AUTONOMY

"To take away a man's freedom of choice, even his freedom to make the wrong choice is to manipulate him as though he were a puppet and not a person." L'Engle, American Writer.

Autonomy is defined as having the freedom to make personal choices about issues that affect one's life without interference from others (Burkhardt *et al.*, 2015). When it comes to health care choices, Wright and Leahey (2005) describe autonomy as the freedom to make independent choices about one's health care. Honouring client autonomy is also closely associated with the view that all persons possess value and that their choices need to be respected.

Threats to Client Autonomy

Many aspects of medical care can threaten client autonomy. For instance, when a person is admitted to hospital they are placed in a gown that sometimes has an open back and often the client's undergarments are removed. Being half naked, while being cared for by strangers can undermine the confidence of even the most self-assured individual. Fear of the unknown, experiencing pain and being in a foreign environment may also result in a feeling of vulnerability.

Sometimes the client's need for autonomy is lost in the power differential that exists between the health care professional and the client, especially in a teaching hospital where a physician or nurse talk *over* or *about* the client within their hearing distance as if they do not exist. Behaviours of this sort threaten the individual's sense of personhood and self-control. Within the practice of the ethic of care, nurses must attend to the individual first and keep them at the center. Each step of the away the person should be informed about the choices that are available to them.

Paternalism which is sometimes referred to as **parentalism** occurs when physicians decide to make decisions for their clients without their consent (Oberle & Bouchal, 2009). The idea behind paternalism is that the doctor knows best, which may or may not be the case. Nurses do not use this moral principle because it violates client autonomy.

Mental Health Clients & Autonomy

In most jurisdictions in Canada there are laws under the title of a Mental Health Act that determines when and how a person who suffers from mental illness can be forced to receive treatment against their will. As a nurse it is imperative that you are familiar with your province or territory's Mental Health Act because specific aspects of the act differ from one jurisdiction to another (Pollard, 2014).

When a client is involuntarily committed (also referred to as certified) under a Mental Health Act, they are hospitalized against their will due to mental illness. What commonly occurs, is that the client who is certified can be given treatment related to their psychiatric diagnosis without their consent. They also cannot leave the hospital until de-certified (Pollard, 2014). These laws follow the principle of paternalism and were created to benefit the client who suffers from a debilitating mental illness. The argument is that due to impairment in cognitive reasoning, the individual is unable to make choices that will assist in their wellbeing or ensure their personal safety or the safety of others (Pollard, 2014). Often clients who suffer from serious mental illness are unaware that they are ill and they subsequently possess no insight and are prone to poor decision making. For instance, a lack of insight may cause a client to make poor choices and render them more inclined to refuse to follow a beneficial treatment plan (Smith, Hull, Israel, & Wilson, 2000).

It is important that the nurse be aware that they can honour client autonomy even when a person is involuntarily committed for treatment. The individual can be given choices in as many aspects of their care as is deemed possible. Increased autonomy may also be granted in stages as the client progresses toward wellness. Respecting client autonomy in small ways increases self-esteem and client empowerment and may enhance their capacity to make better choices when they are discharged back into the community (Pollard, 2014).

MORAL COURAGE: DARING TO BE BRAVE

"Every time we turn our heads the other way when we see the law flaunted, when we tolerate what we know to be wrong, when we close our eyes and ears to the corrupt because we are too busy or too frightened, when we fail to speak up and speak out, we strike a blow against freedom and decency and justice." Robert Kennedy, Politician, Lawyer & Former United States Attorney General.

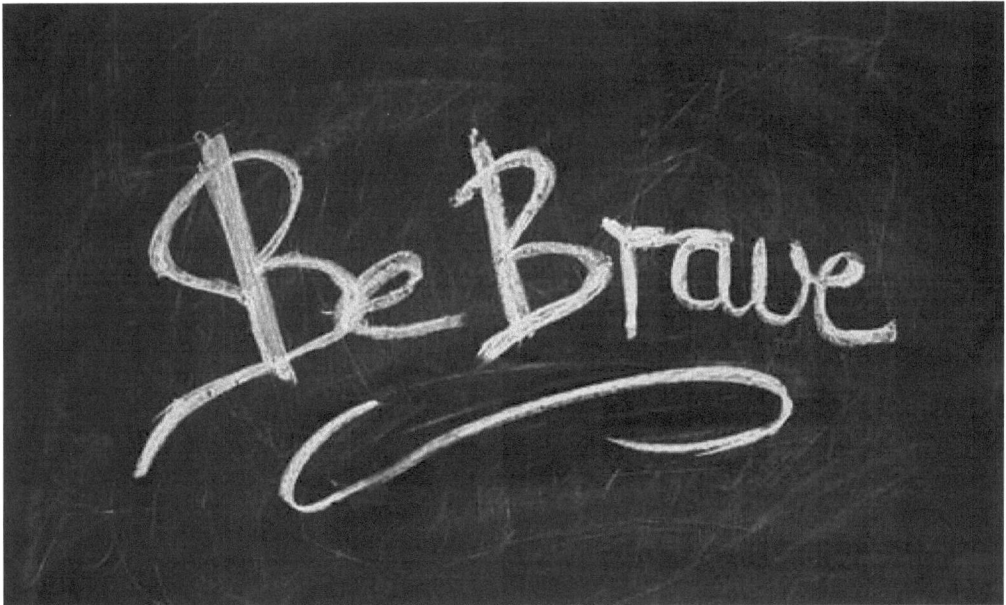

Fig. (2.4). Be Brave. Source: www.pixabay.com.

Box 2:3. MORAL COURAGE DEFINED (Stephany, 2006, p. 56).
Moral courage is the ability to adhere to the fundamental law of integrity, ethics and perseverance even in the face of rejection or opposition.

Moral courage involves being brave (Fig. **2.4**). It consists of "the ability to adhere to the fundamental law of integrity, ethics and perseverance even in the face of rejection or opposition" (Stephany, 2006, p. 56). Box (**2.3**) Being morally courageous involves taking tough stands for what is right, even when it is difficult to do so (Numminen, Repo & Leino-Kilpi, 2017). It is about doing what is morally just especially where client safety is concerned. For example, LaSala and Bjarnson (2010) point out that morally responsible nursing consists of being able to recognize and respond to unethical practices or to address issues that threaten quality client care. In this manner, moral courage is closely aligned with the ethical principles of beneficence and maleficence, which entails doing what benefits the client and preventing undo harm to the client.

Moral Courage, The Ethic of Care & Advocacy

Moral courage is closely affiliated with the ethic of care. LaSala & Bjarnason (2010) remind us that the ethic of care is not concerned with applying rigid rules to ethical issues. Rather, the ethic of care results in action that is attentive, responsible, competent, responsive and made on behalf of the people in our care (LaSala & Bjarnason, 2010). For instance, moral courage begins with the intention of righting wrongs but not without demonstrating empathy, compassion and sensitivity to the needs of others (Cleary & Horsfall, 2014).

The ethic of care and moral courage often result in client advocacy. **Advocacy** entails being the voice for, or acting on behalf of, a client or a cause. Advocacy becomes very important especially when a client is too afraid to speak up for themselves. For instance, nurses who act with moral courage uphold the key attributes of the ethic of care by consensus building and by taking into consideration what the client wants, followed by deliberate action to advocate on behalf of the client's wishes (LaSala & Bjarnason, 2010). The narrative that ensues demonstrates how a brave nurse used moral courage to advocate for her client when she was too afraid and vulnerable to speak up on her own behalf. Box **(2.4)**.

Key Attributes of Moral Courage in Nursing

Numminen *et al.* (2017) conducted an extensive and comprehensive concept analysis to identify the key attributes of moral courage. Their study involved doing a literature review of six extensive databases that examined the concept of moral courage as demonstrated in nursing studies (Numminen *et al.*, 2017). The result of their all-encompassing analysis identified seven attributes of a morally courageous nurse: "true presence, moral integrity, responsibility, honesty, advocacy, commitment and perseverance, and personal sacrifice" (Numminen *et al.*, 2017, p. 883). Box **(2.5)** gives a brief summary of each of these personal characteristics.

Box 2:4. Narrative: Moral Courage & Advocacy.

Mary arrived to the Emergency Room (ER) 26 weeks pregnant with her third child. She was in active labour, the fetal heart rate was strong at 140/minute but there were some signs of imminent birth. Mary's nurse Eva was at her bedside when the attending physician explained to Mary that her baby would be born soon but would likely not survive. The doctor then left to attend to other clients. Mary was extremely upset and crying. Eva stayed with her client to offer compassionate support. Mary told Eva that this was a very wanted child. She and her husband had two sons and she knew that this baby was a girl. Eva informed Mary that there was an option that might increase the chances of her premature fetus's survival. She could request to be urgently transferred to Woman's Hospital where there are neonatal specialists and an intensive care unit for premature babies. Eva asked Mary if she wanted to consider this alternative. Mary said, "*Yes*" but was too afraid to ask the doctor. Eva agreed to make the appeal on Mary's behalf. At first the request for the transfer was denied because a maternity nurse was unavailable to accompany Mary on the transfer. Eva offered to go with Mary and after a bit of convincing, the doctor agreed to the transfer and to notify the specialist at the receiving Tertiary facility. Eva got clearance and coverage from her supervisor to be replaced in the ER. The ambulance rushed to Woman's Hospital with sirens blaring. Mary's labour pains grew stronger. The maternity kit was opened and ready to use but Eva was really hoping that Mary could hold on until they arrived at their destination. Mary gave birth to a tiny girl 16 seconds after they made it to the delivery room. After seven weeks in hospital Mary's daughter was healthy and ready to go home. When a client is too afraid to ask for what they want and need the nurse must be courageous enough to speak up for them, even if it means being criticized. That is the essence of moral courage and advocacy.

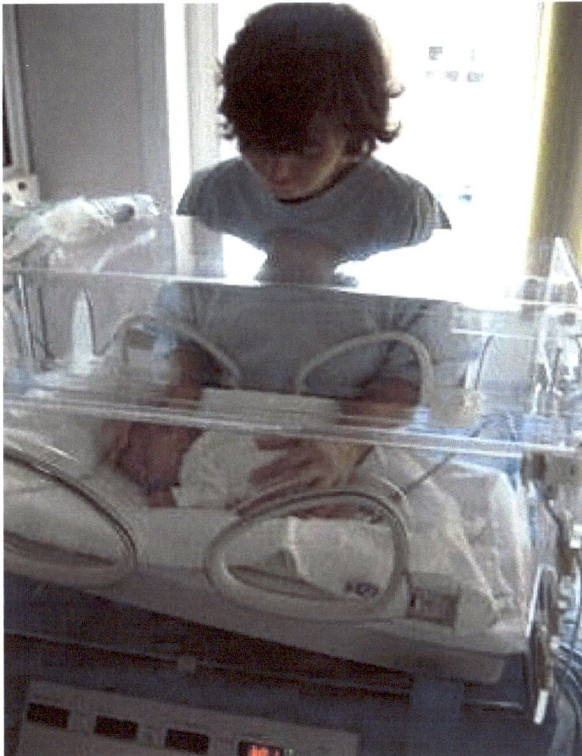

Fig. (2.5). Premature Infant. Source: www.pixabay.com.

Box 2:5. KEY ATTRIBUTES OF MORAL COURAGE IN NURSING (as adapted & summarized from Numminen *et al.*, 2017).
True Presence: Be truly present with the client. View the client as a fellow human being worthy of your care and concern. Dare to be touched by the client's vulnerability and admit to your own vulnerability.
Moral Integrity: Be honest & trustworthy and persevere in defending what is right. Do not compromise or conform with the mainstream. Feel empowered when you take a stand.
Responsibility: Aim for excellence in your work. Commit to the client's well-being and to preserve their dignity. Willingly admit your mistakes & limitations.
Honesty: Speak up and report unsafe practices. Question your own and other's practices. Admit your mistakes and take action to rectify them.
Advocacy: Intervene for and with the client, to preserve their dignity and to ensure that their needs and rights are respected.
Commitment & Perseverance: Be committed to giving good care and endure difficult situations. Avoid the easy way out. Maintain professional boundaries.
Personal Sacrifice: You have to be willing to commit and participate with your whole being in care situations. Take a stand if it is the right thing to do (*e.g.*, to preserve client safety) even when it may cause strain in your relationships.

Impediments to Moral Courage

Acting with moral courage is not without its impediments. Organizational structures, management styles that are autocratic, and fear of retaliation through being bullied or being fired, may inhibit a nurse from taking appropriate action even when they deem it morally necessary to do so (LaSala & Bjarnason, 2010). The following learning activity encourages nurses to come up with ideas on how to overcome obstacles to acts of moral courage. Box (**2.6**).

Box 2:6. LEARNING ACTIVITY: DEVELOP STRATEGIES TO OVERCOME IMPEDIMENTS TO MORAL COURAGE.
As a whole class or in small groups, discuss strategies that nurses can employ either individually or collectively to support each other in pursuing acts of moral courage.
Suggestion: You may want to review the CNA Code of Ethics (2017) and your Professional Nursing Standards of Practice for ideas.

Box 2:7 CASE IN POINT: PRACTICING NON-MALEFICENCE
Mathew is a 44-year-old who is unconscious and ventilated on a respirator in the Intensive Care Unit (ICU) after taking an almost lethal overdose of prescription medication. You come on duty and in report you learn that this man has been accused of the fatal beating of his three-year-old step daughter, although he has not been charged or convicted of the alleged crime. You are assigned to be Mathew's nurse for the next 12-hour shift.

Questions Pertaining to the Case in Point:

1. What emotions were generated when you read this story?
2. Did you think that Mathew deserves to be punished?
3. Can you still practice safe, competent and respectful care in the presence of strong negative emotions?
4. How can you transform negative feelings and judgements into something that is helpful and caring?

REFLECTING BACK

Summary of Key Points Covered in Chapter 2

- Moral principles are a set of ethical values that are used to guide decision making in practice.
- It was made evident how the ethic of care and specific moral principles are closely connected.
- Integrity is consistently acting in honest ways and is the value that guarantees all other values.
- Veracity is the duty to tell the truth and it is a likely ally of integrity.
- Fidelity is the act of keeping promises and was identified as foundational to the nurse – client relationship.
- Respect for self-worth views each person as equal and deserving of dignity.
- Blaming the victim holds people burdened by social conditions as accountable for their own situations and needed solutions.
- Victim blaming poses a barrier to honouring the self-worth of all people.
- Beneficence is the obligation to do what is beneficial for the client.
- Non-maleficence is the duty to prevent harm either intentionally or unintentionally.
- It was pointed out that sometimes medical interventions with known associated risks are utilized prior to considering less harmful options.
- Autonomy is having the freedom to make choices about one's life.
- Paternalism goes against the principle of autonomy because it consists of the doctor making decisions for the client in their best interest without their consent.
- Moral courage was identified as the ability to adhere to the fundamental law of integrity, ethics and perseverance even in the face of rejection or opposition.
- Acts of moral courage often result in client advocacy, which is acting as the voice for the client.
- The following seven key attributes of a morally courageous nurse were identified: true presence, moral integrity, responsibility, honesty, advocacy, commitment and perseverance, and personal sacrifice.
- Impediments to moral courage do exist and nurses are encouraged to develop

strategies to overcome them.

SOMETHING TO PONDER

1. Nurses are human beings. Is it a reasonable expectation that nurses consistently practice unconditional positive regard?
2. Explain how moral principles like veracity and fidelity relate to the integrity of the nurse.
3. What specific actions by a nurse can honour client autonomy when a prescribed treatment is specifically designed from the premise of paternalism?
4. Persons who suffer from a mental illness can be forced to receive treatment against their will, yet clients who suffer from medical problems are seldom treated in this manner. Is this fair?
5. Can you describe an act of moral courage that you have already achieved or would like to initiate?
6. Does anything about acting with moral courage frighten you and if so, why?
7. Which of the moral principles that were introduced in this Chapter are the easiest to follow and which ones are more challenging for you?

CLASSROOM GROUP EXERCISES

1. As a classroom discussion, come up with a list of ways that each of the ethical principles that were introduced in this Chapter align with the ethic of care.
2. Break into groups of four. Discuss the moral arguments for and against forcing clients to adhere to treatment against their will. Do this exercise not only concerning persons who suffer from mental illness but also with people who have a serious medical condition who do not comply with treatment suggestions that would benefit their condition. How would the application of the ethic of care and select moral principles assist you with your discussion?

ON YOUR OWN

1. Pick a moral principle that you find most difficult to adhere to. Journal about how you feel. What can you do to incorporate that value into your way of being? Set clear goals that will help you to integrate that principle into your life and practice, then follow through with your plan.

RECOMMENDED READING

Kidder, R. M. (2005). *Moral courage.* New York: Harper Collins Publishers.

Lachman, V. D. (2009). *Developing your moral compass.* New York: Springer Publishing.

WEB RESOURCE

Web Resource: Integrity & Values: Twenty Leadership Traits

http://www.integrityandvalues.com/leadership-traits/

CONSENT FOR PUBLICATION

Not applicable.

CONFLICT OF INTEREST

The authors confirm that this chapter contents have no conflict of interest.

ACKNOWLEDGEMENTS

Declared none.

REFERENCES

Austin, W & Boyd, MA (2010) Ethical psychiatric and mental health nursing practice.*Psychiatric nursing for Canadian practice* Lippincott Williams & Wilkins, Philadelphia 83-100.

Brammer, LM & MacDonald, G (1999) *The helping relationship: Process and skills.*Allyn and Bacon, Toronto.

Burkhardt, MA, Nathaniel, AK & Walton, NA (2015) *Ethics and issues in contemporary nursing* Nelson, Toronto, Ontario.

Cleary, M & Horsfall, J (2014) Nursing and enacting the courage of one's convictions. *Issues in Mental Health Nursing,* 35, 724-6.
[http://dx.doi.org/10.3109/01612840.2014.938965]

Cooper, M (1991) Principle-orientated ethics and the ethic of care: A creative tension. *Advances in Nursing Science,,* 4, 22-31.

Cutcliffe, JR & Stevenson, C (2007) *Care of the suicidal person.*Elsevier, Toronto.

Hulchanski, D (2017) No, Ottawa has not put forth a national housing strategy. *The Globe & Mail* Retrieved from: https://www.theglobeandmail.com/opinion/-ottawa-has-not-put-forth-a-national-housing-strategy/article37173057/

LaSala, C A & Bjarnason, D Creating work environments that support moral *Online Journal of Issues in Nursing,,* 15Manuscript 4. (2010) Retrieved from: http://ojin.nursingworld.org/MainMenuCategories/EthicsStandards/Resources/Courage-and-Distress/Workplace-Environments-and-Moral-Courage.html
[http://dx.doi.org/10/3912/OJIN]

Numminen, O, Repo, H & Leino-Kilpi, H (2017) Moral courage in nursing: A concept *Nursing Ethics,* 24, 878-91.
[http://dx.doi.org/10.1177/0969733016634155]

Patel, M, Patel, S, Hardy, D, Benzies, B & Tare, V (2006) Should Electroconvulsive therapy be an early consideration for suicidal clients? *The Journal of Electroconvulsive Therapy,* 22, 113-5.

Pollard, C (2014) Ethical responsibilities and legal obligations for psychiatric mental health practice In: C. L., Pollard, S. L. Ray, Haase, (Eds.),   Toronto: Elsevier, Canada, 114-30.

Ray, MA (2016) Transcultural caring dynamics in nursing and health care, 2nd ed. F.A. Davis Company,

Philadelphia.

Salzberg, S (2004) *Lovingkindness: The revolutionary art of happiness.*Shambala, London.

Siegal, B (1989) *Peace, love & healing, body mind communication & the path to self healing: An exploration.*Harper & Row Publishers, New York.

Smith, TE, Hull, JW, Israel, LM & Wilson, DF (2000) Insights, symptoms, and neurocognition in schizophrenia. *Bulletin,* 26, 193-200.

Smolkin, D, Bourgeois, W & Findler, P (2010) *Debating health care ethics.*McGraw-Hill Ryerson, Canada.

Stephany, K (2012) *Each day is a new creation: Guidelines on living a life of purpose*IN: Balboa Press, Bloomingdale,.

Stephany, K (2017) *How to help the suicidal person to choose life: The ethic of care and empathy as an indispensable tool for intervention.*Bentham Science Publishing Ltd, United Arab Emirates.

Wright, L M & Leahey, M (2005) Nurses and families: A guide to family assessment and intervention, 4th ed. Philadelphia.

CHAPTER 3

The CNA Code of Ethics Part I: Integrating Nursing Ethical Values & Responsibilities into Care

Abstract: Chapter Three begins with exploring the role of Canadian law because nurses who have a working knowledge of the Canadian legal system are better equipped to deal with legal issues that may arise during their practice. A brief overview of *The Canadian Constitution* and *The Charter of Rights and Freedoms* is also undertaken for similar reasons. Key aspects of the role of the Canadian Nurses Association (CNA) are presented followed by a discussion of the purpose and foundation of the CNA Code of Ethics. A connection is drawn between themes from the CNA Code of Ethics and the ethic of care. Nurses are made aware that the ethical values and responsibilities as laid out in Part I of the CNA Code of Ethics are not discretionary and must be followed by all practicing nurses. Each of the seven CNA Code of Ethics values are then discussed in terms of how they play out in actual practice and narratives are used to emphasize important points. Some topics that directly relate to Part I of the CNA Code of Ethics include: safety and nursing research; what to do if a nurse suspects that a health professional is practicing unsafely or unethically; key elements of informed consent; and the role of the nurse practitioner and registered nurse in medical assistance in dying (MAID). The Chapter ends with a Case in Point where a nurse deliberately covers up a mistake that costs a client their life.

Keywords: Accountability, Common law, Case law, Compassion, Criminal law, Civil law, Conscientious objection, Confidentiality, Distributive justice, Ethics, Ethic of care, Injustice, Justice, Knowledge and care, Law, Medical assistance in dying (MAID), Nursing research, Nursing competence, Precedent, Practice standards, Statutory law, Safety, Safety plan, Self-disclosure, Social justice, Social injustice, The Supreme Court of Canada, *The Canadian Constitution*, *The Charter of Rights and Freedoms*, The Canadian Nurses Association (CNA), The CNA Code of Ethics, Values.

LEARNING GUIDE

After Completing this Chapter, the Reader Should be Able to

- Understand that law always supersedes ethics.
- Explain the two key ways that laws are made in Canada.

- Differentiate between common law, case law, precedent, statutory law, criminal law and civil law.
- Define democracy.
- Gain an awareness of the importance of *The Canadian Constitution* & *The Charter of Rights and Freedoms.*
- Describe the role of the Canadian Nurses Association (CNA).
- Explain the purpose and foundation of the CNA Code of Ethics (2017).
- Appreciate the connection between The CNA Code of Ethics & the ethic of care.
- Be aware that the ethical values and responsibilities as laid out in Part I of the CNA Code of Ethics must be followed by all practicing nurses.
- Understand some of the ways in which the seven values of Part I of CNA Code of Ethics and relevant ethical responsibilities are applied in nursing practice.
- Gain a comprehensive understanding of the important legal and ethical issues in relation to the CNA Code of Ethics values.
- Apply what was learned to the Case in Point: What Happens When a Nurse Deliberately Covers up a Mistake.

In this current Chapter the relationship between ethics and the law is presented first. The role of the Canadian Nurses Association (CNA), and the purpose and foundation of the CNA Code of Ethics is then clearly articulated, followed by a discussion of the connection between the CNA Code of Ethics and the ethic of care. Each of the seven core ethical values and some of the responsibilities as laid out in Part I of the new 2017 edition of the CNA Code of Ethics is then carefully delineated, with special attention given to new content. At the close of the Chapter a Case in Point is presented that demonstrates a terrible tragedy that occurs when a nurse deliberately covers up her error.

THE RELATIONSHIP BETWEEN ETHICS & THE LAW

"In law a man is guilty when he violates the rights of others. In ethics he is guilty if he only thinks of doing so." Immanuel Kant, German Philosopher.

Nurses need to be aware that law always supersedes ethics and nurses are obligated to obey the law. Box **(3:1).** Although **ethics** is the study of ideal conduct, **law** is concerned with the rules and regulations formed by government. In fact, nurses who have a working knowledge of the Canadian legal system are better equipped to deal with legal issues that may arise, especially in trying situations (Keatings & Smith, 2016). Although laws are meant to be derived from ethics, debate exists around how some of these laws are administered. For instance, a law that makes it an offence to touch another person without their consent is based on the ethical principles of autonomy and non-maleficence (Keatings & Smith, 2016). Laws that intentionally restrict a competent person's freedom to make an informed choice are not based on ethics. An example may be a court ruling to allow food producers to exclude some important nutritional information on the labels of processed foods. Such a law would be intended for the purpose of allowing certain industries to make more money but may cause harm to the consumer.

Box 3:1 LAW SUPERSEDES ETHICS (Source: K. Stephany)
Nurses need to be aware that law always supersedes ethics and nurses are obligated to obey the law.

How Laws are Made in Canada

In Canada, there are two ways in which laws are created: through the judicial system as in the practice of common law, which is referred to as case law; and through government and the legislative system, which is referred to as statutory law. Common laws are formed by the judicial system, where courts and judges make decisions and each level is answerable to a more superior court. In lower courts, decisions made in one province are not legally binding in another province (Burkhardt, Nathaniel & Walton, 2015).

The Supreme Court of Canada is the highest court in Canada as well as the final court of appeals within the Canadian justice system (Government of Canada: Department of Justice. (n.d.) (Fig. **3.1**). The Canadian Supreme Court's rulings are enforceable across Canada, however the Supreme Court of Canada prefers to instruct governments to form statutory laws, particularly on controversial issues.

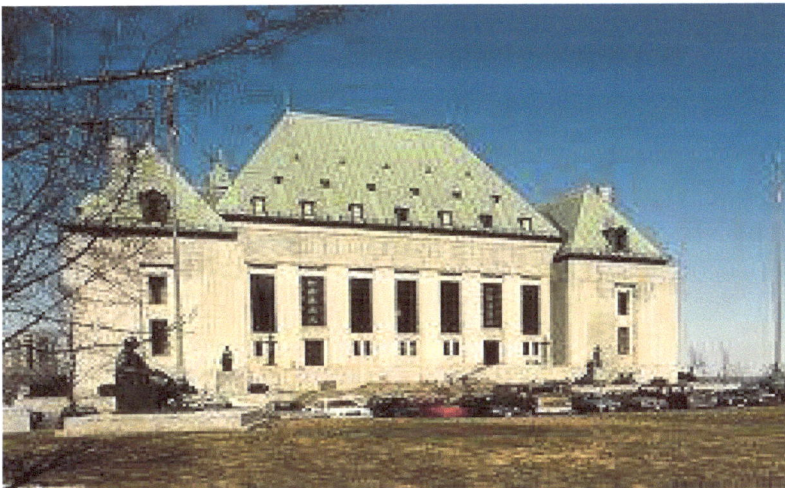

Fig. (3.1). The Supreme Court of Canada. Source: www.thecanadianencyclopedia.ca

Common law (sometimes called case law) is a system based on rules, principles, and doctrine developed by English judges over the centuries that are meant to be based on common sense (Keatings & Smith, 2016). Within the common law system laws of conduct are not formally written down. Instead a judge follows **case law**, or decisions made from past legal cases. A **precedent** is an aspect of a previous case where a judge writes out the reasons for a decision in a specific legal matter. Similar cases that come before the courts can then site such former rulings.

Statutory laws are laws that politicians make such as acts, or statutes (Burkhardt *et al.,* 2013). An example of a statutory law is a law which makes it illegal to drink alcohol and drive. In Canada, such laws can be made by either the federal parliament or provincial or territorial legislatures. **Criminal law** is derived from statutory law. It regulates the arrest, charging, and trying of suspected offenders. Criminal law includes decisions that are made regarding the punishment of individuals convicted in the courts of committing a criminal act (Burkhardt *et al.*, 2015). While non-criminal matters are resolved in courts between two or more entities, criminal cases can only be brought before a court by a government lawyer, called Crown Counsel. In Canada, what courts can consider as crimes is defined by *The Canada Criminal Code*, which is a piece of federal legislation. It is the job of police and crown counsel to bring cases before a court if they suspect a piece of legislation, has been breached (Burkhardt *et al.*, 2015).

The Province of Quebec & Civil Law

Civil law is based on Roman law which is prevalent in Europe and in the province of Quebec where civil law is practiced instead of common law (Fig. **3.2**). Civil law is a body of laws that deal with disputes between individuals and does not deal with criminal cases or legal cases that relate to government. In civil law, legal principles and rules are written in an organized fashion into a central statute or code (Keatings & Smith, 2016). Civil law is primarily concerned with the rights of individuals in society in the form of contracts and torts. A legal **contract** is an agreement between two or more people that can be enforced by law whereas a **tort** consists of an   alleged wrong doing or harm done to   another (Burkhardt *et al.*, 2015).

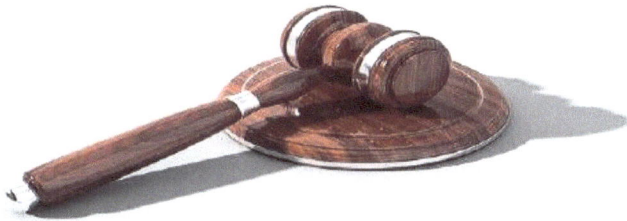

Fig. (3.2). Civil Law. Source: www.pixabay.com

CANADIAN DEMOCRACY & THE CANADIAN CONSTITUTION

Canada is a democratic country. Democracy was defined by the 16th United States President, Abraham Lincoln as government of the people, by the people and for the people (In the Democracy Center, n.d.). The term was derived from the Greek language and means rule by simple people. Democracy was created as a reaction to abuse of power by rulers. In modern times **democracy** is a form of government where a constitution guarantees basic personal and political rights, fair and free elections, and independent courts of law (In the Democracy Center, n.d.).

In our Canadian democracy, persons, institutions and even governments are subject to a higher law known as *The Canadian Constitution*. *The Canadian Constitution* establishes the fundamental rules and principles of how the country of Canada is ordered, how its laws are made and the extent of the power of its government and its courts (Keatings & Smith, 2016). *The Canadian Constitution* includes *The Charter of Rights and Freedoms* which conveys the basic legal and democratic rights of all Canadians (Keatings & Smith, 2016). The rights as set out by the Charter cannot be infringed upon by government unless justifiable and any government measure or created law that violates a person's constitutional rights is deemed illegal and invalid according to the Charter (Keatings & Smith, 2016). Note that, this discussion of the law in this current Chapter has been very basic because an in-depth discussion of the practice of law in Canada is beyond the scope of this textbook. Nurses are encouraged to become keenly aware of laws that pertain to the practice of health care delivery in their specific jurisdiction and are obligated to follow the law.

The Canadian Nurses Association (CNA)

"When CNA speaks on a public health issue, governments and citizens listen. The

level of respect is in large part due to its strong, credible voice." Donna Brunskill, Nurse Advocate & Former Executive Director of the Saskatchewan Registered Nurses Association.

The Canadian Nurses Association (CNA) serves as the national regulatory body for registered nurses. A key role of the CNA includes ensuring that the professional designation of Registered Nurse (RN) and Nurse Practitioner (NP) are recognized by the public as gold standards (Brunskill, 2010). Registration and certification exams, standards of practice and a Code of Ethics are just a small part of what the CNA is involved in. The CNA is an organization that embodies nursing leadership. For example, the CNA influences legislation, government programs and national and international advancement of health policy (Keatings & Smith, 2016). The CNA is also a member of the International Council of Nurses. The following are a few examples as pointed out by Brunskill (2010), of how the CNA has served the public interest. The CNA follows Canadian values of peace, order and democratic views of conduct. The CNA was involved in ensuring that the values of equity and solidarity were included in *The Canada Health Act*. The CNA also has been instrumental in ensuring that public access to health care is honoured (Brunskill, 2010).

The CNA (2018) has a long history in Canada. For instance, since 1908 the CNA has served as the national and professional voice of RNs. The CNA has recently expanded its membership beyond RNs and NPs by inviting Licensed/Registered Practical Nurses (LPNs) and Registered Psychiatric Nurses (RPNs) to be members of the Association (CNA, 2018). The reason for this decision is based on the goal of increasing the collaboration within and across health-care and due to the rise of interprofessional care models becoming the norm (CNA, 2018).

THE CNA CODE OF ETHICS

The Purpose of the CNA Code of Ethics

The Canadian Nurses Association **(CNA)** *Code of Ethics for Registered Nurses* is a declaration of the ethical values of nurses and of nurse's responsibilities to people with health-care needs and those requiring care (CNA, 2017). The purpose of the Code is both aspirational and regulatory (CNA, 2017). Specific values and ethical responsibilities are set out in Part I of the Code. Part II outlines how nurses can work toward ending social inequities. There are several key aspects to the purpose of the CNA Code of Ethics that are summarized in Box (**3:2**).

Box (3:2) THE PURPOSE OF THE CNA CODE OF ETHICS (as adapted & summarized from CNA, 2017, p. 2).
1. The CNA Code of Ethics provides guidance for ethical relationships, behaviours and decision-making.
2. The CNA Code of Ethics coincides with professional standards, best practices, research, laws and regulations that guide practice.
3. It guides nurses on how to work through ethical challenges that arise with persons receiving care & with colleagues in nursing and other fields of health care.
4. The CNA Code of Ethics is intended for nurses in all contexts and domains of practice and at all levels of decision-making.
5. It is not based on one particular philosophy but arises from different schools of thought such as: relational ethics, the ethic of care, principle-based ethics, feminist ethics, virtue ethics and values.
6. Self-evaluation, feedback and peer review is the basis for advocacy.
7. The CNA Code of Ethics is the ethical basis for nurses to advocate for quality practice environments.
8. Due to the fact that the societal context in which nurses work is constantly changing, which can influence practice, the CNA Code of Ethics is periodically revised.

The Foundation of the CNA Code of Ethics

The CNA (2017) requires that nursing ethics prioritize and advocate for changes in broad societal issues that negatively affect the health and well-being of Canadian residents. Therefore, the foundation of the Code expects that nurses maintain an understanding of key aspects of social justice that affect social determinants of health (CNA, 2017). These actions are expected of nurses as part of their ethical practice and are deemed important (CNA, 2017).

The CNA Code of Ethics & The Ethic of Care

As aforementioned, the CNA Code of Ethics (2017) draws from a whole stream of philosophical underpinnings which includes the ethic of care. The CNA Code of Ethics and the ethic of care share many common concerns and values. For example, both provide guidance for ethical relationships and direction and assistance to nurses working through the ethical challenges that they face in practice. The CNA Code of Ethics and the ethic of care also equate human connectedness, the caring motif, respect for diversity and advocacy as central to the role of the nurse. Part II of the CNA Code of Ethics requires that nurses maintain awareness of social justice issues and outlines how nurses can act to end social inequities. Similarly, the ethic of care condemns exploitation or the deliberate hurting of others and calls nurses to take action to stop or prevent all deliberate mistreatment of persons (Gilligan, 1982). Further links between the ethic of care and the CNA Code of Ethics will become more evident in the dialogue that ensues.

Part I of the CNA Code of Ethics: Nursing Values & Ethical Responsibilities

"Peace requires that you do what in your heart you know – that your chosen values guide your actions" Peggy Chin, Nurse & Author.

Values are standards that are esteemed, desired important or have merit or worth (Fry & Johnstone, 2002). Burkhardt *et al.*, (2015) describe values as principles, beliefs, traditions, behaviours, characteristics, or goals that are highly prized or preferred by individuals, groups, or society. The CNA as a national nursing regulatory body has identified seven key values in their Code of Ethics (2017) followed by a set of ethical responsibilities that are closely related to each specific value. The ethical responsibilities are intended to help nurses apply The Code of Ethics values. It is important to note that the values and ethical responsibilities as stated in the Code are not discretionary. Nurses cannot pick and choose which ones they will or will not follow. The underlying expectation is that all of these values and responsibilities will be incorporated into the practice of nursing. However, sometimes there are actual challenges in the implementation of these values. For instance, in the delivery of health-care services, values may be sometimes conflict. The CNA Code of Ethics advises that any value conflict needs to be carefully evaluated in relation to specific situations (CNA, 2017). When conflicts do occur, nurses are encouraged to use an ethical decision-making model for guidance (CNA, 2017). Two specific ethical decision-making models will be introduced in Chapter Five. The seven primary CNA Code of Ethics values are listed in Box (**3:3**).

Box 3:3 THE SEVEN PRIMARY CNA CODE OF ETHICS VALUES (CNA, 2017, p. 3).

A. Providing safe, compassionate, competent and ethical care
B. Promoting health and well-being
C. Promoting and respecting informed decision-making
D. Honouring dignity
E. Maintaining privacy and confidentiality
F. Promoting justice
G. Being accountable

Value A: Providing Safe, Compassionate, Competent & Ethical Care
Safety First

Value A of the CNA Code of Ethics (2017) instructs nurses to consistently provide safe, compassionate, competent and ethical care. Safety is noted to be a priority. Nurses are directed to question and intervene, when necessary, to address unsafe conditions (CNA, 2017). Nurses are also mandated to act with integrity and to take any needed action to prevent or minimize incidents that jeopardize client safety, which includes near misses (CNA, 2017). The following narrative illustrates how a student nurse took the initiative to act on behalf of her client's safety regardless of opposition from a staff nurse. Box (**3:4**).

Box 3:4 Narrative: Advocating for a Mental Health Client's Safety

Sasha was in the final semester in a Bachelor of Science in Nursing (BSN) Program. Sasha was doing a clinical rotation in the area of mental illness and addictions. She was assigned to care for clients who were admitted to hospital in acute adult psychiatry. On one particular clinical day Sasha was assigned to a 21-year-old woman, Anna, who had been admitted to hospital several days after an intentional and almost lethal overdose of prescribed medications. This was Anna's third attempt at suicide in one year. Eighteen months ago Anna's brother committed suicide. On this particular clinical day Anna's psychiatrist had just written an order for her to go out on a four-hour pass. Sasha did a suicide risk assessment and concluded that Anna was not currently contemplating hurting herself, but because of her history, Sasha was aware that Anna was still at risk. Anna herself stated that she was nervous about leaving and that she was worried about how she would cope when away from the unit. Sasha reassured Anna that a friend was going to pick her up and stay with her during the pass. Sasha thought that another intervention would help keep Anna safe. She had learned in one of her previous classes how to conduct a safety plan. A safety plan usually includes a minimum of two features. First, the client writes down five positive ways in which they will cope if they become stressed, which includes reasons for living. Secondly, they record the phone numbers of five persons and/or agencies that they will call, in order of priority, if they start to experience suicidal thoughts. Sasha consulted with her nursing instructor and they both agreed that a safety plan was a good idea. Anna really enjoyed developing the safety plan with Sasha. She told Sasha that it helped her to think differently and to focus on helpful modes to deal with stress. However, when a staff nurse noted the safety plan at Anna's bedside she removed it and informed Sasha that she should not be performing this task because, "It is not our policy to do safety plans." The staff nurse may have felt insecure with new best practices coming onto the unit, which may mean more work for her already overburdened caseload. Sasha went to her clinical instructor for help. Her instructor spoke to the nurse and informed her that although developing a safety plan may not be hospital policy, it does fall under best practices when assisting a person who is at risk of self-harm to remain safe. The staff nurse became angry at Sasha and her instructor and went to summon the psychiatric nurse clinician. The psychiatric nurse clinician met with the nurse, student nurse and clinical instructor and asked to examine the contents of the safety plan. After reviewing the plan the psychiatric nurse clinician stated that she thought that the tool was useful and that she would look into using it in the future. Meanwhile, Anna was able to take the safety plan with her on her pass. Client safety comes before all else, but sometimes it requires moral courage to do the right thing in the face of opposition.

Safety & Nursing Research

Another specific ethical responsibility under Value A of the CNA Code of Ethics (2017) stresses the importance of nurses supporting, utilizing and engaging in research and other related activities and that they use guidelines to conduct ethical research. The research process consists of a series of steps that include but are not limited to: choosing the topic, reviewing the literature, forming a question, design & methodology, data collection, analysis, interpretation, dissemination of results, which may or may not include publication (Barker, Pistrang & Elliott, 2015). The rights, dignity and welfare of human research subjects must be safe guarded (Barker *et al.*, 2015). The safety of research subjects must be planned for in the design & methodology step but should also be considered in each phase of research. There are at least five major ethical issues that nurses need to be aware of in any research that involves human participants. Box (**3:5**).

Box 3:5 THE ETHICAL SAFETY OF HUMAN RESEARCH PARTICIPANTS (as adapted from Barker *et al.*, 2015).
1. **Informed Consent:** Participants must enter the study freely which means they cannot be coerced into becoming involved in research. The researcher must give each subject full disclosure about the study that includes potential risks and benefits and must ensure that the participants understand what the risks *versus* benefits entail. 2. **Freedom to Leave the Study:** Participants must be made aware that they can drop out of the study at any point in time for any reason. 3. **Avoidance of Harm:** Although there may be a trade-off between the potential harm to individual participants and the potential benefit to humanity, harm should be avoided as much as possible. The subjects must also be made aware of any potential harm that they may encounter prior to consenting to be a part of the study. 4. **Privacy & Confidentiality:** Subjects have the right to confidentiality concerning any of their personal data. 5. **External Review:** All research involving humans should be reviewed and approved by an external ethics committee or review panel before the study is started.

Compassionate Care

Compassion consists of identifying with the suffering of another person. The notion of compassion was introduced in Chapter One as a component of the Mosaic of Care and nurses are mandated by Value A of the CNA Code of Ethics (2017) to practice compassion. Acts of compassion consists of identifying with the human condition of vulnerability with sincere, caring actions and the compassionate nurse does not criticize or judge (Ray, 2016; Rosenberg, 2003). In fact, the compassionate nurse seeks to do whatever they can to alleviate suffering and they make it their intention to enrich another person's life in some way (Rosenberg, 2003). In this manner compassion is a process of giving from the heart (Fig. **3.3**).

Competent Nursing Care & Client Safety

Competent and ethical care are crucial parts to Value A of the CNA Code of Ethics (2017) and they are closely related to Chapter One's explanation by Mayerhoff (1971) of the application of knowledge & care. **Knowledge and care** refer to acquired learning as competence and skillfulness in practice. **Nursing competence** is essential and implies that nurses draw from evidence-based data, that they are life-long learners and that they maintain competency in their field of expertise. Nurses must be cautioned not to work outside of their scope of practice. For instance, a nurse who has just graduated from nursing school and who does not have any additional training in a specialty area should refrain from working in that area until they obtain the appropriate additional education and training.

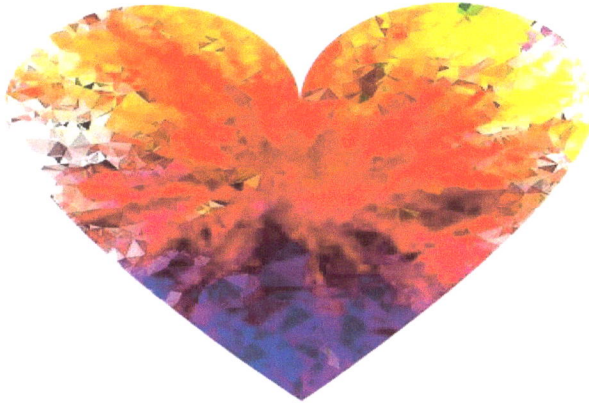

Fig. (3.3). Heart. Source: www.pixabay.com

Practice standards guide nursing practice and the scope of nursing is legally legislated (Oberle & Bouchal, 2009). A nurse who breaches practice standards that does not cause harm to a client will be disciplined by their regulatory body. However, a nurse who causes harm to a client can be disciplined by their regulatory body and legally charged under the Criminal Code. A person is **criminally negligent** when doing anything or omitting to do anything, that is his duty to do, shows wanton or reckless disregard for the lives or safety of other persons (Criminal Code (R.S.C., 1985, C. C-46). Subsequently, a nurse can be charged with criminal negligence if they have intentionally acted in a reckless or malicious manner and demonstrated blatant disregard for the rights and safety of others who might reasonably be expected to suffer harm or injury due to such conduct (Keatings & Smith, 2016). A nurse who is accused of a mistake will have the care that was provided judged from what can be reasonably expected of a prudent nurse with the same training, under similar circumstances (Oberle & Bouchal, 2009). For example, if something goes wrong in a critical care setting that implicates the nurse, then the care that was provided will be judged according to what can be reasonably expected from a prudent nurse who is also trained in critical care. This rule stands for when a nurse is being disciplined by a nursing regulatory body and/or if being tried by a court of law for an offence (Keatings & Smith, 2016).

When You Suspect that a Member of the Health Care Team May be Practicing Unsafely or Unethically

Nurses need to report unsafe working conditions or situations that may jeopardize the safety and welfare of the clients in their care, which may include reporting any Health Professional (HP), not just a nurse (CNA, 2009; CNA, 2017). It is crucially important that nurses are aware of provincial or territorial legislation as well as nursing practice standards and guidelines regarding exposure and reporting of alleged or imminent harm (CNA, 2017). When harm is not immediate but there is risk for harm, nurses must work to resolve the issue as directly as possible in ways that benefit all of those who are involved (CNA, 2017). What that means is that nurses should seek to consult other members of the team, their professional nursing associations or colleges, their collective agreement, union representatives, and any other party who are able to help address and resolve the problem (CNA, 2017). What follows is list of some possible situations that may oblige a nurse to report a HP, followed by suggestions on how best to proceed (CNA, 2009; CNA, 2017; British Columbia College of Nursing Professionals (BCCNP), 2018). Box (**3:6**) & Box (**3:7**).

Box 3:6 TYPES of SITUATIONS THAT MUST BE REPORTED (as adapted & summarized from CNA, 2017; BCCNP, 2018)

1. Suspicion that a Health Professional's (HP) behaviour indicates that they are working while impaired by substances (*e.g.*, alcohol or drug use).
2. Incompetence (*e.g.*, not being able to apply or integrate knowledge to administer appropriate safe, competent and ethical care).
3. Inappropriate relationship between a HP and client (*e.g.*, touching or behaviour that is of a sexual nature).
4. Unethical Conduct (*e.g.*, theft, fraud, breach of trust, inappropriate relationship with a client or former client & abusing or abandoning a client).
5. An employer has not reported that a HP's employment has been terminated or changed in any way because of unsafe or incompetent practice.

Box 3:7 HOW TO PROCEED WHEN A HEALTH PROFESSIONAL'S CONDUCT IS SUSPECT (as adapted & summarized from CNA, 2009; CNA, 2017; BCCNP, 2018)

1. Make detailed notes of the situation. The behaviour must be carefully described with as much detail as possible. Is the HP's behaviour indicative of unsafe or unethical conduct, what is the proof and is someone likely to be harmed if no action is taken?
2. Decide what is the most appropriate course of action. Do you need to discuss your concerns with the HP involved, or do you need to consult with a colleague, a member of your professional association or regulatory body, or someone else?
3. When in doubt report to your manager or the person to whom you normally report to in your workplace.
4. If the matter is not reported by your Manager (or designate) you must proceed to report the matter to the HP's specific regulatory body. Find out which regulatory body governs the HPs conduct then determine who it is you should contact.
5. When in doubt seek guidance from your professional regulatory body.
6. Note that in many jurisdictions in Canada you are not legally liable (or likely to be sued by the HP in question) as long as your report was made in good faith. However, seek legal advice as needed.

Value B: Promoting Health & Wellbeing

"The health of the people is really the foundation upon which all their happiness and all their powers as a state depend" Benjamin Disraeli, British Statesman who served twice as the Prime Minister of the United Kingdom.

The World Health Organization (WHO) (2018) defines **health** as a state of complete physical, mental, and social wellbeing and not merely the absence of disease or infirmity. Value B of the CNA Code of Ethics (2017) advises that, nurses work with people who have health-care challenges or are under medical care to enable them to achieve their highest possible level of health and wellness. What this means is that nursing practice is not only concerned with caring for the sick, which is a crucial part of what nurses do, but nurses also promote health and wellbeing in other ways. **Health promotion** teaches people to envelope healthier life-styles that will help ward off some disease processes. For example, incorporating exercise into one's daily routine and better food choices are two small but effective avenues for health promotion.

Empowerment is the process of assisting and encouraging another person to find the strength to pursue their goals (Oberle & Bouchal, 2009). Client empowerment is not always that easy to achieve, especially when people are living in impoverished conditions. For instance, how does a person eat healthy food when there is so little money? How can someone readily recover from a pneumonia when they are homeless and constantly exposed to the elements and have not received any medical attention? Just surviving sometimes takes precedence over everything else. This discussion brings us to importance of socio-economic determinants of wellbeing as big influencers of health. For example, health was once narrowly defined as the absence of illness. However, as previously stated, new and expanded views of health include a high-level of wellness that takes into consideration physical and life style choices, as well as social and economic conditions (Oberle & Bouchal, 2009). Therefore, nurses can impact health by working to improve the plight of the poor and this action aligns perfectly with the ethic of care and Part II of the CNA Code of Ethics (2017). We will explore some of the specific actions that nurses can take to accomplish this worthy task when we review aspects of Part II of the CNA Code of Ethics in the subsequent Chapters of this textbook.

Value C: Promoting & Respecting Informed Decision-Making

Value C of the CNA Code of Ethics (2017) affirms that, nurses must identify, recognize, respect and promote their clients right to make informed decisions **Informed consent** is defined as consent that is given with a full understanding of available treatment options and the likely effects of those treatments if their effects are known (Smolkin, Bourgeois & Findler, 2010). Informed consent also includes a capable person's right to treatment or to refuse or withdraw from treatment at any time (CNA, 2017). Informed consent is closely aligned with the principle of autonomy. **Autonomy** involves the individual freedom to make choices about situations that will impact a person. However, a client must have the cognitive capacity to fully understand the risks and benefits of the suggested treatment before they can give informed consent for or against the proposed remedy. Therefore, informed consent is related to mental competence. **Mental competence** measures the capacity for informed choosing and whether or not an individual is capable of rational self-determination. Is the person mature enough to choose? Are their reasoning powers intact? Are they capable of choosing their own medical treatment? Individuals may be cognitively proficient relative to some tasks, but not to others (Smolkin *et al.,* 2010). If a client is incapable of giving consent, the nurse must uphold the law in their particular jurisdiction and what the law advises in regard to a capacity assessment and substitute decision-making (Canadian Protective Society (CNPS), 2009). There are key elements that need to be considered when ensuring that informed consent occurs when informing mentally competent person of their choices Box (**3:8**).

Box 3:8 KEY ELEMENTS OF INFORMED CONSENT (as adapted from Burkhardt *et al.*, 2015). The following elements need to be explained to a mentally competent client to ensure that they are adequately informed before consenting to treatment.)

1. A description of the health concern, diagnosis, and prognosis.
2. Details about the consequences/prognosis associated with each option for treatment as well as with no treatment.
3. A description of the treatment or intervention.
4. Details about the potential risks for harm (*e.g.*, physical, emotional, psychological & social).
5. Information about the voluntary notion of consent.
6. Consent information should be provided at a level of understanding appropriate to the client with limited use of medical or legal terms and full explanation, in lay language, of each term.
7. Consent processes should not be rushed except in emergency situations.
8. Ideally before reaching a decision, clients should be given time to reflect on the available options and discuss the choices with their support network or significant others.

The Sensitive Issue of Deferred Decision-Making

The CNA Code of Ethics (2017) advises that nurses must also be aware that capable persons receiving care may sometimes choose to defer the decision making to a member of their family. However, nurses must also be cognizant of the risk of some clients being taken advantage of by factors beyond their control. Nurses are therefore, obligated under the Code of Ethics to advocate for clients, including situations when family members disagree with the decisions made by a person with health-care needs (*e.g.*, when a person chooses experimental treatment over traditional medicine). In these specific situations nurses are obligated to assist families in gaining an understanding of the client's point of view (CNA, 2017).

Advance care planning as described by the CNA Code of Ethics (2017) consists of a process of reflection, communication and documentation that considers a person's values and wishes for future health challenges and personal care if they become incapable of consenting to or refusing treatment or other forms of care. A client's advance directives should be regularly reviewed and updated and clarification needs to occur on an on-going basis with family and friends of the client (CNA, 2017). Due to the fact that laws vary in different jurisdictions in Canada, nurses need to be aware of what their specific provincial/territorial legal and health guidelines advise concerning this sensitive issue (CNA, 2017). When in doubt, nurses should solicit advice from their regulatory body and/or legal counsel in how best to proceed, keeping in mind that these decisions are often emotionally loaded for those closest to the client, especially when it concerns end of life decisions.

Value D: Honouring Dignity

"If I can stop one heart from breaking, I shall not live in vain. If I can ease one life from aching, or cool one pain, or help one fainting robin into his nest again, I shall not live in vain." Emily Dickinson, American Poet.

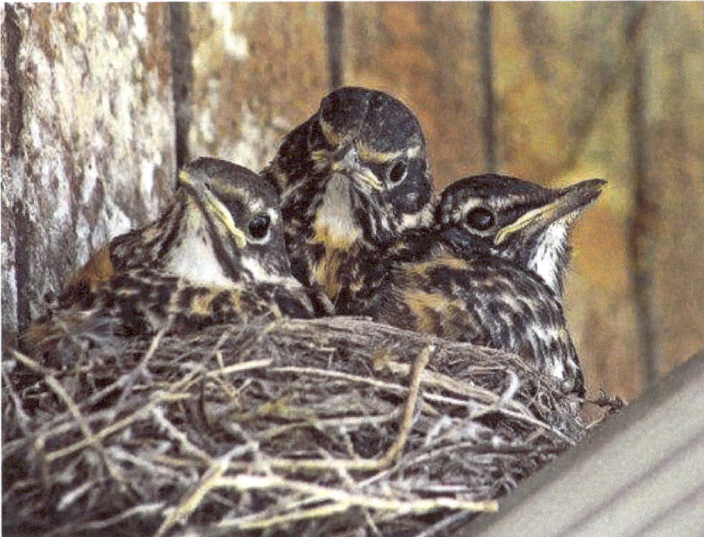

Fig. (3.4). Baby robins in a nest. Source: www.pixabay.com

Value D of the CNA Code of Ethics (2017) urges nurses to identify the intrinsic worth of every person, without exception and that they strive to ensure that people receiving care are able to maintain their dignity. This theme was emphasized in the first two Chapters of this textbook and continues to surface as an example of how the ethic of care plays out in everyday life. To teach a person their loveliness involves telling them in word and in deed that they are worth caring about. The following narrative illuminates this point Box (**3:9**).

Box 3:9 Narrative: A Hunger for Respect

Elvis was a nursing student of Indigenous descent. His goal was to become a registered nurse, complete a master's degree as a Nurse Practitioner and then return to his home native reserve to practice. Elvis used the public transit system daily to and from class. On one particular morning, as Elvis walked toward the bus station he was approached by a street person. The man seemed older, he was unshaven and his clothes were tattered and soiled. He came up to Elvis with his hand held out and pleaded, "Any money for food or food to share?" Elvis pulled out an apple from his back pack and told the man that he could have his apple but that he needed his money for the bus. As Elvis handed the man his apple he smiled. The man smiled back and said, "God bless you, you are the first person in days to acknowledge me. Thank-you for the apple but also thank-you for treating me like a human being." Elvis said good-bye and ran to the bus stop so he wouldn't be late. On the ride to school Elvis couldn't stop thinking about the man on the street. In his heart he concluded that perhaps people who are down on their luck or homeless are just as hungry for respect as they are for food and wondered why so many people ignore them. Myss (2004) point out that, "each time you reach out to another person, whether you decide to do a small or because you feel compelled to help, you perform an invisible act of power" (p. 31).

Dignity in Death

Preserving dignity also relates to people who are terminally ill or dying. An important message that I want to convey to all of my clients, family and friends is to help them to realize that sickness and death are not failures, they are simply a part of the human experience (Stephany, 2015). Nurses who are caring for the ill or dying are expected to give comfort, decrease suffering, advocate for adequate pain relief and help people to achieve their goals of culturally and spiritually suitable care (CNA, 2017). As nurses ensuring that dignity in death occurs entails making sure that no one dies alone and that they receive comfort in their passing (Gilligan, 1982). This means that if a client who is dying does not have family or friends present, it is the nurse who can fulfill that role of assisting them in passing from this life.

The Role of the Nurse Practitioner (NP) & Registered Nurse (RN) in Medical Assistance in Dying (MAID)

Over the past several years, Canadian law has been undergoing changes to end-of-life decisions that directly impacts the way in which nurse's practice. In June of 2016 Bill C-14, *An Act to Amend the Criminal Code and to Make Related*

Amendments to Other Acts (Medical Assistance in Dying) was passed. The act's amendments allow eligible persons to receive medical assistance in dying (MAID) under specific circumstances (CNA, 2017a). Subsequently, medical assistance in dying is now legal in Canada. **Medical assistance in dying** is defined as:

(a) the administration by a medical practitioner or nurse practitioner of a substance to a person, at their request, that causes their death; or (b) the prescribing or providing by a medical practitioner or nurse practitioner of a substance to a person, at their request, so that they may self-administer the substance and in doing so cause their own death (*An Act to Amend the Criminal Code*, s.241.1 (a) (b) as cited in CNA, 2017, p. 24).

The CNA Code of Ethics is clear in its advice to nurses and the issue of MAID. Nurses are obligated to ensure that they understand the law concerning MAID and be aware of their own beliefs and values about MAID (CNA, 2017). Nurses may have a wide range of personal views on the issue of MAID. The role of the registered nurse (RN) in MAID differs somewhat in the various provinces and territories. Therefore, nurses are strongly advised to consult their specific regulatory body for guidance on what their respective role is. It is also within the rights of a nurse to conscientiously object to being involved in MAID. A **conscientious objection** occurs when a nurse informs their employer that they possess a conflict of conscience and that they feel compelled to refrain from providing care because a practice or procedure conflicts with their personal moral beliefs (CRNBC, 2017 as cited in CNA, 2017). Nothing in the Criminal Code compels nurses to aid in the provision of medical assistance in dying. However, as is clearly articulated in CNA (2017a), although a nurse may harbour beliefs and values around death and dying that differ from those of their client, a nurse cannot just abandon a client who has chosen to end their life through MAID even though they consciously object to participating. Box **(3:10)** carefully explains how the process of a conscientious objection to MAID plays out in actual reality.

Box 3:10 CONSCIENTIOUS OBJECTION TO MAID (CNA, 2017a, p. 16)

If nurses can anticipate a conscientious objection to MAID, they have an obligation to notify their employers as soon as possible or, in the case of self-employed nurses, inform persons seeking MAID that they do not provide this service so alternative arrangements can be made. NPs who do not personally provide MAID may have a professional duty in accordance with professional standards in their jurisdiction to refer the person who requests it to another NP or medical practitioner who provides this service. Nurses with a conscientious objection are required to take all reasonable steps to ensure that the quality and continuity of care for clients are not compromised. If MAID is unexpectedly proposed or requested without an arrangement in place for alternative providers, nurses must inform those most directly involved of their conscientious objection. Nurses must also ensure a safe, continuous and respectful transfer of care to an alternate provider that addresses the unique needs of a client.

The CNA has also undertaken the responsibility to provide nurses with direction on their role as it pertains to each of the CNA Code of Ethics Values and Ethical Responsibilities and end of life care, which includes the sensitive subject matter of MAID (CNA, 2017a). The Values and Ethical Responsibilities associated with preserving and honouring dignity during end of life is listed in Box **(3:11)**. For a comprehensive guide on all of the remaining CNA Code of Ethics Values and Ethical Responsibilities concerning the nurse's role in MAID, please refer to *The CNA National Nursing Framework on Medical Assistance in Dying in Canada* (2017a). A web resource link to this document is listed at the end of this Chapter.

Box (3:11) CNA Code of Ethics Value D. Preserving & Honouring Dignity at End of Life (CNA, 2017a, p. 10)
i. Nurses work with the person inquiring about or requesting MAID, and with family members, groups and communities, in accordance with the person's consent while respecting the person's values, beliefs and decision. ii. Nurses work to prevent or eliminate discrimination toward all those involved — persons, family members, health-care staff — in end-of-life care decisions and provisions, including MAID. iii. Nurses listen actively to persons' concerns, experiences and requests for information to identify opportunities for clarifying their goals of care, education needs, alterations in care and access to resources. iv. Nurses foster comfort and support a dignified death. v. Nurses provide support for the family during and following the death. vi. Nurses treat each other and all members of the health-care team respectfully, whether or not they choose to be involved in providing or aiding in MAID.

Value E: Maintaining Privacy and Confidentiality

Value E if the CNA Code of Ethics (2017) asserts that, nurses must recognize the importance of privacy and confidentiality and that they work to protect personal, family and community information that has been obtained in the milieu of the professional relationship. **Confidentiality** is concerned with keeping medical information about a client private. It protects a person from harm that may occur if information about their diagnosis or treatment is shared with others. One clear example of harm that may occur when confidentiality has been breached occurs when someone who suffers from a mental illness experiences discrimination after their diagnosis is shared with persons who have no right to know. The media is sometimes guilty of this breach. When confidentiality is ensured clients are more willing to speak frankly about their problems with health care providers without the fear of a breach of trust. Maintaining confidentiality in modern times can sometimes prove to be challenging. Many people have access to medical records and the confidentiality of computerized records can easily be violated at any computer station, especially if a health care professional forgets to log off after accessing a record. Box **(3:12)** outlines some directives from the CNA Code of Ethics for keeping client information private.

> **Box 3:12 KEEPING CLIENT INFORMATION PRIVATE** (CNA Code of Ethics, 2017, p. 14).
>
> 1. When nurses are conversing with persons receiving care, they take reasonable measures to prevent confidential information in the conversation from being overheard.
> 2. Nurses collect, use and disclose health information on a need-to-know basis with the highest degree of anonymity possible in the circumstances and in accordance with privacy laws.
> 3. When nurses are required to disclose information for a particular purpose, they disclose only the amount of information necessary for that purpose and inform only those necessary. They attempt to do so in ways that minimize any potential harm to the persons receiving care or colleagues.
> 4. Nurses respect policies that protect and preserve the privacy of persons receiving care, including security safeguards in information technology.

Ensuring that Clients Have Access to Their Own Records

In addition to preserving privacy, The CNA Code of Ethics (2017) requires that nurses advocate for clients to have access to their own health records in a timely manner. However, clients need to be aware that they must gain access to their own record by following the protocols that are in place in their specific medical institution. The same applies to nurses who wish to access their own health records.

When Breaching Confidentiality is Necessary

Although confidentiality is extremely important, it is not an absolute value. There are some specific circumstances that require that a nurse breach confidentiality (Canadian Nurses Protective Society, 2008). For example, in some situations, overriding confidentiality might be justified in order to provide important benefits to clients or to prevent serious harm to third parties (Keatings & Smith, 2016). Refer to Box **(3:13)** for a summary of some of the exceptions to the duty to maintain confidentiality. Note that this list is not exactly the same for every jurisdiction in the country. The need to do your own research into the laws governing confidentiality within your own jurisdiction, cannot be overemphasized (Canadian Nurses Protective Society, 2008). A good place to begin with your inquiries is to consult with your specific regulatory body or legal counsel. It is important for nurses to be aware that they are not allowed to disclose health records or information to a police officer upon request. When a police officer requests information the nurse must refer them to the appropriate administration or the police can obtain a court order giving them legal access to a client's records (Canadian Nurses Protective Society, 2008).

Understand that there are consequences to unauthorized disclosure of client information. A client may take legal action, and a nurse may be sued for negligence, breach of confidentiality or privacy or defamation (Canadian Nurses

Protective Society, 2008). Your professional nursing licensing body may also instigate disciplinary proceedings (Canadian Nurses Protective Society, 2008).

Box 3:13 EXCEPTIONS TO THE DUTY TO MAINTAIN CONFIDENTIALITY (as adapted from Canadian Nurses Protective Society, 2008)

1. It is okay to disclose relevant health information, both verbally and written within the health care team that is caring for the client.
2. A family connection or friendship does NOT entitle a person to a client's information. Written authorization from the client may be required prior to disclosure of health information to a third party.
3. Legal Legislation may require that a nurse disclose otherwise, confidential information. Common examples include child protection legislation and communicable disease legislation, and other mandatory reporting legislation (*e.g.*, gunshot wounds). In some jurisdictions privacy legislation may authorize disclosure to protect public health and safety (*e.g.* Alberta).
4. Involvement in legal proceedings, either as a party or as a witness, can justify disclosure of health information relevant to the legal issues. If you are a party, your lawyer will advise you. If you are a witness, disclosure may be made under the direction of a court order or subpoena.
5. In rare circumstances a nurse may be justified in divulging confidential client information for the purpose of warning others of possible danger from a client or if a client is in danger. In some jurisdictions (*e.g.*, British Columbia) a nurse can share confidential information concerning a committed mental health client who has left the hospital without permission, who may be at risk of self-harm.
6. When in doubt as to whether to disclose information it is advisable to consult legal counsel for direction.

When is Self-disclosure Okay & When is it Not Appropriate?

Although nurses are encouraged to be kind and respectful it is important that they ensure that they uphold appropriate professional boundaries with those in their care and that their relationships are consistently focused on the benefit of the client (CNA, 2017). Nurses must be consciously aware of the possible vulnerability of those in their care. They therefore, must take precautions to ensure that they do not ever abuse their relationship with clients for personal or financial gain and do not enter into personal relationships them. For example, romantic, sexual, or other personal relationships with those under their care is strictly prohibited (CNA, 2017).

A specific example that comes to mind where boundaries may become blurred concerns the issue of self-disclosure. **Self-disclosure** occurs when a nurse shares some personal information about themselves that they believe may help the client. The ethical advice dictates that if it serves the client then you can use limited self-disclosure, but if you want to feel understood, then ethically you should refrain from proceeding. Also be reminded that in your professional role you have to keep what the client tells you confidential, they however do not have to follow the same rules.

Value F: Promoting Justice

The ethical principle of **justice** is based on the notion of fairness and theories of justice focus on how we treat individual and groups within society (Keatings & Smith, 2016). Value F of the CNA Code of Ethics (2017) maintains that, nurses must preserve the principles of justice by protecting human rights, equity and fairness and by promoting good for the public. According to Aristotle justice is a lived virtue. **Justice** as a moral virtue includes lawfulness (universal justice) and fairness (particular justice) (Scott, 2015). **Injustice** equals unlawfulness and/or unfairness.

As mentioned earlier, **social justice** emphasizes the relative position of specific social groups in relation to others in society. **Social injustice** is a relative concept that consists of the claimed unfairness or injustice of a society. In some societies social injustice concerns the distribution advantages for some and distribution disadvantages of others. In other societies it may include repression of people's rights and freedoms (Definitions.net, n.d.). Fairness requires that the privileges of people in given situations be distributed proportionately and equally which is referred to as **distributive justice**. The fair and equitable delivery of health resources in a Canadian publicly funded health care system can often be challenging. For example, people who live in distant rural communities often do not have ready access to all of the same sort of services as people who live in high density cities.

There is Never a Right Time to Discriminate

Nurses are advised that there is no right reason to ever discriminate against another person. Nurse must refrain from lying, judging, labelling or demeaning or stigmatizing other persons, other professionals and each other (CNA, 2017). Providing ethical care without discrimination to everyone all of the time is something that most nurses understand on an intellectual level. In reality, however, it is not always easy to do, especially when dealing with a client who has harmed others or who follows a creed that endorses violence. In Chapter Four of this textbook I will speak in detail about how personal values and values which conflict with clients' choices play out in real life. Therefore, I will rely on brevity here, by sharing the candid advice of Siegel (1993). Dr. Bernie Siegel, a surgeon, points out that we do not have to love everyone or even like them. We are not obligated to like criminals or what they have done, but we do need to try and understand them. Dr. Siegel speaks about the fact that all people possess a shadow side and a light side. We each have the inherent potential of becoming a criminal or a saint. Often times we project parts of us that scare us onto others because it is easier to judge others than to face the potential that our own darkness exists.

However, in actuality, accepting our own shadow makes it easier to accept someone's else's. Dr. Siegel concludes his discussion on this issue by quoting an excerpt from *The Human Comedy* by William Saroyan.

The evil do not know they are evil and are therefore innocent, the evil man must be forgiven every day. He must be loved because something of each of us is in the most evil man in the world, and something of him is in each of us. He is ours and we are his. None of us is separate from any other. The peasant's prayer is my prayer, the assassin's crime is my crime (Siegel, 1993, p. 190).

Value G: Being Accountable

A later Chapter will thoroughly cover the topic of accountability in nursing practice, therefore this current discussion is brief. Value G of the CNA Code of Ethics (2017) declares that, nurses must be completely accountable for their actions and answerable for their professional practice. **Accountability** is concerned with responsible action and being answerable to someone outside yourself for what you do. Accountability also aligns with the ethic of care because it is relational in focus. For instance, a nurse's relationship to their client is built on undeniable trust and being accountable is about our commitment to doing our very best to help others.

Accountability is also closely associated with nursing competence and professionalism. The CNA Code of Ethics ethical responsibility as given under Value G, is very clear in their direction that nurses refrain from practicing outside their scope of practice and that they always practice within the limits of their competence. When aspects of care are beyond their level of competence they are advised to seek out additional information, report to their supervisor or another competent health professional, or request a different work assignment (CNA, 2017). The following Case in Point is an example of how badly things can go wrong when a nurse takes on a work assignment that is clearly beyond her expertise. See Box **(3:14).**

Questions Pertaining to the Case in Point

1. What was Sandeep's first mistake?
2. What CNA Code of Ethics Value & ethical responsibilities were not followed in this case?
3. What should Sandeep have done to ensure client safety before administering an IV anti-coagulant?
4. The Coroner's Report concluded that Mr. Chang may have lived if Sandeep had immediately told someone about the error. Fresh frozen plasma could have been given IV to avert bleeding. Why do you think Sandeep kept quiet?

5. What do you think should happen to Sandeep?

Box 3:14 CASE IN POINT: WHAT HAPPENS WHEN A NURSE DELIBERATELY COVERS UP A MISTAKE

Sundeep was a newly graduated registered nurse from a reputable school of nursing. Sandeep was called by staffing to work a shift on a Renal Dialysis Unit, even though it was a specialty area and she had not yet received the extra training needed to safely work on this unit. Sandeep was getting her client, Mr. Chang, ready for dialysis. Sandeep prepared an intravenous (IV) push dose of an anti-coagulant to ensure vessel patency prior to the treatment. The anti-coagulation medication that was ordered to be given was Heparin 5,000 units. Sandeep drew up the Heparin and did not double check the dosage with another nurse before administration occurred. After Sandeep administered the Heparin IV push, she looked at the label on the vial and noticed that she had inadvertently given 50,000 units of Heparin instead of the 5,000 units that was ordered. Sandeep was really worried about the error she had made but she didn't tell anyone. After dialysis was completed, Mr. Chang seemed fine, his vital signs were within normal range and he was discharged home. However, that same evening Mr. Chang developed a severe head-ache and went to bed after taking Tylenol for his head pain. Mr. Chang's wife woke up the next morning to find her husband lying dead beside her. A post-mortem was ordered by the Coroner who was assigned to investigate the death. Cause of death was deemed to be from a massive brain bleed. The Coroner's investigation also revealed that Mr. Chang had received a lethal dose of anti-coagulation medication the day prior to his death.

REFLECTING BACK

Summary of Key Points Covered in Chapter 3

- Nurses were made aware that law supersedes ethics and although some laws are derived from ethics, this is not always the case.
- Nurses must obey the law and nurses who have a working knowledge of the Canadian legal system are better equipped to deal with legal issues when they arise.
- The Supreme Court of Canada is the highest court in this country as well as the final court of appeals within the Canadian justice system.
- In Canada, laws are created in two ways: through the judicial system (case law) and through government (statutory law).
- Common law (also called case law) is a system developed by English judges of rules, principles and doctrine based on common sense.
- Statutory laws are laws that politicians make, such as acts or statutes.
- In Canada common law is practiced everywhere except for in Quebec, where civil law is practiced.
- Civil law is based on Roman law which is prevalent in Europe and consists of principles and rules written in a central code or statute.
- Canada is a democratic country and democracy is government of the people, by the people and for the people.
- All governments and institutions in this country are subject to *The Canadian Constitution* and *The Charter of Rights and Freedoms*, which articulates the

basic legal and democratic rights of Canadians.

- The role of the Canadian Nurses Association (CNA) was briefly presented. The CNA serves as the national regulatory body for registered nurses and influences legislation, government programs and national and international advancement of health policy.
- The purpose and foundation of the CNA Code of Ethics (2017) was reviewed. The CNA Code of Ethics provides guidance for ethical relationships, behaviours and decisions. Specific values and ethical responsibilities are set out in Part I of the Code, which was the focus of this particular Chapter. Part II of the Code outlines how nurses can work toward ending social inequities.
- The commonalities between the CNA Code of Ethics and the ethic of care were pointed out. Both were derived from the same stream of thought and equate human connectedness and the caring motif as central to nursing practice.
- Each of the following seven primary CNA Code of Ethics Values were reviewed individually.
  - A. Providing safe, compassionate, competent and ethical care
  - B. Promoting health and well-being
  - C. Promoting and respecting informed decision-making
  - D. Honouring dignity
  - E. Maintaining privacy and confidentiality
  - F. Promoting justice
  - G. Being accountable
- Safety was noted to be a priority and nurses were admonished to ensure that they protect research subjects by making them aware of their rights prior to participating in any study.
- It was pointed out that a nurse who breaches practice standards that does not cause harm to a client will be disciplined by their regulatory body. However, a nurse who causes harm to a client can be disciplined by their regulatory body and legally charged under the Criminal Code.
- Nurses were made aware that they must report unsafe working conditions or situations that may jeopardize the safety and wellbeing of clients, which may include reporting any Health Professional (HP).
- Health is no longer regarded as the mere absence of disease. The definition is expanded to include a state of complete physical, mental, and social well-being.
- In informed consent the risks *versus* benefits of any advised treatment must be clearly explained and a mentally competent person has the right to refuse or withdraw from treatment at any time.
- Honouring dignity consists of nurses recognizes the worth of each person which includes preserving dignity in death.
- The role of the nurse practitioner (NP) & Registered Nurse (RN) in Medical Assistance in Dying (MAID) was explored. By law a NP can be involved in

MAID, however, the role of the RN differs in the various provinces and territories. Nurses are strongly advised to consult their specific regulatory body for guidance in this sensitive and legal matter.

- Nothing in the criminal code compels nurses to aid in the provision of MAID. However, a nurse cannot abandon a client who has chosen to end their life through MAID.
- Nurses must protect client information but they must also be aware of the particular circumstances that may warrant a breach of confidentiality.
- Nurses are admonished to uphold the principles of justice by safeguarding human rights, equity and fairness and by promoting the public good.
- Nurses are reminded that there is no right reason to ever discriminate against another person.
- Nurses are accountable for their actions and answerable for their practice.

SOMETHING TO PONDER

1. It was argued that the law supersedes ethics and that nurses must obey the law even when the law contravenes solid ethical values. In what sort of situations would this prove problematic in nursing practice and how would you deal with it?
2. You want to advocate on behalf of one of your clients who really needs someone to speak up for them, but you are afraid to act because you are a student. What would you need in the way of support to be more willing to act in an advocacy capacity?
3. Does it bother you that you have been told that as a practicing registered nurse you cannot pick and choose which of the Code of Ethics Values or ethical responsibilities to follow and which ones to ignore. Do you think that the mandate to follow all of them is a violation of your personal autonomy? Why or why not?
4. What would you do if you discovered that a mental health client was given experimental medications without being informed of the possible risks or benefits? Does this client have the right to informed consent if they are mentally ill? What does your Provincial or Territorial Mental Health Act have to say about the use of experimental drugs being administered for clients who are committed under a Mental Health Act?

CLASSROOM GROUP EXERCISES

1. Either as a whole class or in smaller groups, discuss the following two questions.
   a. Why do you think so many people find it difficult to acknowledge a homeless person?
   b. In this age of internet social networking (*e.g.* Facebook, twitter &

Instagram) how can nurses prevent violations of client privacy? What sort of things should nurses avoid sharing and why?

ON YOUR OWN

1. It was pointed out that providing ethical care without discrimination to everyone all of the time is something that most nurses understand on an intellectual level. In reality, however, it is not always easy to do, especially when dealing with a client who has harmed others or who follows a creed that endorses violence. How do you ensure that you provide competent, compassionate & ethical care to everyone?

Recommended Readings

Siegel, B. (1993). *How to live between office visits: Guide to life, love and health.* New York: Harper Collins.

Walsh, E., & Norman, A.E. (2014). *Nursing in the criminal justice services.* USA: M & K Publishing.

Web Resources

Web Resource: Canadian Nurses Association (CNA). (2018a). Site Home Page https://www.cna-aiic.ca/en

Web Resource: CNA Code of Ethics (2017 Edition) https://www.cna-aiic.ca/-/media/cna/page-content/pdf-en/code-of-ethics-2017-edition-secure-interactive.pdf

Web Resource: CNA Client Safety Position Statement https://www.cna-aiic.ca/-/media/cna/page-content/pdf-en/ps102_client_safety_e.pdf?la=en&hash=D8A2EB 457C43622A6284F14F1B40E25AC6BA412F

Web Resource: The Canadian Judicial System https://www.scc-csc.ca/court-cour/sys-eng.aspx

Web Resource: The CNA National Nursing Framework on Medical Assistance in Dying in Canada https://www.cna-aiic.ca/~/media/cna/page-content/pdf-en/cna-national-nursing-framework-on-maid.pdf

CONSENT FOR PUBLICATION

Not applicable.

CONFLICT OF INTEREST

The authors confirm that this chapter contents have no conflict of interest.

ACKNOWLEDGEMENTS

Declared none.

REFERENCES

An act to amend the Criminal Code and to make related amendments to other acts. S. C. c. 3.

Barker, C, Pistrang, N & Elliot, R (2015) *Research methods in clinical psychology: An introduction for students and practitioners* (Third Edition). Wiley-Blackwell, England. [http://dx.doi.org/ 10.1002/9781119154082]

British Columbia College of Nursing Practitioners (BCCNP) (2018) https://www.bccnp.ca/Standards/ RN_NP/PracticeStandards/Pages/dutytoreport.aspx

Brunskill, D (2010) A time for unity and a strong voice. *Canadian Nurse,* 106, 36.

Burkhardt, MA, Nathaniel, AK & Walton, NA (2015) *Ethics and issues in contemporary nursing* Nelson Education Limited, Toronto, Ontario.

Canadian Nurses Association (CNA) (2009) *CNA Client Safety Position Statement* https://www.cna-aiic.ca/-/ media/cna/page-content/pdf-en/ps102_client_safety_e.pdf?la=en&hash=D8A2EB457C43622A6284 F14F1B40E25AC6BA412F

Canadian Nurses Association (CNA) (2017) *CNA Code of Ethics for Registered Nurses.* Revised Edition). Ottawa: Author.

Canadian Nurses Association (CNA) (2017a) *CNA National Nursing Framework on Medical Assistance in Dying in Canada* https://www.cna-aiic.ca/~/media/cna/page-content/pdf-en/cna-national-nursing-framework-on-maid.pdf Ottawa: Author.

Canadian Nurses Association (CNA) (2018) CNA proposes membership expansion to represent all nurses: What members need to know about the proposed changes, its context and the decision that lies ahead. *Canadian Nurse,* 114, 35-6.

Canadian Nurses Association (CNA) (2018a) *Site Home Page.*Retrieved from. https://www.cna-aiic.ca/en

Canadian Nurses Association (CNA) (2018b) *Policy & advocacy.* Retrieved from. https://www.cna-aiic.ca/en/policy-advocacy

Canadian Nurses Protective Society (October 2008) *Confidentiality of health information InfoLAW* https://www.cnps.ca/upload-files/pdf_english/confidentiality.pdf

Canadian Nurses Protective Society (CNPS) (2009) *Consent for the incapable adult InfoLaw* 1-2.

College of Registered Nurses of British Columbia (CRNBC) (2017) *Consent Practice Standard* https://www.crnbc.ca/Standards/PracticeStandards/Pages/consent.aspx

Criminal Code (R.S.C., 1985, C. C-46) (1985) *Criminal Negligence.* http://laws-lois.justicegc.ca/ eng/acts/C-46/section-219.html

Democracy. (n.d.). In the Democracy Center https://democracyctr.org/build-real-democracy/

Fry, S & Johnstone, M J (2002) Ethics in nursing practice: A guide to ethical decision-making (2nd ᵉᵈ.). *International Council of Nurses.* Blackwell, Oxford.

Gilligan, C (1982) *In a different voice: Psychological theory and women's development.*Harvard University Press, Cambridge: MA.

Keatings, M & Smith, OB (2016) *Ethical & legal issues in Canadian nursing (Kindle ed) Canada: Saunders*

Mayerhoff, M (1971) *On caring.*Harper & Row, New York.

Myss, C (2004) *Invisible acts of power: Channeling grace in your everyday life.*Free Press, Toronto.

Oberle, K & Bouchal, SR (2009) *Ethics in Canadian nursing practice.*

Ray, MA (2016) Transcultural caring dynamics in nursing and health care. 2nd edF.A. Davis Company, Philadelphia.

Scott, D (2015). Levels of argument: A comparative study of Plato's Republic & Aristotle's nichomachean ethics. Notre Dame Philosophical Reviews: An electronic Journal. https://ndpr.nd.edu/news/levels-of-argument-a-comparative-study-of-plato-s-republic-and-aristotle-s-nicomachean-ethics/

Siegel, B (1993). *How to live between office visits: Guide to life, love and health.* New York: Harper Collins.

Supreme Court of Canada *In The Canadian Judicial System* https://www.scc-csc.ca/court-cour/sys-eng.aspx n.d.

Rosenberg, MB (2003) *Nonviolent communication: A language of life,* 2nd ed. California: Puddle Dancer Press.

Smolkin, D, Bourgeois, W & Findler, P (2010). *Debating health care ethics.* Canada: McGraw-Hill Ryerson.

Stephany, K (2015). *Cultivating empathy: Inspiring health professionals to communicate more effectively.* United Arab Emirates: Bentham Science Publishing Ltd.

CHAPTER 4

Values Clarification: Identifying what Matters to Nurses and Clients & Respecting the Differences

Abstract: The purpose of Chapter four is to inform nurses to learn how to respect differences in opinions through the process of values clarification. When a nurse is unaware of their values, especially when it comes to precarious subject matter, they may inadvertently impose their point of view onto others. From an ethical perspective, this type of response can be extremely problematic. It is recommended that nurses go through the process of uncovering their hidden values by increasing self-awareness. Nurses are also encouraged to use empathetic listening to respect client beliefs that differ from their own. Moral agency, moral residue and moral disengagement are explained. Unresolved moral conflicts can sometimes lead to moral residue that causes a nurse to become morally disengaged. Nurses are advised to get help before this occurs. Self-care strategies are highly recommended. In the Case in Point a client's right to choose results in moral residue for the nurse.

Keywords: Attitudes, Beliefs, Empathetic listening, Respect, Moral agency, Moral disengagement, Moral residue, Moral outrage, Reflective journaling, Self-awareness, Values clarification, Values.

LEARNING GUIDE

After completing this Chapter, the Reader Should be Able to:

- Contemplate where values come from.
- Understand the association between values, beliefs and attitudes.
- Recognize that values are deeply rooted and that they cannot be easily changed.
- Learn how to uncover hidden values.
- Understand that the purpose of values clarification is to identify what matters to nurses and clients and to respect the differences.
- Learn how to unlock your hidden values and how to respect client values that differ from your own.
- Discern the association between moral agency, moral residue and moral disengagement.
- Perform an exercise to determine your inherent worth.

• Apply what was learned to the Case in Point: When a Client's Right to Choose Results in Moral Residue for the Nurse.

In Chapter four nurses gain an appreciation of the fact that personal values are deeply rooted and are not easily changed. They are encouraged to go through the process of uncovering their hidden values through a values clarification process that enhances self-awareness by reflective journaling. Empathetic listening is recommended to respect client values that conflict with their own. Nurses are also made aware that they may encounter morally challenging situations in their practice and that they may become emotionally impacted by this process. Self-care is encouraged as a strategy to combat the negative effects of this problem. The Chapter ends with an exercise that assists nurses in being reminded of their inherent value followed by a Case in Point where a nurse develops moral residue when their values differ from their client's.

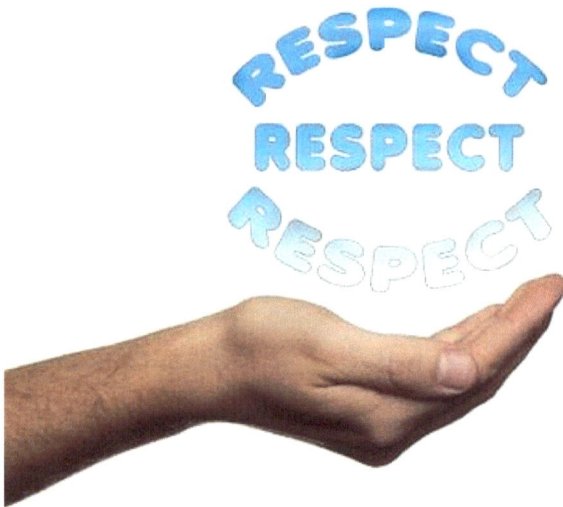

Fig. (4.1). Respect. Source: www.pixabay.com.

When Nurse & Client Values Differ: Respecting Client Autonomy

"I must respect the opinions of others even if I disagree with them." Hebert H. Lehman, Former Governor of New York & US Senator.

The values and ethical responsibilities as laid out in the CNA Code of Ethics (2017) must be followed by all practicing registered nurses. In addition to values that are associated with a specific profession, persons and/or groups possess their own set. Nurses have the right to follow their own personally chosen array of morals and to live according to them. However, a nurse's private repertoire of ideals will sometimes conflict with the outlook of the client. When this occurs the nurse must be cautioned not to willingly or inadvertently interfere with their client's values or choices. Respect for client autonomy takes precedence over a nurse's personal views (Fig. **4.1**). Box (**4:1**) The importance of a nurse identifying personal belief systems and any values which conflict with clients' values will be a vital focus of the following dialogue.

Box 4:1 RESPECT FOR CLIENT AUTONOMY (Source: K. Stephany)
Respect for client autonomy takes precedence over a nurse's personal views.

WHAT ARE VALUES?

"What is firmly established cannot be uprooted. What is firmly grasped cannot slip away. It will be honoured from generation to generation." Lao Tsu, Chinese Philosopher & Author of the Daodejing.

In Chapter three, **values** were defined as standards that are esteemed, desired important or have merit or worth and may consist of principles, beliefs, traditions, behaviours, characteristics, or goals that are highly prized or preferred by individuals, groups, or society (Fry & Johnstone, 2002; Burkhardt, Nathaniel & Walton, 2015). Values are also central, enduring appraisals of what is important to us, our lives and our larger world (Galanti, 2004). Examples of commonly held universal axioms, or values include truth, beauty, goodness, righteousness, charity, generosity and love.

Where do personal values come from? A person is not born with them, they are learned. People usually acquire their belief system early on in life from parents, family, school, society, religion, and culture. Some values are chosen consciously and others we incorporate uncritically and unconsciously into our way of being (Daniels & Horowitz, 1998). Consequently, many people are unaware of what some of their values are. They become so entrenched into how a person thinks and behaves that an individual may operate on them in an automatic fashion.

WHAT IS THE RELATIONSHIP BETWEEN VALUES, BELIEFS & ATTITUDES?

What is the association between values, beliefs and attitudes? Values are deeply rooted and cannot be easily changed and beliefs are derived from our values. Beliefs are usually more apparent to us than our values. **Beliefs** are defined as having confidence in the existence of something that is not necessarily susceptible to actual verification that it exists (Dictionary.com, n.d.). Beliefs are derived from our viewpoint and opinion on matters that we care about and are often action orientated. **Attitudes** stem from our beliefs and consist of our opinion on a particular subject, person or matter (Dictionary.com, n.d.). Attitudes are a bit more flexible than either values or beliefs and have to do with preferences (*e.g.*, liking something *versus* disliking it).

Consider the analogy of a tree to clarify the fine link between the three concepts (Fig. **4.2**). Values are like the roots of the tree. Although the roots are not necessarily visible to the eye, they are strongly embedded in the earth and cannot be easily pulled out. Beliefs are like the trunk of the tree. The tree trunk is joined to the root system and obtains water and nutrients from the soil but grows upwards and is visible to the eye. Attitudes resemble branches. They are still a crucial component of the tree but they are more easily swayed by the wind because branches are much thinner than the trunk of the tree.

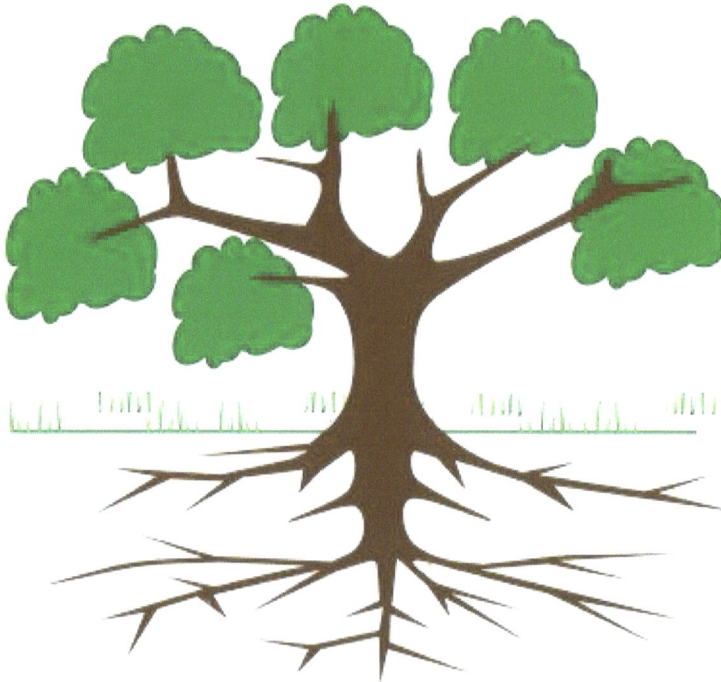

Fig. (4.2). Tree with Deep Roots. Source: www.pixabay.com

The following explanation may help make the connection between the three concepts clearer. The *value* of the ethic of care as a lived virtue in nursing practice is likened to the root of a tree, because it is foundational. The *belief* that all persons are created equal is derived from the value of the ethic of care. It is akin to the trunk of the tree. The *attitude* that all people should be respected resembles the branches of the tree. The key thing to remember is that because values are deep-seated, they are sometimes invisible or remain unknown, but they will be played out in a person's action/beliefs and attitudes. If you want to get a glimpse of what hidden key values are playing out in your life without you being aware of them, think back to a time when you got into an argument with someone on a specific life issue and you were convinced that your opinion was right and theirs was wrong. This is an example of how your unconscious values play out in real time.

THE IMPORTANCE OF VALUES CLARIFICATION

Keatings and Smith (2016) describe **values clarification** as a progressive process where persons seek to understand what values are important to them and why. Identifying what matters to nurses and clients and respecting the differences is the purpose of values clarification. Subsequently, nurses who make a conscious effort to identify and understand their own key values are more likely to recognize and respect the values of others, even if they differ from their own (Oberle & Bouchal, 2009).

What is the danger of nurses not gaining knowledge of their inherent values on controversial topics? If you do not take the time to become aware of your values, especially when it comes to precarious subject matter you may inadvertently impose your point of view onto your clients. Box (**4:2**).

Box 4:2 LEARNING ACTIVITY: DO YOU KNOW WHY YOU BELIEVE WHAT YOU BELIEVE?
Consider journaling why you believe certain values or morals are ones that you should live by, and why you believe that other values are not worthy of your consideration. Brain-storm where your beliefs and ideas come from.

Using Self-awareness to Unlock Hidden Values

The primary way to help to bring hidden values to the surface is by increasing self-awareness. **Self-awareness** is the act of looking at oneself as the observer in order to gain a clearer understanding of the motives behind our actions. It consists of the process of learning how to watch and study our actions without being directly involved in them (Daniels & Horowitz, 1998). Deliberate self-awareness also entails becoming acquainted with emotions as they are experienced in the moment, then taking a step back before acting on those feelings.

You need to be cognizant of the fact that every personal value that you hold dear is emotionally charged. What many people do not understand is that a thought always precedes a feeling. Sometimes a person's thoughts are so automatic and so quick to evoke emotion that the individual is unaware of the thought that triggered their visceral reaction (Beck, 1995). As previously stressed, if you experience strong feelings about a specific topic, chances are you are closing in on a deeply held value.

Reflective Journaling is the Key to Self-awareness

We are incredibly good at suppressing our emotions but emotions surface to try and tell us something. If you push them away they will keep re-surfacing until you pay attention to what they want you to address (Stephany, 2006). One of the best ways to increase self-awareness and to uncover hidden motives is through reflective journaling (Fig. **4.3**). **Reflective journaling** involves writing about your experiences while they occur or afterwards. I recommend that you keep a notebook with you at all times and Siegal (1993) suggests that you put your feelings down on paper every day.

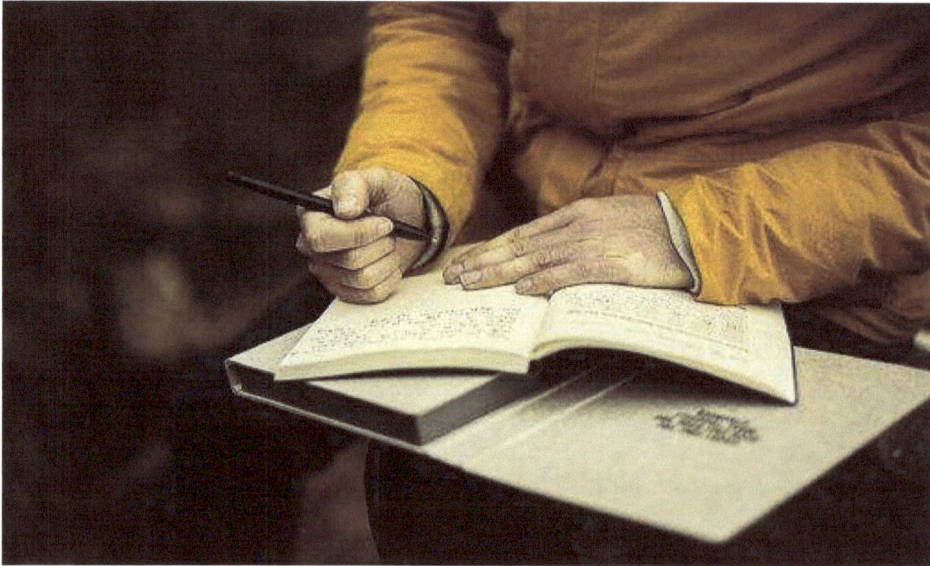

Fig. (4.3). Reflective Journaling. Source: www.pixabay.com

Journaling for Answers

In order to get better acquainted with your feelings and hidden values I suggest that you consider using a technique that I adapted from Day (1996) and the book called, *Welcome to Your Crisis*. After a few days of writing in your journal about everything that you have been experiencing, take out a highlighter pen and re-read what you have written. Highlight whatever stands out for you, then go back and read the highlighted sentences on their own. There will likely be some answers to your questions in there for you. Do this exercise often and it will likely help you to unveil some of your unknown beliefs. The subsequent narrative illustrates how what we feel is connected to our underlying values. Box (**4:3**). The story also demonstrates how an emotional outburst based on covert values may interfere with the nurse-client relationship.

Box 4:3 Narrative: When a Client's Situation Unveils a Nurse's Past Trauma

Jane was a registered nurse working in a Public Health Unit. Her first client of the day was a 23-year-old woman, Lan, who was 36 weeks pregnant with her second child. Lam was at the clinic for a routine pre-natal check-up. Jane took Lan's vital signs and noted that her blood pressure was slightly higher than on the past visit. However, when Jane lifted the client gown to listen to the fetal heart, Jane noticed something quite alarming. Lan's groin and upper thighs were badly bruised. Her abdomen was not injured. When Jane questioned Lan about the bruising, Lan became defensive and stated that she had fallen. Jane started feeling very angry and yelled out, *"Tell me the truth? You were beaten by someone weren't you?"* Lan refused to comment and looked away. She then requested to have another nurse attend to her because she did not like Jane's tone of voice. Jane stormed off to get a colleague to finish doing the assessment. Jane went on a break and could feel her anger escalate. When one of the nurses in the staff room, Peter, asked Jane what was wrong, Jane admitted that she was very angry at a client for trying to cover up possible abuse. Peter asked Jane if the rage she was feeling was out of the ordinary for her. Jane admitted that she did get very emotional quickly and that her client likely felt judged by her. Jane asked if she could be left alone for a few minutes to sort through what she was feeling. Peter agreed that this was a good idea and left to go for a walk. When Jane was sitting quietly by herself her wrath turned to sadness and tears. She recalled how her mother had been beaten by her step father when she was young and how terrible it was to see her mother put up with the abuse. Jane realized that her strong emotional reaction toward the bruising on her client's body was based on her childhood experiences and her belief that all violence is wrong. Jane felt angry at herself for not being able to control her feelings. She knew in her heart that if she was going to be able to help persons who are victims of abuse she would first of all need to get a handle on her feelings so they do not interfere with the care she provided. However, Jane was unsure how exactly to do that.

Utilizing Empathetic Listening to Respect Values that Differ from Your Own

"If you are going to start helping people, you're going to have to start doing the following things. First, you've got to stop imposing yourself on others, and your value systems upon them. You've got to learn to listen." Dr. Leo Buscaglia, Psychologist, Author and Teacher

One way that a nurse can learn to respect clients' values that may differ from their own is through the act of empathetic listening. **Empathetic listening** is listening with the deliberate intention of wanting to understand what the other person is really experiencing. Rosenberg (2003) points out that empathy for others can only happen when we have diligently made a conscious effort to set aside our pre-conceived ideas and judgments. Yet, what often occurs is, instead of offering a listening ear we feel an overwhelming urge to jump in with our own opinion, as if we know what is best. Offering advice never results in personal connection. It is direct means to push others away. What does the art of empathetic listening entail? Box (**4:4**) contains a list of suggested actions recommended by Rosenberg (2003) that really work.

Box 4:4 ACTIONS THAT FACILITATE EMPATHETIC LISTENING (as adapted from Rosenberg, 2003)

1. Don't jump into action, stand there and be fully present.
2. Empty your mind and listen with your whole being.
3. Ask before offering advice or reassurance.
4. Remind yourself that intellectual understanding (or logical inferences) block empathy.
5. Be aware that what lies behind intimidating messages is merely a person who is appealing to us to meet their emotional needs.
6. A difficult message often becomes an opportunity to enrich someone's life by listening to them and not judging them.
7. When we sense that we are going to a place of judgment or becoming defensive, we need to stop, breathe, give ourselves empathy, or take a time out.

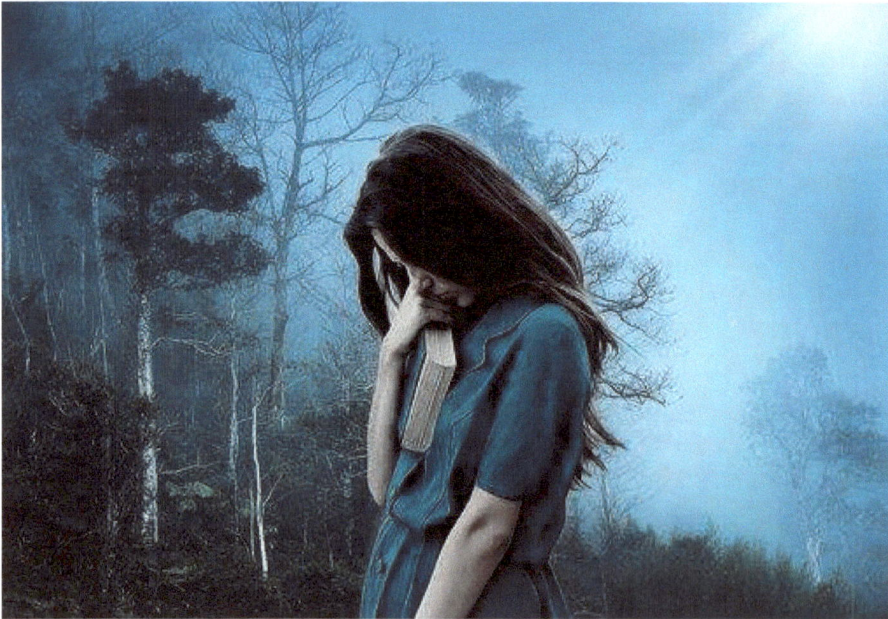

Fig. (4.4). Sad & Distressed Nurse. Source: www.pixabay.com

Moral Agency, Moral Residue, Moral Disengagement: When Caring Becomes Challenging

Moral agency is the ability of a nurse to act on their moral beliefs (Oberle & Bouchal, 2009). When a client's beliefs or decisions conflict with that of the nurse, the nurse may experience **moral residue**, which consists of feelings of guilt or remorse (Oberle & Bouchal, 2009) (Fig. **4.4**). Sometimes, for nurses who experience moral residue caring may become challenging which may develop into moral disengagement. **Moral disengagement** consists of distancing oneself from relational aspects of nursing and resorting to merely performing tasks (Oberle & Bouchal, 2009). Moral disengagement is not in alignment with the ethic of care but it does occur. When it does happen it is imperative that the nurse seek to find ways to reconcile their moral residue, such as reaching out to other colleagues for support or seeking professional counselling (Fig. **4.5**).

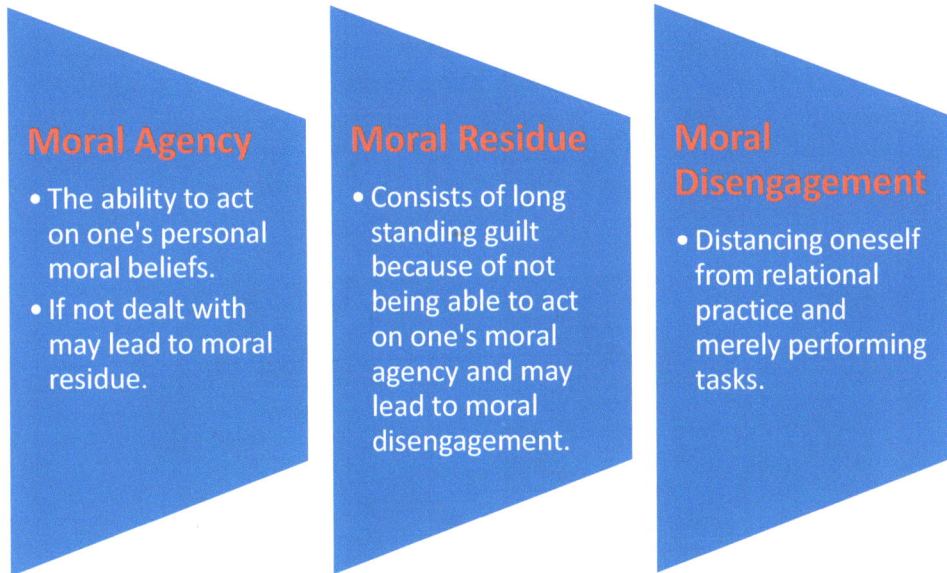

Moral Agency
- The ability to act on one's personal moral beliefs.
- If not dealt with may lead to moral residue.

Moral Residue
- Consists of long standing guilt because of not being able to act on one's moral agency and may lead to moral disengagement.

Moral Disengagement
- Distancing oneself from relational practice and merely performing tasks.

Fig. (4.5). How moral agency leads to moral residue and moral disengagement. Source: Oberle & Bouchal, 2009.

When Client's Moral Decisions Conflict with Your Own: The Importance of Self-care

Self-care is one important way for nurses to deal with the emotional labour associated with caring for clients whose moral decisions conflict with their own. Making self-care a priority involves nurses learning to treat themselves with the same respect, kindness and patience that they so willingly offer their clients. Schmidt (2002) explains that self-care should be a priority because it ultimately makes nurses better caregivers. Box (**4:5**).

Box 4:5 Caring for Ourselves Helps Us to Be Better Caregivers (Schmidt, 2002, p. 83)

A universal goal in all helping relationships is encouraging our clients to take care of themselves. Therefore, it must be an expectation for ourselves. . . . Caring about ourselves on a personal level helps maintain emotional, physical, and spiritual health that is vital to caring relationships. Caregivers who are emotionally capable, physically fit, and spiritually at peace are more able to have the psychological strength, physical stamina, and inner calmness to care about and for other people.

Moral Outrage

Moral Outrage is more distressful than moral residue. It is experienced when someone in the health care setting performs an act the nurse believes to be immoral but they feel somewhat disempowered likely because of being on the fringes of the moral situation rather than directly involved in it (Burkhardt *et al.*, 2015). A situation where moral outrage could occur is when a new graduate nurse who works on a medical ward accidentally discovers that on the Adult Psychiatric Unit clients have been prescribed an experimental anti-psychotic medication without giving consent or even being informed of the potential risks associated with the drug. The nurse is aware that this contravenes *The Mental Health Act* in her province and that this action may cause undo harm to extremely vulnerable clients. However, because the nurse is a new graduate and works on a different ward they may feel reluctant to act for fear of being ridiculed, reprimanded or bullied.

Fig. (4.6). Positive Character Traits. Source: www.pixabay.com

Determining Your Inherent Value

"Seek respect mainly from thyself, for it comes first from within." Steven Coogler, Successful Businessmen.

The famous Psychologist, Dr. Leo Buscaglia (1986) clearly articulated a sad truth, that too often we are our own worst critics and that we are not very inclined to point out what is good about ourselves (Fig. **4.6**). Yet, learning how to revere your own inherent value is the starting point to respecting what is wonderful about other people. A view of others as persons of value begins with a healthy self-esteem. The following exercise has been adapted from the seminal work of Diane Uustal (1978) who is very well known for her pioneer work on values clarification in nursing practice. Box (**4:6**). The goal of this exercise is for nurses to own their personal and inherent value.

Box 4:6 Determining Your Inherent Value (as adapted from Uustal, 1978)
1. Take a full page of blank paper and write your name in the middle of the page.   2. In the area that immediately surrounds your name write down at least six positive adjectives that describe your strengths or character attributes that make you a good person.   3. In each of the four corners of the page write your responses to these questions:
a. What two things would you like your colleagues to say about you?   b. What single most important thing do you do to make your nurse-client relationships positive?   c. What do you do on a daily basis that indicates that you value your health?   d. What are three values that you believe in most strongly?
Evaluation Process:
Take a closer look at your responses and the way in which you describe yourself along with your answers to the previous questions. Now consider the following questions.   1. Was it difficult to focus on your strengths or to identify six of them?   2. What have you realized about yourself?   3. Were any of the questions especially difficult to answer?   4. What values were exposed in the answers you gave?   5. What additional questions would you ask?

Questions Pertaining to the Case in Point:

1. What (ideally) could have occurred to help Graham and the other health care team members to better deal with Mrs. Jones' tragic death?
2. What would you do if you were Graham?
3. If Graham does want help, who can he turn to or where can he get the help that he needs?
4. What could potentially happen to Graham is he doesn't get help?

REFLECTING BACK

Summary of Key Points Covered in Chapter 4

- Nurses were made aware that they cannot force their personal set of values onto their clients.
- Values are learned and people acquire them early on in life from parents, family, school, society, religion and culture.
- People can be unaware of what some of their values are. Values are so entrenched into how a person thinks and behaves that often they are acted upon in an automatic fashion.
- Values, beliefs and attitudes were deemed to be closely connected.
- Values are deeply rooted. Beliefs are derived from values and consist of our opinion on matters. Attitudes stem from beliefs and are more flexible than either values or beliefs.
- It is important to remember that, because values are deep-seated they are sometimes invisible, but they will be played out in a person's actions, beliefs and attitudes.
- The purpose of the values clarification process is to assist nurses to identify what matters to them and clients and to respect the differences.
- If a nurse is not aware of their values, especially when it comes to precarious subject matter, they may inadvertently impose their point of view onto their clients.
- A way to help bring hidden values to the surface is through increased self-awareness. Reflective journaling was recommended to facilitate this process.
- Empathetic listening was recommended as a means to learn how to respect client values that conflict with yours.
- The association between moral agency, moral residue and moral disengagement was explained.
- Nurses were advised to get help when moral residue leads to moral disengagement.
- It was pointed out that self-care should be a priority for nurses because taking better care of ourselves makes us better caregivers.
- It was pointed out that moral outrage is more distressful than moral residue. It is experienced when someone in the health care setting performs an act the nurse believes to be immoral but they feel somewhat disempowered likely because of being on the fringes of the moral situation.
- An exercise was recommended as a way for nurses to discover and own their inherent value.

Box 4:7 CASE IN POINT: WHEN THE CLIENT'S RIGHT TO CHOOSE RESULTS IN MORAL RESIDUE FOR THE NURSE

Mrs. Jones was booked for a laparoscopic hysterectomy. Graham was the operating nurse (OR) nurse assigned to her case. Graham was going through the pre-operative check list when he noted that Mrs. Jones had signed a form that indicated that she would not receive blood products for any reason because it was against her religion. Graham asked Mrs. Jones if she was aware of the risks of refusing blood products in an emergency situation. She informed Graham that the surgeon and anesthetist had gone over the risks in detail but that her mind was made up. Once the pre-operative check was completed, Graham, the surgeon and assisting physician scrubbed and gloved in preparation for the procedure. When they entered the OR theatre Mrs. Jones was anesthetized and the surgeon began the laparoscopy. Midway through the procedure Mrs. Jones began to bleed. The surgeon proceeded to cauterize all visible bleeding vessels and to apply pressure but the bleeding continued and worsened. The anesthetist did everything he could to try and stabilize Mrs. Jones' vital signs with IV fluids and medications but she was still progressing toward shock. The anesthetist summoned the circulating nurse to urgently speak with Mrs. Jones' husband to see if he would over-ride her request to not receive blood products. Meanwhile a second surgeon was asked to assist and a laparotomy was performed. The pelvis was noted to be full of blood and it was extremely difficult to determine the source of the bleeding. The circulating nurse returned a few moments later and stated that Mrs. Jones' husband refused to consent to have blood products administered to his wife. Unfortunately, Mrs. Jones when into cardiac arrest. A Code Blue was called and the team worked on Mrs. Jones for over an hour before stopping. Mrs. Jones was pronounced dead and the Coroner was notified. Graham was extremely upset about Mrs. Jones' death, especially because he believed that her demise may have been prevented if blood products could have been given. Graham was angry at Mrs. Jones and her spouse for choosing to abstain from receiving a possible life saving measure. Graham became even more distraught when he learned that Mrs. Jones had a four-year-old daughter at home that no longer had a mom. No one in the OR talked about the death the remainder of the shift. Graham was having a difficult time concentrating on his work. With his supervisor's permission, he went home after all of the paper work associated with the critical incident was completed but before his shift was over. The next day Graham booked off work because he still could not shake the anger and sadness that he was feeling. He didn't seem concerned at first because he thought that it was normal to be gloomy after a client dies, but when he was still feeling despondent three weeks later, he knew that something was definitely wrong.

SOMETHING TO PONDER

1. Is it really possible to suspend your point of view?
2. It appears that there is a great deal of pressure on nurses to do the right thing all of the time. Is that fair or even plausible?
3. Is moral disengagement such a bad thing? After all, nurses do have an obligation to ensure that their relationships with their clients are professional and they have a lot of tasks that need tending to.
4. Why is it sometimes easier to pick out personal weaknesses and not as simple to identify and own individual strengths?

CLASSROOM GROUP EXERCISES

Pose the following questions for open classroom discussion.

1. Have you ever seen a nurse inadvertently pass judgment on a client and no one on the team address it?
2. What is the ethically correct action that should be undertaken by a nurse if they witness another nurse or health professional ridicule or unfairly judge a client?

ON YOUR OWN

1. It was pointed out that self-care should be a priority for nurses because taking better care of ourselves makes us better caregivers. So how do we do this? Consider implementing some of the following strategies for self-care into your daily round Box (**4:8**).

Box 4:8 SELF-CARE STRATEGIES (as adapted from: Stephany, 2006; Stephany, 2012; Elgin, 2015; Stephany, 2015; Stephany, 2017)

1. Start a daily routine of writing in a gratitude journal. Write in your journal (either in the morning or at the end of the day) a list of five things you are grateful for. **Rationale:** Gratitude makes what we already have a reality and helps us to change our focus.

2. Start your day by reading something positive. Daily devotionals are a good idea, either in paper or electronic form. **Rationale:** What you focus on grows. Starting the day with reading something encouraging helps to set the tone for the whole day and assists you in reminding yourself of what is truly important.

3. Spend less time on social media. Either take planned breaks or a prolonged holiday from social media. **Rationale:** Social media offers instant gratification but can also be too time consuming and even addicting. It acts on our pleasure centers in our brains in the same way that other addictions do, and it draws us away from more intimate ways of communicating.

4. When distressed seek out the company of those who support you. Rationale: We all need support especially when things are not going well.

5. Stay away from negative people. Rationale: Negative people drain your energy.

6. Make one change in your diet that is life enhancing and stick to it. Rationale: Sometimes it is just one small change that can make a difference in your health and it is much easier to do one thing then to try to make many drastic changes. If we try to do too much, we set ourselves up for failure because we become overwhelmed.

7. Make one change in your physical activity regime that increases your well-being and stick to it. Rationale: Trying something easy like deciding to walk more every day, perhaps on your lunch break, is a huge benefit, decreases stress and it doesn't cost you anything.

8. Work on making your connection to others more personal. Consider talking directly to others in person or and/or by phone. Avoid communicating solely through Facebook, Instagram, Twitter and texting as substitutes for direct human contact because they are too impersonal. **Rationale:** Human beings are social creatures and are meant to feel connected to other people. When we feel a lack of connection we feel alone and are more prone to depression. The opposite is also true. Feeling understood by another human being can make a huge difference in our ability to cope with life's stressors.

Recommended Readings

Fida, R., Tramontano, C., & Paciella, M. (2015). Nurse Moral Disengagement. *Sage Journals, 23* (5), 547 – 564 Retrieve from: https://journals.sagepub.com/doi/10.1177/0969733015574924

Uustal, D. B. (1998). *Caring for yourself – caring for others: The ultimate balance*. East Greenwich, USA: Educational Resources in Healthcare.

Web Resources

Web Resource: Exploring Values & Beliefs to Create a Shared Purpose: Values Clarification Exercise https://www.fons.org/resources/documents/Creating-Caring-Cultures/Values-Clarification-Exercise.pdf

Web Resource: Ways of Working (WOW) in Nursing Resource Packaging: Conduct a Values Clarification Exercise https://www.health.nsw.gov.au/nursing/projects/Documents/wow-values.pdf

CONSENT FOR PUBLICATION

Not applicable.

CONFLICT OF INTEREST

The authors confirm that this chapter contents have no conflict of interest.

ACKNOWLEDGEMENTS

Declared none.

REFERENCES

Attitudes (n.d.). In Dictionary.com https://www.dictionary.com/browse/attitude

Beck, JS (1995) *Cognitive therapy: Basics and beyond.* The Guilford Press, London.

Beliefs. (n.d.) In Dictionary.com https://www.dictionary.com/browse/beliefs

Burkhardt, MA, Nathaniel, AK & Walton, NA (2015) *Ethics and issues in contemporary nursing* Nelson Education Limited., Toronto, Ontario.

Buscaglia, LF (1986) *Bus 9 to paradise.* Leo F. Buscaglia Inc., USA.

Canadian Nurses Association (CNA) (2017) *CNA Code of Ethics for Registered Nurses.* Ottawa: Author.

Daniels, V & Horowitz, L J (1998) *Being and caring: A psychology for living.* Long Grove, Illinois.

Day, L (1996) *Welcome to your crisis.* Little Brown and Company, New York.

Elgin, M (2015) Social media addiction is a bigger problem than you think. *Computerworld Newsletter.* https://www.computerworld.com/article/3014439/internet/social-media-addiction-is-a-big ger-problem-th-n-you-think.html?page=2

Fry, S & Johnstone, M J (2002) *Ethics in nursing practice: A guide to ethical decision-making,* 2nd ed. International Council of Nurses. Oxford: Blackwell.

Galanti, G (2004). *Caring for clients from different cultures*, 3rd ed. Philadelphia: University of Pennsylvania Press.

Keatings, M & Smith, OB (2016). *Ethical & legal issues in Canadian nursing* (Kindle ed.). Canada: Saunders.

Oberle, K & Bouchal, SR (2009). *Ethics in Canadian nursing practice.* Toronto: Pearson.

Rosenberg, MB (2003). *Nonviolent communication: A language of life.* California: Puddle Dancer Press.

Schmidt, J J (2002). *Intentional helping: A philosophy for proficient caring relationships.* Columbus, Ohio: Merrill Prentice Hall.

Siegel, B (1993). *How to live between office visits: Guide to life, love and health.* New York: Harper Collins.

Stephany, K (2006). Honour yourself: Inspiring lessons to enrich your life. Ontario, Canada: Volumes Publishing.

Stephany, K (2012). *Each day is a new creation: Guidelines on living a life of purpose.* Bloomingdale, IN: Balboa Press.

Stephany, K (2015). *Cultivating empathy: Inspiring health professionals to communicate more effectively.* United Arab Emirates: Bentham Science Publishing Ltd.

Stephany, K (2017). *How to help the suicidal person to choose life: The ethic of care & empathy as an indispensable tool for intervention.* United Arab Emirates: Bentham Science Publishing Ltd.

Uustal, DB (1978) Values clarification in nursing: application to practice. *Am J Nurs,* 78, 2058-63. [http://dx.doi.org/10.1097/00000446-197812000-00029] [PMID: 251399]

CHAPTER 5

Utilizing Tools for Ethical Decision Making

Abstract: Chapter Five begins with an overview of the association and differences between ethical problems, ethical dilemmas, moral distress, moral agency and moral residue. Two specific tools for nurses to use when confronted with moral issues in practice are presented: *The Mosaic Model for Ethical Decisions* by Stephany (2012) and *A Framework for Ethical Decision Making* by Oberle and Bouchal (2009). An open discussion of the strengths of each strategy is presented. The Mosaic Model differs from other models in that it emphasizes care and caring relationships; keeps the person in the center; is non-linear and is applicable in many settings. The Framework is recommended by the CNA (2017). Tt focuses on the client's best interests; it encourages reflection; offers items to consider in practice; and is very applicable in a variety of ethical situations. The aforementioned model and framework are each presented in a series of five steps. In the Case in Point a client's decision conflicts with some members of the health care team. Nurses are encouraged to use the model or framework presented in this Chapter to sort through the ethical issues in this case.

Keywords: A Framework for Ethical Decision Making, Ethical problems, Ethical dilemmas, Ethical decision-making models, Ethical decision-making frameworks, Moral distress, Moral agency, Moral agency violation, Moral residue, The Mosaic Model for Ethical Decisions.

LEARNING GUIDE

After completing this Chapter, the Reader Should be Able to:

- Determine the association and differences between ethical problems, ethical dilemmas, moral distress, moral agency and moral residue.
- Be aware how moral agency is not the same as moral distress.
- Explain why ethical decision-making models or frameworks are useful.
- Describe the strengths of *The Mosaic Model for Ethical Decisions*.
- Gain an understanding of the Five Parts of The Model along with the rationale for each step.
- Explain why *A Framework for Ethical Decision Making* is recommended.
- Describe the five steps that are associated with this Framework and summarize some of the questions best suited to each step.

• Apply *The Mosaic Model for Decisions* or *A Framework for Ethical Decision Making* to the Case in Point: When Opinions Conflict.

Chapter Five opens with an overview of the association and differences between ethical problems, ethical dilemmas, moral distress, moral agency and moral residue. An argument is made in favour of the use of ethical models and frameworks as tools to assist nurses in moral decision-making in practice (Fig. **5.1**). Although there are many ethical models and frameworks, two are explored in this Chapter in considerable detail: *The Mosaic Model for Ethical Decisions* (Stephany, 2012) and *A Framework for Ethical Decision Making (*Oberle & Bouchal, 2009). When they are first introduced there is an open discussion of the strengths of each strategy. The aforementioned model and framework are presented in a series of five steps. At the closing of the Chapter the Case in Point illustrates how conflict can occur when opinions differ.

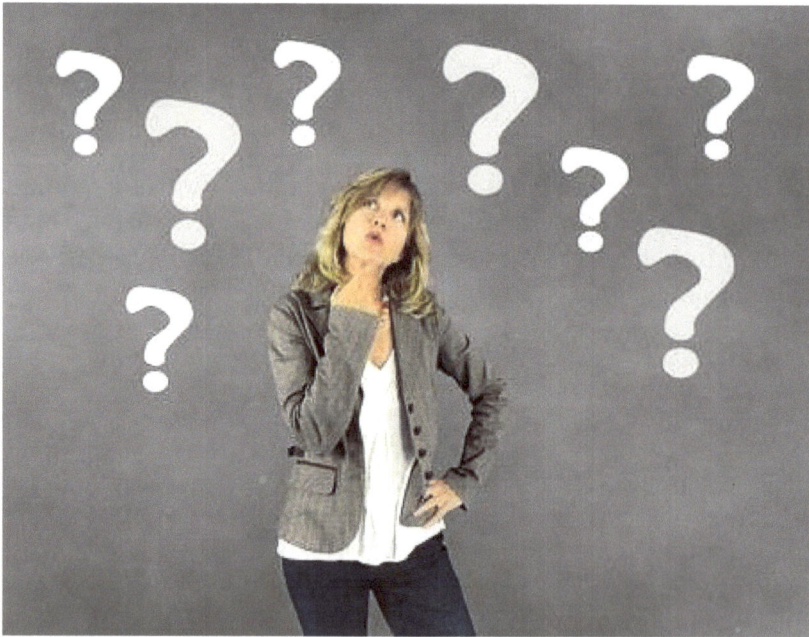

Fig. (5.1). Decision-making. Source: www.pixabay.com

Setting the Stage: Determining the Association & Differences between Key Ethical Terms

In order to create a foundation for using either an ethical model or framework, it is imperative that important associations and differences between key ethical concepts are clarified. A **problem** is a perceived gap between what is happening and what we would prefer to happen (Business Dictionary.com, n.d.). An **ethical**

problem is a basic statement of the key moral issues as they currently appear and sets the stage for further inquiry (Stephany, 2012). It gives us a brief view of what is seen as the basis of the predicament before further action is taken. At the ethical problem stage there are still gaps in knowledge.

With an **ethical dilemma** there are two or more morally defensible courses of action that can be taken but in actuality only one can be played out in practice (Burkhardt, Nathaniel & Walton, 2015). An example of an ethical dilemma is a situation where a client develops a foot that is badly infected and there is a concern that the client may develop sepsis. The surgeon recommends that the affected foot be amputated, but the client wants to have the foot treated medically. The ethical dilemma is stated as: to amputate the infected limb or to treat the limb medically. Both actions are morally defensible.

Moral distress occurs when there is only one ethically right avenue of action that can be taken but institutional or other constraints prevent that right action from happening. An example of moral distress is a situation where a nurse is working on a rehabilitation ward for clients who have suffered from a stroke. Many of the clients are bed ridden and prone to skin ulcers, yet none of them are on proper air mattresses because administration refuses to fund this crucial intervention. Furthermore, because administration also chooses to staff the ward with an inadequate number of nurses the bedridden clients cannot be turned often enough. Subsequently, many of them develop skin ulcers. Moral distress occurs for the nurses because they know what treatment modalities are needed yet they are unable to provide those treatments because of obstacles set out by administration.

Moral agency differs from moral distress yet nurses often confuse the terms. **Moral agency** is the ability of the nurse to act on their own moral beliefs which may or may not coincide with what is ethically right. A **moral agency violation** occurs when the nurse is unable to act on what they believe to be morally right. Moral distress happens when an ethically correct course of action is apparent but it cannot be carried out because of external obstacles Box (**5:1**).

Box 5:1 Moral Agency & Moral Distress are Different
Moral agency is the ability of the nurse to act on their own moral beliefs. Moral distress happens when an ethically correct course of action is apparent but cannot be carried out because of external obstacles.

The Utility of Ethical Decision-Making Models & Frameworks

"The ultimate purpose of collecting data is to provide a basis for action or a recommendation." Dr. W. Edwards Deming, American Engineer, Statistician & Professor.

Why should nurses resort to using an ethical decision-making model or framework when confronted with moral issues in practice? The CNA Code of Ethics (2017) points out how these tools help nurses to organize their approach to an ethical problem and can guide them in how to best proceed. The CNA Code of Ethics also advises that when utilizing one of these tools, some of the following be included in the discussion: ethics committees or boards; ethicists, professional nursing associations and colleges; and other experts. Standards of practice, legal legislation, and nursing unions may also be drawn into the dialogue (CNA, 2017). How do ethical frameworks and models differ? Ethical models tend to be viewed as more theoretically focused and less concrete than frameworks (Oberle & Bouchal, 2009). The following five key points outlines why ethical models and frameworks are useful Box (**5:2**).

Box 5:2 Why Ethical Models & Frameworks are Useful (as adapted from the CNA Code of Ethics, 2017; Keatings & Smith, 2016; Stephany, 2012)

1. Often more than one proposed ethical intervention may be applicable.

2. There is room within the profession of nursing for disagreements concerning the importance of different moral values and principles.

3. Ethical models or frameworks help to enhance communication and discussion between nurses and the rest of the interprofessional team because they allow everyone a chance to contribute to the dialogue.

4. Open discussion is very helpful in resolving ethical problems and situations.

5. Models and frameworks are useful in putting all that is happening into perspective so that the issues that need tending to first become clearer, as do the ones that were not so evident before applying the suggested ideas.

THE MOSAIC MODEL FOR ETHICAL DECISIONS

"It does not take much strength to do things, but it requires great strength to decide what to do." Elbert Hubbard, American Writer & Philosopher

The first tool for ethical decision-making presented in this Chapter is, *The Mosaic Model for Ethical Decisions* (Stephany, 2012) (Fig. **5.2**). It is important to understand some unique components of this specific model. This model aligns well with the ethic of care because it emphasizes care and caring relationships, keeps the person at the center, and begins with the client's story (Stephany, 2012). The goal is to ensure that during the process of ethical reasoning nothing essential gets left out especially what is crucially important to the individual who is at the center of the issue being explored (Benner, 2000).

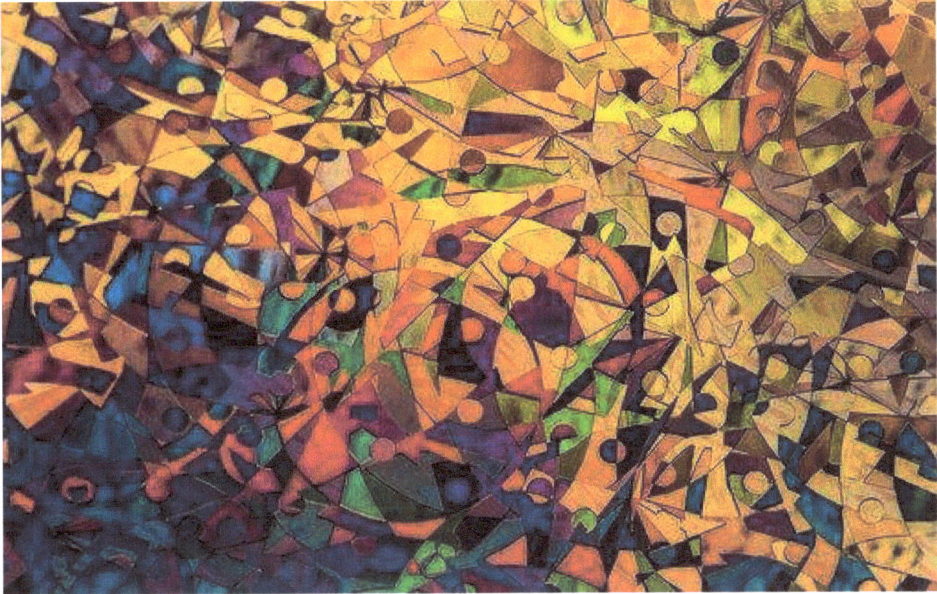

Fig. (5.2). Mosaic. Source: www.pixabay.com

This model consists of five parts, yet it is non-linear, which means that you do not need to proceed through Parts one through five in exact order. You can use some parts and exclude others depending on the situation at hand. Sometimes when new information becomes available you may consider revisiting an earlier part of the model to re-consider how to proceed. For example, what appears valid at one instance may no longer be defensible especially when new facts become available, when the client's condition changes, or if the client has changed their minds about key matters. A strength of this model is that it is applicable in many ethical situations that involve the individual client, community and societal issues. *The Mosaic Model for Ethical Decisions* also ensures that nothing important is left out and considers the law, sound moral principles, the CNA Code of Ethics and any other additional knowledge as deemed appropriate (Stephany, 2012) Box (**5:3**).

Box 5:3 KEY STEPS OF THE MOSAIC MODEL FOR ETHICAL DECISIONS (as adapted from Stephany, 2012)
Part 1: Identifying what Matters to Clients & Others
a) Briefly state the ethical problem. b) Have the client tell their story. c) Identify other players and their views/values.

Cont.....

Part 2: Determine the Key Ethical and/or Legal Issues
a) Identify if there is an ethical dilemmas or moral distress.
b) Is there a law that mandates how the health team should proceed? If yes, obtain legal advice and follow it.

Part 3: Make Use of Other Sources of Knowledge
a) Draw upon the following for guidance in decision-making: MAYERHOFF'S (1971) MULTIFACETED ASPECTS OF CARE, PERLMAN'S (1979) INVENTORY OF CARING TRAITS, STEPHANY'S (2012) COMPONENTS OF THE MOSAIC OF CARE, SOUND MORAL PRINCIPLES or THE CNA CODE OF ETHICS PART 1 NURSING VALUES. Consider any additional knowledge as deemed appropriate. Identify how some of these notions apply to each side of the dilemma or to an issue involving moral distress.

MAYERHOFF'S MULTIFACETED ASPECTS OF CARE (as adapted from Mayerhoff, 1971)
Knowledge & care: applying skillfulness and competency in practice.
Alternating rhythms of care: being flexible and spontaneous when helping.
Demonstrating patience: offering tolerance and encouraging personal growth.
Being honest & trustworthy: nurses need to be consistently honest or trust will be violated.
Showing humility: the willingness to admit when you have made a mistake or when you do not have the answer.
Having hope: the belief that beneficial outcomes are possible.
Maintaining courage: improving the situation for others with perseverance even when faced with opposition.
PERLMAN'S INVENTORY OF CARING TRAITS (as adapted from Perlman, 1979)
Warmth: ability to connect with others.
Acceptance: taking people as they are.
Caring-concern: genuine interest in the welfare of those in our care.
Genuineness: being human and free from self-importance.
Empathy: identifying and understanding the experiences of others.
STEPHANY'S COMPONENTS OF THE MOSAIC OF CARE (as adapted from Stephany, 2007)
Compassion: identification with the suffering of others.
Generosity & care: going above and beyond with our time and efforts.
Unconditional positive regard: there are no conditions or obstacles to your capacity to care for another person.
Presencing: being fully with a person, offering them caring thoughts and is best done in silence.
SOUND MORAL PRINCIPLES (as adapted from Burkhardt *et al.*, 2015; Oberle & Bouchal, 2009; Wright & Leahey, 2005)
Integrity: acting with honesty.
Veracity: truth telling.
Fidelity: keeping promises and being loyal.
Respect for self-worth: all persons as equal and worthy of care.
Beneficence: the obligation to do what will benefit the person.
Non-Maleficence: derived from the concept of beneficence and is the duty to prevent harm.
Hope: the belief that positive outcomes are possible.
Autonomy: the right to make meaningful choices about one's life.
Advocacy: being the voice for another person.
THE CNA CODE OF ETHICS PART 1 NURSING VALUES (as adapted from CNA, 2017)
The expectation is that all of these values and the corresponding responsibilities will be incorporated into the practice of nursing, especially when dealing with ethical issues. For a copy of the CNA Code of Ethics visit www.cna-aiic.ca/ethics

Cont.....

A. Providing Safe, Compassionate, Competent and Ethical Care.   B. Promoting Health and Well-Being.   C. Promoting and Respecting Informed Decision-Making.   D. Honouring Dignity.   E. Maintaining Privacy and Confidentiality.   F. Promoting Justice.   G. Being Accountable.
Part 4: Consider Possible Courses of Action as well as the Benefits & Risks
a) Promote Informed Decision-making.   b) Reflect on the ethical action.
Part 5: Additional Considerations
a) Consider situations that may arise and create problems for any family member and/or healthcare professional who are involved such as: moral distress, moral agency violations, moral residue, moral disengagement & moral outrage.   b) Who requires help with dealing with what transpired?   c) Consider societal issues that may be relevant.

A FRAMEWORK FOR ETHICAL DECISION MAKING

"The most important thing is, whatever you decide to choose, take it seriously and do your best." Tom Sturridge, English Actor.

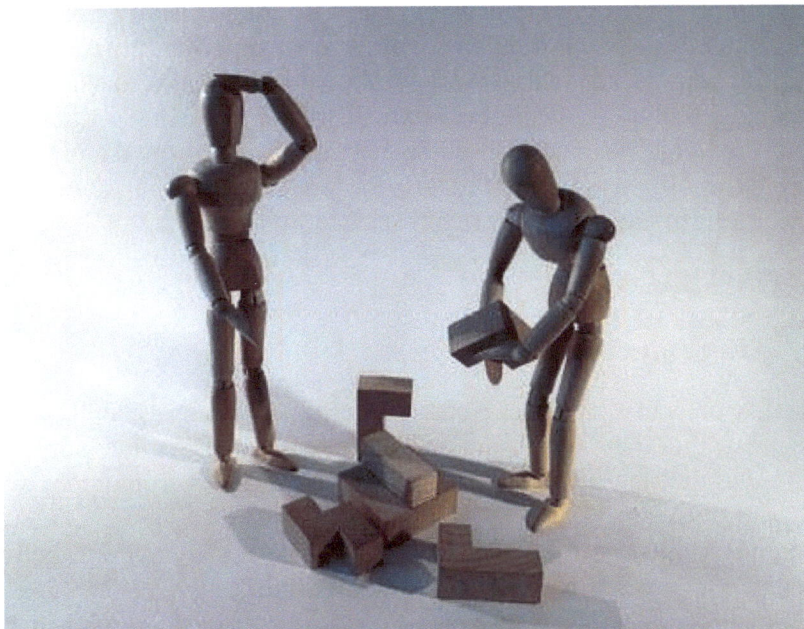

Fig. (5.3). Decisions. Source: www.pixabay.com

The second tool for decision-making presented in this Chapter is, *A Framework for Ethical Decision Making* (Oberle & Bouchal, 2009) (Fig. **5.3**). There are several advantages to this framework. It is recommended by the CNA Code of Ethics (2017) because it encourages reflection; it is very applicable in a variety of ethical situations; it takes into consideration the law, institutional and societal values; and includes professional and family values (Oberle & Bouchal, 2009). The framework can also be used to assist nurses both in actual ethical dilemmas and in day to day encounters between patients and nurses (Oberle & Bouchal, 2009).

The framework is organized into a series of five steps (Oberle & Bouchal, 2009). The five steps are listed below followed by a summary of framework questions to consider under each step. For a detailed copy of the Framework please refer to the textbook: *Ethics in Canadian Nursing Practice,* by Oberle and Bouchal (2009) which is included in the Recommended Reading List at the end of this Chapter. Box (**5:4**).

APPLY AN ETHICAL DECISION-MAKING MODEL OR FRAMEWORK TO THE CASE IN POINT:

It is now one day after Mrs. Brayer received the bad news. Michelle, Mrs. Brayer's daughter is expected to arrive at the hospital later that same day. You are the chair of the ethics committee and you have arranged an urgent meeting with the rest of the health care team in preparation for Michelle to visit her mother. You personally feel very strongly about always honouring a client's right to choose, but the Social Worker and nurse Maria argue that the daughter has rights too. Apply either *The Mosaic Model for Ethical Decisions* or *A Framework for Ethical Decisions* to address the ethical issues in this case.

REFLECTING BACK

Summary of Key Points Covered in Chapter 5

• The association and differences between ethical problems, ethical dilemmas, moral distress, moral agency, moral violation and moral residue were reviewed.
• It was pointed out that nurses often confuse the terms moral agency with moral distress.
• Moral agency is the ability of the nurse to act on their own moral beliefs which may or may not coincide with what is ethically right.
• Moral distress happens when an ethically correct course of action is apparent but it is not carried out.
• The CNA Code of Ethics (2017) points out that tools in the form of ethical decision-making models and frameworks help nurses to organize their approach

to an ethical problem and assists them in how to proceed.

- Two specific tools in the form of a model and a framework were introduced: *The Mosaic Model for Ethical Decisions* (Stephany, 2012) and *A Framework for Ethical Decision Making (*Oberle & Bouchal, 2009).

- Unique components of *The Mosaic Model for Ethical Decisions* include that: it emphasizes care and caring relationships; keeps the person in the center; is non-linear and is applicable in many settings.

- Advantages to utilizing *A Framework for Ethical Decision Making* are that: it focuses on the client's best interests; it encourages reflection; offers items to consider in practice and is very applicable in a variety of ethical situations.

- The aforementioned model and framework are each presented in a series of five steps.

- In the Case in Point a client's right to choose causes a moral conflict for some members of the health care team. Nurses are encouraged to use the model or framework that were presented in this Chapter to sort through the ethical issues in this case.

BOX 5:4 A FRAMEWORK FOR ETHICAL DECISION MAKING (as adapted and summarized from Oberle & Bouchal, 2009; CNA Code of Ethics, 2017)

1) Assessing the Ethics of the Situation: Relationships, Goals, Beliefs, and Values

What relationships are involved?
Who is significant in this situation and how should they be involved?
What are the goals of care?
Are these goals shared by the patient, nurse & others?
What are my beliefs and values?
What Values from the CNA Code of Ethics apply?
What values are important for others?
Do the people in the situation have different values and is there a values conflict?

2) Reflecting on and Reviewing Potential Actions: Recognizing Available Choices and How Those Choices are Valued

What expectation do the patient/family or community have for the care? What do they suppose would do the most good? Have I helped them understand what they value?
What actions(s) will result in the smallest amount of values conflict?
What values are important to society in this case?
Are there economic or political factors to consider?
Is there legal legislation that directs my actions?

3) Selecting and Ethical Action: Maximizing Good

What do I believe is the best course of action?
Am I able to support the patient/ family or community with their choices?
Are there any obstacles that might prevent me from taking ethical action?
Do I possess the moral courage to take the action that I believe is best and am I supported in what I have decided to do?

Cont.....

4) Engaging in Ethical Action
Am I acting in alignment with the CNA Code of Ethics for Registered Nurses? Am I practicing as a reasonable prudent nurse would in similar circumstances? Am I practicing with care and compassion in my relationships in this case? Am I meeting both professional and institutional expectations?
5) Reflecting on and Reviewing the Ethical Action
Were the outcomes in this case acceptable? What was the process of decision-making and action acceptable and did everyone involved feel respected and valued? How were the patient/family and community and health care providers affected? What did I do well? What might I have done differently?

Box 5:5 CASE IN POINT: WHEN OPINIONS CONFLICT
Maria was the nurse assigned to care for Mrs. Brayer, a 72-year-old retired school teacher who was admitted to hospital for tests after she became quite short of breath. In morning report Maria learned that the initial test results indicated that Mrs. Brayer had a pneumonia as well as an aggressive form of leukemia. Shortly after morning report was completed, Mrs. Brayer's family physician, Dr. Gordan, arrived to do rounds. He approached nurse Maria and asked her to accompany him to see Mrs. Brayer. They proceeded to the client's room together. Maria stood at Mrs. Brayer's bedside and remained silent. She gently placed her hand on Mrs. Brayer's back as a means of offering caring touch and her client smiled at Maria in approval. Dr. Gordan greeted his client in a polite manner. "Good Morning Mrs. Brayer, how are you feeling today?" "Not too bad. The oxygen is helping but I had terrible night sweats last night." "The test results have come in and I have some not so good news. Would you like to have someone here with you before we talk about it? "No, I am a tough lady. Tell me what it is." "Well I am afraid that not only do you have a pneumonia, you also have an aggressive form of leukemia." "What does that mean?" "Well, it means that we will have to treat you with blood transfusions and then refer you to the Cancer Agency for follow-up, but there is no real cure for this type of leukemia. You will eventually die from the disease. Meanwhile your pneumonia may become worse and you are at risk of developing further infections. "Well, then I don't want any more treatments. I have lived a good life and I want to leave this world in dignity. My husband died three years ago and life has not been the same since. I hate living alone. My only daughter, Michelle, is a successful lawyer and she lives in the Maritimes. She is busy with her career and doesn't have time for her old mother. Call my daughter and have her come and see me so I can arrange for my funeral." Dr. Gordan advised that Mrs. Brayer spend some time thinking about the decision before making up her mind. In his opinion Dr. Gordan thought that Mrs. Brayer should wait until the Cancer Agency had an opportunity to discuss all of the options with her, but in the end he informed Mrs. Brayer that he would respect her wishes. The physician then left the patient's room. Nurse Maria remained with Mrs. Brayer who

Cont.....

was crying. Maria asked Mrs. Brayer if she wanted to talk more about what had just happened. Mrs. Brayer informed Maria that she preferred to be alone right now but that she could return a bit later to perhaps just sit with her for a while. Dr. Gordan placed a telephone call to Mrs. Brayer's only daughter, Michelle. He informed Michelle of her mother's diagnosis and that her mother was refusing further treatment. Michelle became angry with Dr. Gordan and demanded that her mother receive all treatment options available to help her. Michelle explained that she had already lost her Dad and she wasn't about to lose her mother so quickly. Dr. Gordan told Michelle that because her mother was mentally competent she could decide for herself. Michelle stated that she would take the first plane available to come and see her mother and then hung up the phone. Nurse Maria went on to perform her other nursing duties with her other assigned clients.

However, Maria felt emotionally distressed by Mrs. Brayer's choice not to receive treatment. Maria's mother had died from breast cancer a few years ago and she always felt cheated out of quality time with her mother because her mother had refused chemo-therapy. Maria was tearful but she didn't know what to do.

SOMETHING TO PONDER

1. Have you ever experienced moral residue after dealing with a situation in the clinical setting? If yes, how did you sort through it? What would you do differently now?
2. Have you encountered a situation that provoked moral outrage? Did you understand what was happening? Did you get help with dealing with it? If not, why not?

CLASSROOM GROUP EXERCISE

1. Break into groups of four. Each group pick a case situation that has occurred in the clinical setting that had ethical issues. Use *The Mosaic Model for Ethical Decisions* or *A Framework for Ethical Decision Making* to sort through the issues in the case and then share your findings with the other members of the class for feedback and discussion.

ON YOUR OWN

1. Journal about an ethical issue that was troubling for you. Rather than focusing primarily on what went wrong, reflect on what you learned from what transpired and how you will be better informed to act in a similar situation in the future.

Recommended Readings

Davis, A. J., Fowler, M., & Arosker, M. (2010). *Ethical dilemmas and nursing practice* (5th edition). USA: Pearson.

Oberle, K. & Bouchal, S. R. (2009). *Ethics in Canadian nursing practice: Navigating the journey*. Toronto: Pearson.

Canadian Nurses Association (CNA) (2017). *The CNA Code of Ethics for*

Registered Nurses (Revised Edition), *Appendix A. Ethical Models*. Ottawa: Author, pp. 28 – 31.

Web Resources

Moral Distress: A Case Study
https://www.nursingcenter.com/journalarticle?Article_ID=4345476&Journal_ID=54016&Issue_ID=4345459

Ethical Challenges: Building an Ethics Toolkit
http://ethicsunwrapped.utexas.edu/wp-content/uploads/2017/01/Ethical-Challenges-PDF-1-Elliott-1.pdf

REFERENCES

Benner, P (2000) The role of embodiment, emotion and the life world for rationality and agency in nursing practice. *Nurs Philos,* 1, 5-19.
[http://dx.doi.org/10.1046/j.1466-769x.2000.00014.x]

Burkhardt, MA, Nathaniel, AK & Walton, NA (2015) *Ethics and issues in contemporary nursing* Nelson, Toronto, Ontario.

Oberle, K & Bouchal, SR (2009) *Ethics in Canadian nursing practice: Navigating the journey.* Pearson, Toronto.

Perlman, HH (1979) *Relationship: The heart of helping people.* The University of Chicago Press, Chicago.

Problem. (n.d.). In Business Dictionary.com. Retrieved from: http://www.businessdictionary.com/definition/problem.html

Smolkin, D, Bourgeois, W & Findler, P (2010) *Debating health care ethics.* McGraw-Hill Ryerson, Canada.

Stephany, K (2007). Suicide intervention: The importance of care as a therapeutic imperative (unpublished doctoral dissertation). Breyer State University, Alabama, USA.

Stephany, K (2012) *The ethic of care: A moral compass for Canadian nursing practice.* Bentham Science Publishing Ltd., United Arab Emirates.
[http://dx.doi.org/10.2174/97816080530491120101]

Wright, LM & Leahey, M (2005) Nurses and families: A guide to family assessment and intervention, 4th ed. F. A. Davis Company, Philadelphia.

CHAPTER 6

Professionalism & Accountability: Inspiring Nurses to Act Responsibly

Abstract: Professional behaviours and accountability are the key focus of Chapter Six. Some of the professional nursing standards that were discussed include: professional responsibility & accountability, knowledge-based practice, competent application of knowledge, a code of ethics, provision of services in the public interest and self-regulation. Strategies to ensure that the practice of nursing be lived as a call to care were included in the discussion of professionalism. The discussion then focusses more definitively on accountability and begins by drawing a connection between accountability, the ethic of care and CNA Code of Ethics key ethical responsibilities. A crucial order of priorities in nursing accountability is clearly articulated and it is asserted that a client's welfare supersedes all other responsibilities. Explicit tools are suggested for nurses to follow when they encounter an ethical conflict with institutional policy. At the end of the Chapter, two Cases in Point are presented. One involves a client record being intentionally altered. The other features an alarming situation where a nurse is ordered to withhold crucial information from clients who are at risk of harm.

Keywords: Accountability, Affirmative action, Boundary violations, Code of ethics, Communities of practice, Conflict of interest, Ethics committees, Ethic of care, Fiduciary relationship, Fitness to practice, Professional, Professional boundaries, Professional standards, Responsibility, Self-regulation, Synergism, Scope of practice.

LEARNING GUIDE

After completing this Chapter, the Reader Should be Able to:

- Define the term professional.
- Describe some key components of the profession of nursing.
- Recite the nine rules that apply to proper documentation.
- Understand the importance of setting boundaries in professional relationships.
- Demonstrate simple ways that a nursing career can be lived as a call to care.
- Explain how nursing accountability is linked to the ethic of care.
- Gain an understanding of the CNA Code of Ethics key ethical responsibilities associated with accountability.
- Explain the order of priorities of accountability in nursing practice.

• Apply what was learned to the following two Cases in Point: When a client record is altered & When a nurse is ordered to withhold crucial information.

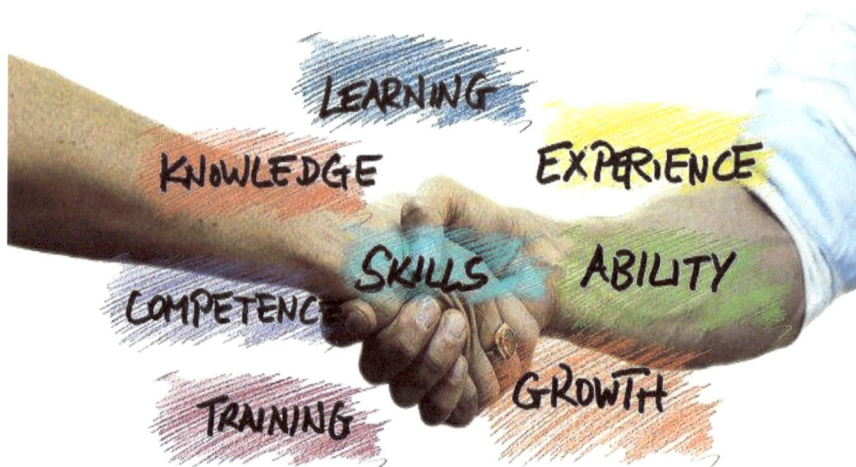

Fig. (6.1). Nursing & Professional Values. Source: www.pixabay.com

"It is not the job you do, it's how you do the job." Frank Tyler, American Architect.

Chapter Six covers the essential topics of professionalism and accountability in nursing as it relates to responsible action. Fig. (**6.1**). The first part of the Chapter begins with describing the four criteria of any profession followed by a brief discussion of some key components associated with the profession of nursing. The rules of proper documentation, the importance of setting professional boundaries, and the significance of embracing the profession of nursing as a call to care are also presented.

The second portion of the Chapter focusses more definitively on specific criteria associated with accountability. For example, it explains how nursing accountability is closely connected to the ethic of care followed by an overview of the CNA Code of Ethics (CNA) key ethical responsibilities that are associated with accountability. A crucial order of priorities in nursing accountability is clearly articulated and the argument is made that a client's welfare supersedes all other responsibilities. Explicit strategies are suggested for nurses to follow when they encounter an ethical conflict with institutional policy. Two Cases in Point are presented. The first involves a client record being intentionally altered. The second one is concerned with a nurse being ordered to withhold crucial information from clients who are at risk of harm.

PROFESSIONALISM

A **professional** is an educated, skilled and knowledgeable individual who offers a particular service to the community and professions exist for the purpose of meeting the needs of society (Burkhardt, Nathaniel & Walton, 2015). The public has an expectation that professionals will practice within their professional mandate. Therefore, both the scope and limitations of practice are established through legal legislation. Similarly, professional behaviours are monitored by government and respective professional bodies (Oberle & Bouchal, 2009).

Key Components of The Nursing Profession

For any group of individuals to call themselves a profession there are four aspects that must be present: they must possess a specialized body of knowledge, they must be accountable, they must be self-governing, and they must abide by a code of ethics (Stephany, 2012). The profession of nursing requires a bit more of their members than just the basic criteria. Nurses must abide by their regulatory body's standards of practice. Every Canadian nurse needs to be aware of the specifics of their own professional standards as laid out by their licensing body. What exactly is a **professional standard**? It is the minimal level of performance expected of nurses in their practice (British Columbia College of Nursing Professionals (BCCNP), n.d.). Although standards differ somewhat from one jurisdiction to another in Canada, some common standard themes include but are not limited to: responsibility & accountability, knowledge-based practice, competent application of knowledge, code of ethics, provision of services in the public interest and self-regulation.

I. Professional Responsibility and Accountability

Within the profession of nursing, **accountability** is concerned with a nurse taking responsibility for their own nursing actions and professional conduct (BCCNP, n.d.). The later portion of this Chapter will give a more extensive overview of accountability, therefore, this current discussion on this topic is brief. Ultimately nurses are not only accountable to the clients that they serve but also to society. For instance, in a profession such as nursing, ideas of right and wrong or our perceptions of our duty as professionals are largely shaped by the mandate of the profession of nursing but also by what the public requires of us (CNA, 2017). The community expects nurses to act responsibly. For example, nurses have consistently been judged as top rate when compared to a list of trusted professionals and rank very highly in the minds of Canadians (Insights West Survey, 2017).

II. Knowledge-Based Practice

Professional nursing practice must be guided by information that is evidence based and derived from either nursing or other relevant sciences or humanities (BCCNP, n.d.). Nurses need to know where and when to look up important information and are obligated to communicate their knowledge with clients and the public (BCCNP, n.d.). My view is supported by the BCCNP (n.d.) that a nurse is a nurse 24 hours a day and nursing knowledge should be shared when appropriate circumstances arise. I believe that every occasion presents itself as an opportunity to teach. I recall an instance when a nurse was compelled to impart nursing information. She was shopping for Thanksgiving dinner. She noticed a new mother with a tiny infant strapped to her chest in a snugly. The woman was handling the fresh turkeys on display looking for the right one to buy. The nurse politely approached the mother and informed her to make sure that she washed her hands thoroughly before touching her baby because fresh turkeys may be a source of salmonella that could make her baby very ill. The new mom thanked the nurse and headed off to the restroom to wash her hands.

This nurse made it her intention to be authentic and caring which can include sharing nursing knowledge when it is indicated. Bishop and Scudder (1996) describe integral care as a means of being with other people with the purpose and desire to demonstrate genuine care through action. The nurse in this scenario spoke her mind because she was concerned for the welfare of that baby.

III. Competent Application of Knowledge

Nursing professional duties entail identifying and making use of information from varying sources in order to inform decision-making. Attending conferences and educational forums; being published in nursing journals; and involvement in research clubs and communities of practice; are just a few examples of competent application of knowledge. **Communities of practice** consist of a group of people who share a common concern or interest in a topic and who come together to achieve individual and mutual goals. Within the profession of nursing they are often associated with creating new knowledge to advance the domain of practice.

Evaluating the effectiveness of any action that is taken is also a crucial component of competent application of knowledge (BCCNP, n.d.). Developing plans of care and timely, accurate and appropriate documentation are included in this process (BCCNP, n.d.). The following short but distressing story demonstrates an attempted violation of documentation rules and in fact was illegal. Box (**6:1**) The Nine Rules of proper nursing documentation are listed following the narrative. Box (**6:2**).

Box 6:1 Narrative: A Serious Attempted Violation of Documentation Rules
Dr. Ferguson was on-call on the weekend. Nurse Watson from a surgical ward telephoned Dr. Ferguson at home and requested that she write a Do Not Resuscitate Order (DNR) on one of her clients. Dr. Ferguson requested background data because she was not familiar with this particular client. After asking a few questions Dr. Ferguson refused to comply with the DNR order and hung up the phone. It turns out that the client that nurse Watson was requesting a DNR order for, had died suddenly post operatively and unexpectedly the previous day. By mistake, it was assumed that this client had a DNR order, but they did not have one, yet resuscitation efforts did not occur. Nurse Watson was attempting to cover up the serious mistake by soliciting a retroactive DNR order from a doctor after the person had died.

BOX 6:2 THE NINE RULES OF PROPER NURSING DOCUMENTATION (as adapted from Keatings & Smith, 2016).
1. **Record Contemporaneously:** Charting should occur at the time of the event. If not, the record should be made as soon as possible after the event. Late entries are often deemed by the courts as less accurate because memory fades with time
2. **Record Only Your Own Actions:** Nurses must document only what they have done or observed (*e.g.*, record facts or observations and not opinions).
3. **Record in Chronological Order:** All entries should be made in sequential order.
4. **Record Clearly and Concisely:** Entries should be clear, concise, factual, and as objective as possible. Subjective entries potentially create confusion in communication.
5. **Make Regular Entries:** The nurse should make sure that the record contains regular entries. Even writing, "status unchanged" indicates that the nurse is checking up on the client's condition. If there are significant gaps in the record, this poses a problem in court or at a Coroner's Inquest. What is not documented is assumed not done.
6. **Record Corrections Clearly:** Any alterations, corrections, or deletions to the record should be carefully documented, dated (including the hour) and initialed by the nurse who makes the change.
7. **Record Accurately:** Vague terms should be avoided and include as much detail as is necessary when describing client assessment. "*Slept well, had a good day,*" is of limited use because it is open to speculation and debate as to what it means.
8. **File Incident Reports:** Sometimes a patient falls, or a mistake is made in administering medication. In these situations, a report should be prepared that documents and describes the incident, all relevant facts, any injuries sustained by the client and any remedial action.
9. **Record Legibly:** The records and any corrections should be legible, illegible entries may be misinterpreted.

IV. Professional Code of Ethics

A code of ethics is an essential piece of each profession and professional codes of ethics guide what professionals ought to do, and what not to do when they are dealing with moral issues in practice. In addition to guiding conduct ethical codes influence public perceptions of the profession (Oberle & Bouchal, 2009). As already emphasized in Chapter three, nurses are required to adhere to the ethical standards of nursing by upholding the values and ethical responsibilities as outlined by the CNA Code of Ethics (2017).

Ethics Committees

In ideal circumstances ethical issues and dilemmas should be resolved by the client, the client's family and the health care professionals who are most involved in the client's care (Keatings & Smith, 2016). However, sometimes the moral concerns are more global in nature or are complex and may have larger implications for the community, society or agency. **Ethics committees** or panels exist for the purpose of providing education, advice, guidance and support in relation to ethical issues (Keatings & Smith, 2016). They also serve the purpose of investigating and adjudicating complaints of unethical conduct made by members of the public (Ford, 2006). Although nurses spend a great deal of time with clients, especially in the hospital setting, they are often excluded from membership on ethics committees (Keatings & Smith, 2016).

V. Provision of Services in the Public Interest

The provision of services in the interest of the public involves nurses working together with other members of the health care team to provide quality care. The administration of excellent care includes delegating duties to qualified personnel and acting in the form of advocacy (CNA, 2018a). The New Health Professionals Network is an integral player in ensuring that advocacy concerning the provision of services is an interdisciplinary effort. The New Health Professionals Network was first formed in Canada in 2004 and represents thousands of Canadians in seven professions: nursing, medicine, pharmacy, social work, occupational therapy, physical therapy and chiropractic medicine (CNA, 2006). The role of this network includes: advocating for sustainability of Medicare; maintaining interdisciplinary, team-based health care; and developing new ways of working together to improve access to health services (CNA, 2006). Chapter Seven will deal primarily with the advocacy role of nurses.

VI. Self-Regulation

Self-regulation of any profession is a privilege, not a right. In Canada self-regulation of the nursing profession is granted by the provincial or territorial governments. **Self-regulation** allows nursing members to set requirements for entrance into the profession, devise educational requirements, set standards of practice, investigate complaints and instigate disciplinary action when indicated (Keatings & Smith, 2016). For some background history to self-regulation of Canadian nurses see Box (**6:3**).

In many but not all jurisdictions, separate classes of nurses are regulated by different regulatory bodies, but that is rapidly changing. For instance, in British Columbia (BC) as of September 2018, the newly named BC College of Nursing

Professionals (BCCNP) now regulates registered nurses (RNs), Nurse Practitioners (NPs), Registered Psychiatric Nurses (RPNs), and Licensed Practical Nurses (LPNs) (CNA, 2018). Following the BC initiative, made by the BCCNP, the CNA has also recently expanded its membership beyond RNs and NPs by inviting RPNs and LPNs to be members of the Association (CNA, 2018) (Fig. (**6.2**).

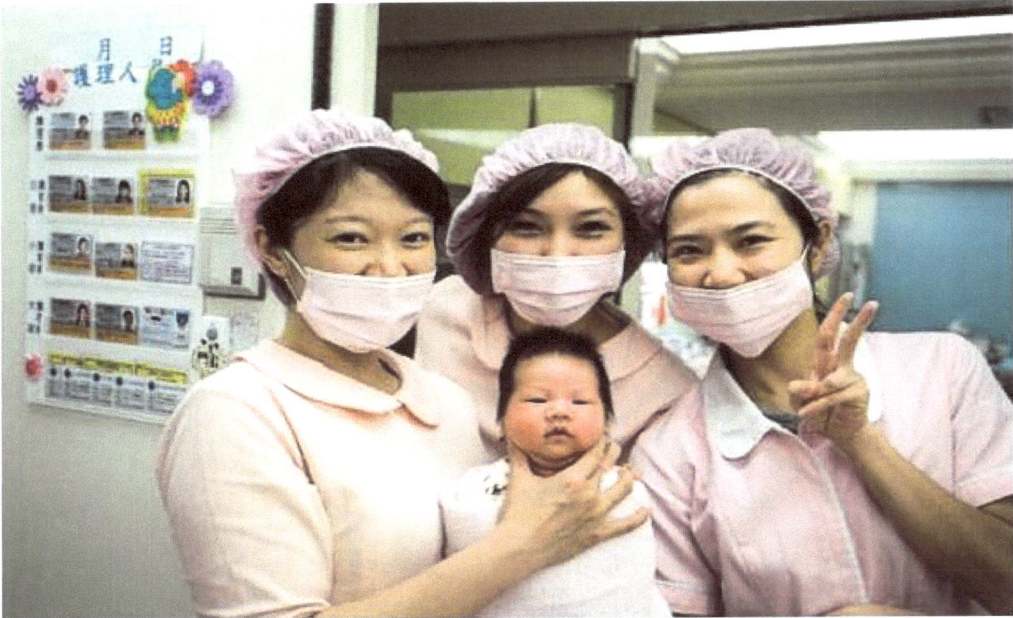

Fig. (6.2). All nurses working as a Team: Source: www.pixabay.com

---

Box 6:3 Some Background to Self-Regulation (as adapted from Coburn, 1988; CNA, 2006).

Canadian nurses have a lengthy history of evolving self-regulation that resulted in close ties with labour trade guilds and unions. Some joined unions as early as 1870 with the remainder of the country's nurses become members of unions before 1950. Due to on-going union support nurses were able to achieve progressive improvement in working conditions and equitable pay for services rendered. However, the struggle is never over, especially when health care decision-makers seek to make sweeping changes to reduce health care costs that may directly affect quality work environments.

Setting Boundaries in Professional Relationships

All therapeutic relationships have at their heart a pillar of trust which can be referred to as a fiduciary relationship. A **fiduciary relationship** is a special confidence in a professional, who in good conscience, is obligated to act in good faith and in the interests of the person(s) in their care (Hall, 2001). What does this mean in terms of nursing practice? The fiduciary relationship requires that professional boundaries be set to promote trust and to maintain privacy. Boundary setting is extremely important when there is a power differential between individuals. Nurses have power over their clients, nursing instructors possess authority over students, and it is assumed that physicians have power over clients, nurses and students. When power is unequally distributed between persons then professional boundaries can be put in place to help prevent an abuse of that power. A **professional boundary** is a limit that is set and determines how far a relationship can go and when it is in appropriate for the relationship to proceed. When boundaries are violated the possibility exists for harm to occur which is referred to as a boundary violation. **Boundary violations** consist of intentional or unintentional actions between two people that go against well accepted social expectations (DeWolf Bosek & Savage, 2007). Box (**6:4**).

Box 6:4 The CNA Code of Ethics Directive on Nurses & Professional Boundaries (CNA Code of Ethics, 2017, p. 13)

Nurses maintain appropriate professional boundaries and ensure that their relationships are always for the benefit of the person. They recognize the potential vulnerability of persons receiving care and do not exploit their trust and dependency in a way that might compromise the therapeutic relationship. They do not abuse their relationship for personal or financial gain and do not enter into personal relationships (romantic, sexual or other) with persons receiving care.

The Nursing Profession as a Call to Care

"If your actions inspire others to dream more, learn more, do more and become more, you are a leader." Simon Sinek, Author, Inspirational Speaker & Leadership Consultant.

Box 6:5 OUR NURSING PROFESSION AS A CALL TO CARE (as adapted from Miller-Tiedeman, 1999)

1. **The Importance of Relationship:** Our relationships teach us to listen, care for, and be interested in someone else instead of ourselves. Our greatest sense of fulfillment in our work comes when we learn how to make our finest contribution to others.

2. **What we Leave Behind is Important:** A career becomes a call to care when we are cognizant of the significance of what we leave behind. Our relationships should be left lovelier than when we first arrived.

3. **Our Work should Give us a Sense of Accomplishment:** If we apply ourselves to the tasks at hand each day with enthusiasm, eagerness, thoroughness and by doing our best, we will see progress and feel increasingly useful.

4. **We must Learn to go with the Flow of Life:** Despite all our efforts and planning, surprises and sudden changes do occur in the course of both career and life. Resiliency skills can be developed by learning how to change direction; to cooperate with the flow of life; and to reach out for help when we need it.

5. **Always Demonstrate Kindness:** We can choose to do our work in automatic mode or we can choose a better way, like addressing the needs of others and showing kindness where kindness is absent. What we give is as important as when we do. People, in general, choose to be a part of a caring profession because they want to make a difference.

Although skills, knowledge and accountability are important aspects of the profession of nursing, so is the call to care (Bishop & Scudder, 1996). Miller-Tiedeman (1999) stresses that our life is our career and when we learn how to fully embrace life, ourselves and others, our work becomes the fruit of that labour. Life is not a dress rehearsal, it is the real stage. When we live and work with the understanding that every word or action has the potential to heal or harm we will grasp the true meaning of our power to affect change. Box (**6:5**) demonstrates ways that a professional nursing career can be lived as a call to care.

ACCOUNTABILITY & THE ETHIC OF CARE

"The purpose of life is to serve other people. To do something of benefit for other people." His Holiness the 14th Dalai Lama.

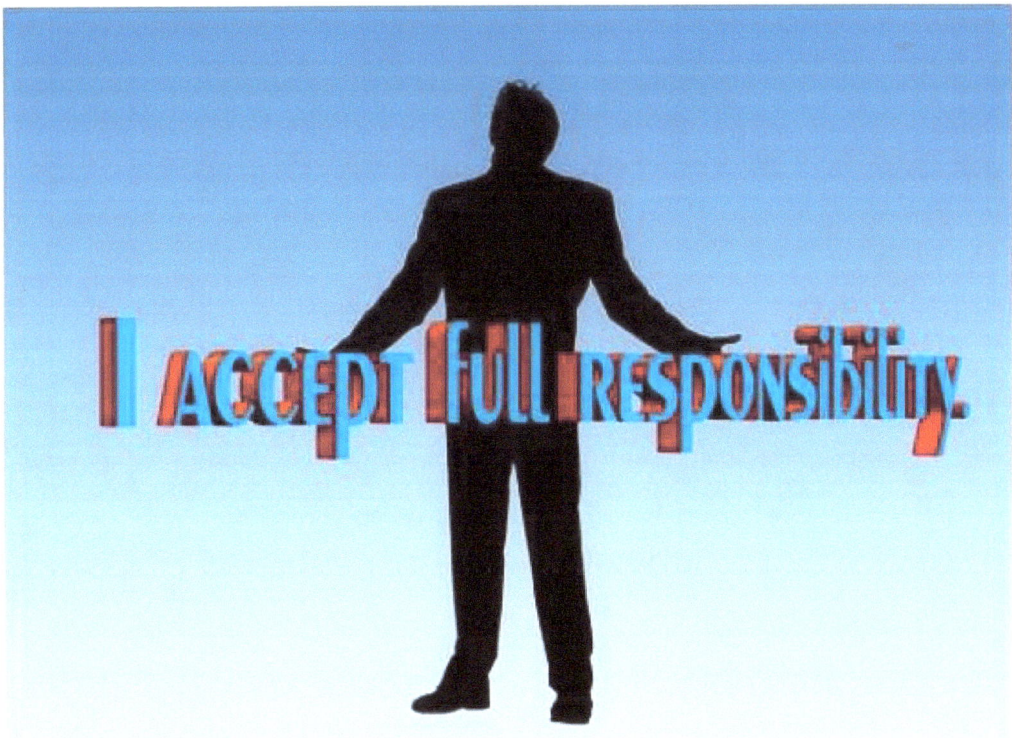

Fig. (6.3). Accountability. Source: www.pixabay.com

This second portion of Chapter six focusses more definitively on specific criteria associated with accountability (Fig.(**6.3**). **Nursing accountability** involves being responsible and answerable to others for what nurses do. Nursing accountability aligns with **the ethic of care** because they each embrace the principle of universal connectedness, caring action, responsibility for others and the protection of vulnerable people.

Universal Connectedness

Connectedness includes a sense of reverence for all of life and all things. It is about a keen awareness that we are universally linked to one another (Watson, 2008; Chopra, 2005). When a pebble is tossed into a still pond the ripples are felt throughout the whole body of water (Fig. **6.4**). The pain or joy that is experienced by one person is felt by all.

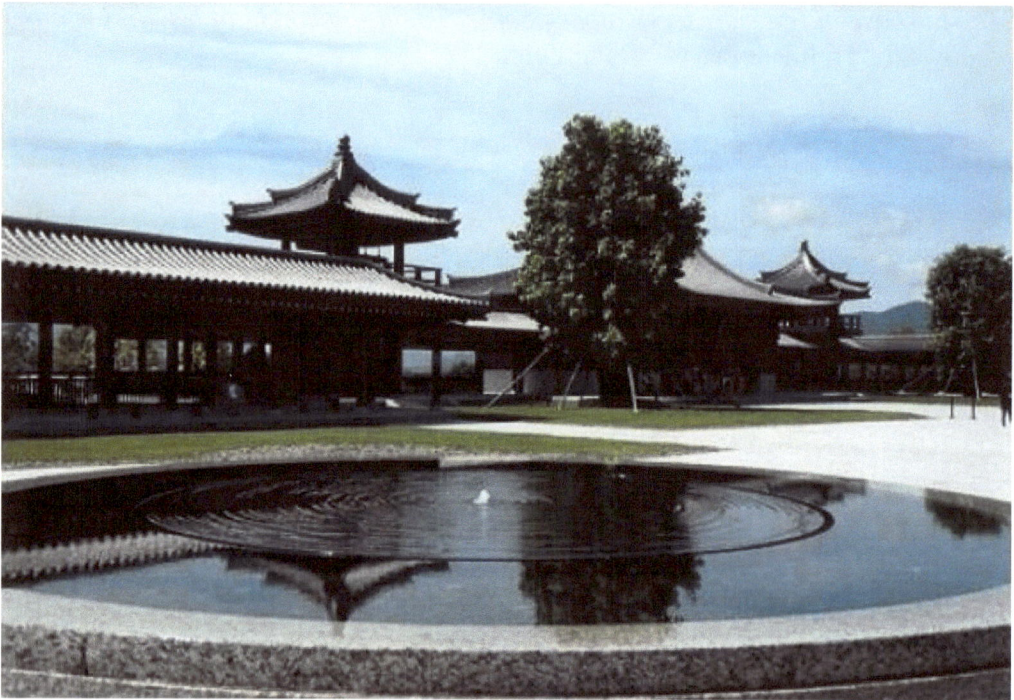

Fig. (**6.4**). Ripples in a Pond. Source: www.pixabay.com

For some nurses caring is a part of spirituality, but even if a nurse does not have a belief in a higher power, caring can still be guided by the assumption that something beyond our physical bodies joins all people in a meaningful way (Gladding, 1996). Covey (1989) referred to this process as **synergism** or the energy in nature that ensures that everything is related to everything else. The whole is deemed to be greater than the sum of the parts, which means that the relationship that the parts have to each other is catalytic, empowering and unifying (Covey, 1989).

Caring Action & Protecting the Vulnerable

Nursing accountability and the practice of the ethic of care are also particularly concerned with protecting vulnerable people which includes denouncing and acting against any intentional exploitation of individuals or groups (Bishop & Scudder, 1990; Gilligan, 1989). For example, not only is a caring nurse one who is concerned for the welfare of people but also keenly aware of the potential for selfish persons to hurt others. Subsequently, the responsible nurse understands the importance of protecting vulnerable people from harm's way (Ray, 2016). Chapter seven of this textbook will address the important role of the nurse in relation to client advocacy.

BEING ACCOUNTABLE: AN OVERVIEW OF CNA CODE OF ETHICS RESPONSIBILITIES

Scope of Practice

As outlined by the CNA Code of Ethics (2017) there are several important ethical responsibilities associated with being an accountable nurse. First and foremost, nurses must abide by their professional standards and the law. They are expected to practice honestly and within the limits of their competence, which includes not practicing beyond their scope (CNA, 2017). Not going beyond one's **scope of practice** means that if a nurse is assigned to care for someone where aspects of the needed care is beyond what they are capable of, they must seek additional information, report to their manager, or ask for a different assignment (CNA, 2017). However, even under these circumstances a nurse must never abandon patient care until they have been relieved of their duties by another more qualified nurse. Furthermore, whenever possible, nurses must strive to work together as a team when caring for clients with increased acuity (CNA, 2017).

Fitness to Practice

In order to be accountable, nurses have to ensure that they maintain their **fitness to practice**, which means that they need to make sure that they are physically, mentally and emotionally able to practice safely and competently (CNA, 2017). If they are unfit to practice nurses are expected to take whatever steps are needed to regain their fitness to practice while consulting appropriate professional resources (CNA, 2017). Likewise, if a nurse notices that a colleague is not able to perform their duties they are obligated to take action to protect the safety of the persons in their care and to report what they are aware of (CNA, 2017).

Conflict of Interest

Being accountable consists of being aware of what to do when a conflict of interest happens in clinical practice. For example, a **conflict of interest** occurs when any aspect of nursing care clashes with a nurse's own moral beliefs but is still in keeping with professional practice. An example of a conflict of interest is when a client who wants medical assistance in dying (MAID) is being cared for by a nurse who strongly believes that MAID violates her religious views. What should the nurse do when such a conflict happens? They must continue to provide safe, compassionate, competent ethical care until they are relieved of their duties. As previously stressed, a nurse must never abandon a client (CNA, 2017).

Mental Health Advocacy & Additional Responsibilities

It is an expectation of the CNA Code of Ethics that an accountable nurse will actively advocate for more comprehensive and equitable services for mental health care across all age groups, socio and cultural parameters and geographic regions (CNA, 2017) Additional responsibilities associated with accountability include nurses sharing their knowledge; offering feedback; and acting as mentors for student nurses, novice nurses, other nurses and other health professionals.

ACCOUNTABILITY & THE ORDER OF PRIORITIES

There is an important order of priorities associated with the practice of nursing accountability. The first priority is to the client, the second is to society, the third is to the profession of nursing and the fourth is to the institutions that nurses work in (Stephany, 2012). We will now review the significance of each of these.

1. Clients Come First

The ethic of care places the client at the center of all that is occurring and ethical practice puts the client first (Benner, 2000; Oberle & Bouchal., 2009). The client's welfare is a priority and supersedes all other responsibilities. In fact, as previously pointed out, nurses are expected to intervene if client safety or respect or dignity is being compromised (CNA, 2017). **Affirmative action** includes taking the necessary steps to protect persons receiving care, which may consist of reporting a safety breach and, at times, admitting when a mistake is made. Appropriate measures must also take place as soon as possible in order to minimize harm (CNA, 2017). The following narrative demonstrates how a nurse had to act quickly to preserve life. Box (**6:6**).

Box 6:6 Narrative: When a Client's Life is Endangered
A young 24-year-old woman, Saja, arrived at a rural hospital Emergency Room (ER) by ambulance after experiencing a fainting spell. Karen, the attending ER nurse learned that Saja was six weeks pregnant and that she experienced sudden onset of severe lower abdominal pain just before she fainted. Karen noted that Saja was extremely pale and diaphoretic. Postural hypotension and a rapid pulse rate of 120/minute was also noted. Examination of the client's belly revealed severe pelvic tenderness and tightness but no external bleeding. It was three in the morning and no physician was on duty, although they were on call. Karen paged the gynecologist who was on the list for that shift and waited for him to respond. She then provided the client with a warm blanket and inserted a large bore intravenous (IV) and began to rapidly infuse a litre of normal saline. Karen explained to Saja that although she was not a doctor she suspected that Saja may be bleeding internally from an ectopic pregnancy. Karen reassured her client that she was in good hands and that help was on its way. Karen asked Saja if she would be willing to receive blood if needed and she agreed. Karen called the laboratory technician who was on call and asked her to come to the ER to do stat blood work and a cross match. The laboratory technician asked if a doctor had seen the client. Karen informed her that she was still waiting for a response from the on-call gynecologist. The laboratory technician refused to come into the hospital explaining that she wasn't going to take orders from a nurse. Karen insisted that she had to come to the ER right away. The laboratory technician reluctantly agreed but informed Karen that she was going to report her. Karen responded with, *"Fine, just get here."* Meanwhile, the gynecologist who was on call still had not responded to the page. Karen paged him again with no answer and then called another gynecologist who was not on call. The second physician picked up the phone. Karen gave him the results of her assessment and he asked her to get the operating room (OR) staff ready to go. Karen concurred. She informed the physician that she had started an IV and ordered a blood cross match without a doctor's order because no doctor was present. He requested that the client be cross matched for six units of blood stat. Within 30 minutes Saja was in the OR. As soon as the blood was ready for transfusion surgery was performed. Surgical laparotomy revealed that the client's pelvis was full of blood. Six units of blood was rapidly transfused and Saja survived without serious complications. The laboratory technician reported Karen to administration, but Karen was not reprimanded. She had filled out an incident report explaining everything in detail and the gynecologist supported all of her actions because her decision to act swiftly saved the client's life.

When nurses are confronted with circumstances where harm is not imminent then they work together with other members of the team to resolve the issue as best as possible and hopefully to the satisfaction of all involved parties (CNA, 2017). However, although it is important to follow the rules, if a person's life is at risk, and no alternative is readily available, then the rules may have to be broken. Client safety supersedes all other responsibilities.

2. Society Deserves to be Protected

"Nurses support the person, family, group, population or community receiving care in maintaining dignity and integrity" Canadian Nurses Association.

Nurses are not only accountable to their clients, they are also answerable to their client's families, their communities and society at large (Oberle & Bouchal, 2009). Nurses are expected to follow the principles of justice by protecting human rights, equity, fairness and by upholding the good of the public (CNA, 2017). The expectation is that nurses will do everything they can to promote health; to prevent needless spread of communicable disease; to prevent harm; to educate the public; to promote social justice and to end social inequities (CNA, 2006; CNA, 2017). Box (**6:7**).

Box 6:7 LEARNING ACTIVITY:
Have an open class discussion of specific clinical examples of how nurses do the following: promote health, prevent spread of communicable disease; prevent harm; educate the public, promote justice & end social inequities.

3. Nurses are Responsible to their Profession

Nurses are responsible to the profession of nursing. Along with other professional members of the health care team, nurses are held to a very high standard of accountability. Mechanisms are in place to ensure that professional regulatory bodies ensure that competent and safe standards of practice are enforced in the following ways: in practice, education, research endeavours and in leadership (Keatings & Smith, 2016).

4. Where do Institution's Policies fit in?

In Canada, although nurses are sometimes employed privately, most nurses work within the publicly funded health care system. Hospitals have policies and rules of conduct that all their employees and nurses are required to follow (Keatings & Smith, 2016). However, when an institutional policy violates nursing values and ethical responsibilities as set out by the CNA Code of Ethics (2017), the delivery of safe, competent, compassionate and ethical care comes first. What should a nurse do if there is an ethical conflict with institutional policy? Wherever possible, the nurse ought to notify their supervisor or employer to try and remedy the situation and diplomacy is of the utmost importance. However, what if that does not work? The nurse can contact a member of their professional regulatory body and request urgent support and guidance. The following narrative illustrates how an issue can sometimes be rectified through good communication and diplomacy Box (**6:8**).

Box 6:8 Narrative: Using Diplomacy to Sort through an Ethical Conflict in Care
A student nurse approached her nursing instructor about a situation that was troubling her. On weekends this student nurse worked in a Care Home for seniors. Recently the new Director had sent out a memo that all clients were to be woken up at 5:30 in the morning, bathed, and seated in a chair in preparation for breakfast. What previously used to happen was that clients were woken up at 8:00, just before breakfast and morning care followed. The student nurse was upset because some of her clients begged her to let them sleep longer and some even cried when woken up so early in the morning. She did not know what to do. The clinical instructor encouraged the student to sort through the dilemma using some of the materials she had learned in her Ethics class and by working it out with the employer. She followed this direction and later emailed her instructor to inform her that the Care Home's Director listened intently to her ideas, particularly after she shared how the new policy negatively impacted the clients. They eventually arrived at a compromise that would allow the clients to sleep a bit longer in the mornings.

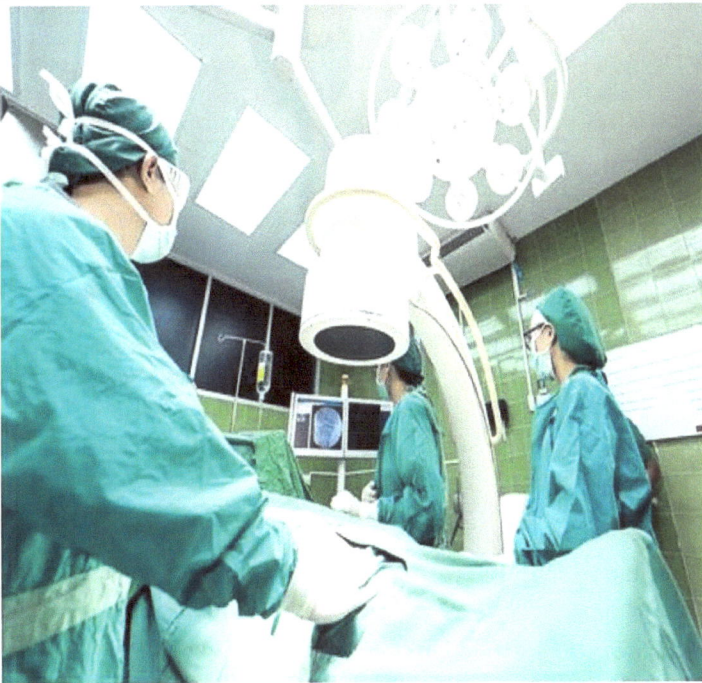

Fig. (6.5). Operating Room. Source: www.pixabay.com

4. Questions Pertaining to the Case in Point:

1. What do you think really happened in the OR that day?
2. Did the OR nurses act responsibly or irresponsibly, when they noticed evidence of a lack of client monitoring?
3. What about the surgeon's role? Should the surgeon have checked on the client's condition earlier? Is the monitoring of the client a shared responsibility?
4. If you were a member of the Coroner's Inquest Jury what recommendations would you make to prevent death under similar circumstances?

Box (6:9) CASE IN POINT: WHEN A CLIENT RECORD IS INTENTIONALLY ALTERED

Kim was a client who had been badly burned in a plane crash. Kim was scheduled to have a debridement of his wounds and skin grafts applied. The operation was performed under general anesthesia. During the procedure the surgeon noted that the blood in the burn areas appeared dark in color and inquired how the client was doing. A Code Blue was immediately called by the anesthetist, but resuscitative efforts were unsuccessful. The Coroner was notified and seized the client record, which was professionally copied, locked and stored for Inquest. After being photocopied the original copy of the chart was returned to the Hospital Records Department. The seized copy of the original record had no documentation of client vital signs, oxygen (O2) saturation levels or fluid balance, even though the client had been under general anesthesia for more than an hour prior to the cardiac arrest being called. The autopsy report revealed that the client had suffered a cardiac arrest due to hypovolemia and electrolyte imbalance as a result of the burns, fluid loss and inadequate fluid and electrolyte replacement. The Operating Room (OR) nursing staff were interviewed by the Coroner at the Inquest. They provided evidence under oath that they suspected that the client was not adequately monitored during the procedure because the cardiac monitoring screen was blank and there was no blood pressure machine or stethoscope in the OR theatre. However, when the original chart was made available at the Coroner's Inquest, unlike the previously seized copy, a series of vital signs and O2 saturation levels were now recorded (as normal) right up until the Code Blue was called. [1]

Box (6:10) CASE IN POINT: WHEN A NURSE IS ORDERED TO WITHHOLD CRUCIAL INFORMATION

Ingrid works as a nurse Risk Manager and because her position is in middle management it is union exempt. Ingrid just discovered that contaminated instruments were used in the Operating Room (OR) in three surgical cases. Ingrid urgently approached her immediate supervisor and requested to notify each of the respective clients so that they could be tested for hepatitis and human immunodeficiency virus (HIV). Igrid's supervisor denied this request because in her opinion this action would lead to an increased risk of legal litigation.

Questions Pertaining to the Case in Point:

1. What would you do if you were Ingrid?
2. Who is Ingrid accountable to? Make a list of priorities.
3. What are the potential repercussions to the person and others if the individuals in this case are not tested for blood borne diseases and have become infected by the contaminated instruments?
4. What could likely happen to Ingrid if she disobeys her supervisor?
5. What are the legal and professional risks to Ingrid if she obeys her supervisor?
6. Where, or to whom, should Ingrid turn to for help and direction?
7. Apply either *The Mosaic Model for Ethical Decisions* or *A Framework for Ethical Decisions* to address the ethical issues in this case. Don't forget to consider the legal aspects of accountability.

REFLECTING BACK

Summary of Key Points Covered in Chapter 6

- A professional is an educated, skilled and knowledgeable individual who offers a particular service to the community and professions exist for the purpose of meeting the needs of society.
- Professional behaviours are monitored by government and respective professional bodies.
- For any group of individuals to call themselves a profession there are four aspects that must be present: they must possess a specialized body of knowledge, they must be accountable, they must be self-governing, and they must abide by a code of ethics.
- The profession of nursing requires a bit more of their members than just the basic criteria. Nurses must abide by a regulatory body's standards of practice.
- Although practice standards differ somewhat from one jurisdiction to another in Canada, some common standard themes include but are not limited to: responsibility & accountability, knowledge-based practice, competent application of knowledge, code of ethics, provision of services in the public interest, and self-regulation.
- Self-regulation of any profession is a privilege, not a right. In Canada self-regulation of the nursing profession is granted by the provincial or territorial governments.
- Self-regulation allows nursing members to set the conditions for entrance into the profession, devise educational requirements, set standards of practice, investigate complaints and instigate disciplinary action when indicated.
- A professional boundary is a limit that is set and determines how far a relationship can go and when it is in appropriate for the relationship to proceed.
- When boundaries are violated the possibility exists for harm to occur which is referred to as a boundary violation.
- The CNA Code of Ethics clearly describes the importance of nurses maintaining appropriate professional boundaries.
- Nursing accountability involves being responsible and answerable to others for what nurses do.
- Nursing accountability aligns with the ethic of care because they each embrace the principle of universal connectedness, caring action, responsibility for others and the protection of vulnerable people.
- The following five CNA Code of Ethics key ethical responsibilities associated with being accountable were presented.
  1. Nurses are obligated to abide by their professional standards and the law.
  2. They are expected to practice honestly and within the limits of their competence which includes not practicing beyond their scope.

3. Nurses must maintain their fitness to practice which consists of being physically, mentally and emotionally able to practice safely and competently.

4. A nurse must never abandon a client not even if there is a conflict of interest. They must remain with the client until relieved of their duties by another competent nurse.

5. Nurses are expected to advocate for equitable services for mental health and to share their knowledge with other nurses and colleagues.

- The following order of priorities in nursing accountability was proposed. The first priority is to the client, the second is to society, the third is to the profession of nursing and the fourth is to the institutions that nurses work for.
- It was argued that a client's welfare is a priority and supersedes all other responsibilities.

SOMETHING TO PONDER

1. Have you ever encountered a situation where you knew that you should share your nursing knowledge with someone but held back due to the fear of being embarrassed? Would you act differently now? Why or why not?

2. You happen to run into a former client at a local pub and the person invites you to have a drink at the bar. It has only been a couple of weeks since you cared for this client on a surgical ward. What is the professional thing to do and how will you ensure that you maintain boundaries in this situation?

3. Have you ever been in a situation where you were asked to do something that you knew would compromise client safety? What did you do? What would you do differently now after what you have just learned about accountability?

CLASSROOM GROUP EXERCISES

1. Break into groups of four. Discuss some of the most common obstacles that occur in health care that interfere with proper nursing documentation. Come up with innovative ideas on how to overcome some of these barriers.

2. Break into groups of four. Think of a situation in your clinical practice where you believe that a nurse you worked with was not acting responsibly in providing client care. How did you and/or the other members of the health care team react? What did you believe impacted the nurse's decision to act in the way that they did? What could you or the other members of the team have done to make things better? Share your stories with the bigger group.

ON YOUR OWN

Spend some time reflecting and writing in your journal about some or all of the following questions:

1. Reflect on a situation where you did not act professionally or responsibly and consider the reasons that governed your choice. What, if anything would you do differently now?
2. How has the value of accountability evolved in your practice, as a nurse or student nurse?
3. What attitudes guide your decisions to act responsibly in day to day endeavours?

Recommended Readings

Dohmann, E. L. (2009). *Accountability in nursing: Six strategies to build and maintain a culture of commitment.* USA: Marblehead.

Merlino, J. (2015). *How to build superior patient experiences the Cleveland clinic way.* USA: McGraw Hill.

Miller-Tiedeman, A. (1999). *Learning, practicing, and living the new careering.* USA: Taylor & Francis Group.

Sinek, S. (2009). *Start with why: How great leaders inspire everyone to take action.* USA: Portfolio/Penguin.

Web Resources

Web Resource: British Columbia College of Nursing Professionals: Professional Standards for Registered Nurses and Nurse Practitioners https://www.bccnp.ca/Standards/RPN/ProfessionalStandards/Pages/Default.aspx

Web Resource: Teaching & Learning Professionalism in Nursing http://www.cno.org/globalassets/4learnaboutstandardsandguidelines/prac/learn/teleconferences/teleconference--teaching-and-learning-professionalism-in-nursing.pdf

Web Resource: Professional Accountability in Clinical Skills Practice http://www.csmen.scot.nhs.uk/media/1318/professionalism_and_professional_accountability.pdf

REFERENCES

Benner, P (2000) The role of embodiment, emotion and the life world for rationality and agency in nursing practice. *Nursing Philosophy,* 1, 5-19.
[http://dx.doi.org/10.1046/j.1466-769x.2000.00014.x]

Bishop, AH & Scudder, JR (1996) *Nursing ethics: Therapeutic caring presence.*Jones and Bartlett Publishers, London.

Burkhardt, MA, Nathaniel, AK & Walton, NA (2015) *Ethics and issues in contemporary nursing* Nelson Education Limited, Toronto, Ontario.

British Columbia College of Nursing Professionals (BCCNP) (n.d.). *Professional Standards for Registered Nurses and Nurse Practitioners*https://www.bccnp.ca/Standards/RPN/ProfessionalStandards/Pages/Default.aspx

Canadian Nurses Association (CNA) (2006) *Social Justice, a means to an end, an end in itself.* . Ottawa: Author.

Canadian Nurses Association (CNA) (2015) *Framework for the practice of Registered Nurses in Canada*https://www.cna-aiic.ca/~/media/cna/page-content/pdf-en/framework-for-the-pracice-of-reistered-nurses-in-canada.pdf

Canadian Nurses Association (CNA) (2017) *CNA Code of Ethics for Registered Nurses (Revised Edition)* . Ottawa: Author.

Canadian Nurses Association (CNA) (2018) CNA proposes membership expansion to represent all nurses: What members need to know about the proposed changes, its context and the decision that lies ahead. *Canadian Nurse,* 114, 35-6.

Canadian Nurses Association (CNA) (2018a) *Policy & advocacy* https://www.cna-aiic.ca/en/policy-advocacy

Chopra, D (2005) *Peace is the way.*Three Rivers Press, USA.

Coburn, D (1988) The development of Canadian nursing: professionalism and proletarianization. *International Journal of Health Science. 18,* (3) 437 – 456.

Covey, S R (1989) *The seven habits of highly effective people: Powerful lessons in personal change.*Simon & Schuster, New York.

DeWolf Bosek, M S & Savage, T A (2007) *The ethical component of nursing education: Integrating ethics into clinical experience.*Lippincott Williams & Wilkins, New York.

Ford, GG (2006) *Ethical reasoning for mental health professionals.*Sage Publications, London.

Gilligan, C (1982) *In a different voice: Psychological theory and women's development.*Harvard University Press, Cambridge: MA.

Gladding, ST (1996) Counseling: A comprehensive profession, 3rd ed. Merril/Prentice Hall, Upper Saddle River, NJ.

Hall, K H (2001) Sexualization of the doctor-patient relationship: Is it ever ethically permissible? *Family Practice,* 8, 511-5.

Insights West Survey *Nurses, doctors and scientists are Canada's most respected professionals* https://insightswest.com/news/nurses-doctors-and-scientists-are-canadas-most-respected-professionals/

Keatings, M & Smith, OB (2016) *Ethical & legal issues in Canadian nursing (Kindle ed).*Saunders, Canada.

Miller-Tiedeman, A (1999) *Learning, practicing, and living the new careering.*Taylor & Francis Group, USA.

Oberle, K & Bouchal, SR (2009) *Ethics in Canadian nursing practice: Navigating the journey.* Pearson, Toronto.

Ray, MA (2016) Transcultural caring dynamics in nursing and health care, 2nd ed. F.A. Davis Company, Philadelphia.

Stephany, K (2012) *The ethic of care: A moral compass for Canadian nursing practice*Bentham Science Publishing Ltd., United Arab Emirates.
[http://dx.doi.org/10.2174/97816080530491120101]

Watson, J (2008) *Nursing: The philosophy of caring (Revised edition).*University Press of Colorado, Boulder, Colorado.

CHAPTER 7

Advocacy: The Heart of Nursing

Abstract: Nursing Advocacy entails acting on behalf of others and Chapter Seven promotes advocacy as the driving force of nursing. Advocacy can occur in the form of being a voice for an individual or by supporting a larger cause. Nurses are expected to maintain quality health care services, preserve public access to health care and ensure health equity. Whistle-blowing is presented as a more drastic form of advocacy that is only to be used as a last resort. Six specific actions are suggested for nurses to seriously consider before whistle-blowing. Nurses are not likely to advocate for a person or group of people that they have a bias toward. Cultural safety and affirmative action are recommended to end discrimination. There are some negative consequences associated with advocacy like that of being morally silenced. The Chapter ends with a Case in Point where a student nurse chooses to be the voice for the client.

Keywords: Advocacy, Autonomy, Affirmative action, CNA Code of Ethics Part II, Cultural safety, Determinants of health, Ethic of care, Ethic of justice, Florence Nightingale, Health equity, Homelessness, Informed consent, Indigenous peoples, Moral silence, Moral residue, Mental illness, Paternalism, Parentalism, Stereotypes, Social justice, Whistle-blowing.

LEARNING GUIDE

After Completing this Chapter, the Reader Should be Able to

- Understand that nurse can advocate for individuals and/or for a cause.
- Define social justice, health equity and social determinants of health.
- Understand three key actions that The CNA Code of Ethics Part II (2017) expects of nurses.
- Become aware of the many ways that nurses can specifically address or eliminate social inequities.
- Gain an understanding of what it means to be Indigenous.
- Become aware of how social determinants of health negatively affect vulnerable populations and ways that nurses can advocate for change.
- Define whistle-blowing and appreciate that it should be used as a last resort.
- Be able to clearly articulate specific actions that nurses should seriously consider before whistle-blowing.

- Be cognizant of the fact that stereotypical biases often impede advocacy efforts.
- Gain an understanding of the risks that are associated with advocacy.
- Apply what was learned to the Case in Point: When the student nurse chooses to be the voice for the client.

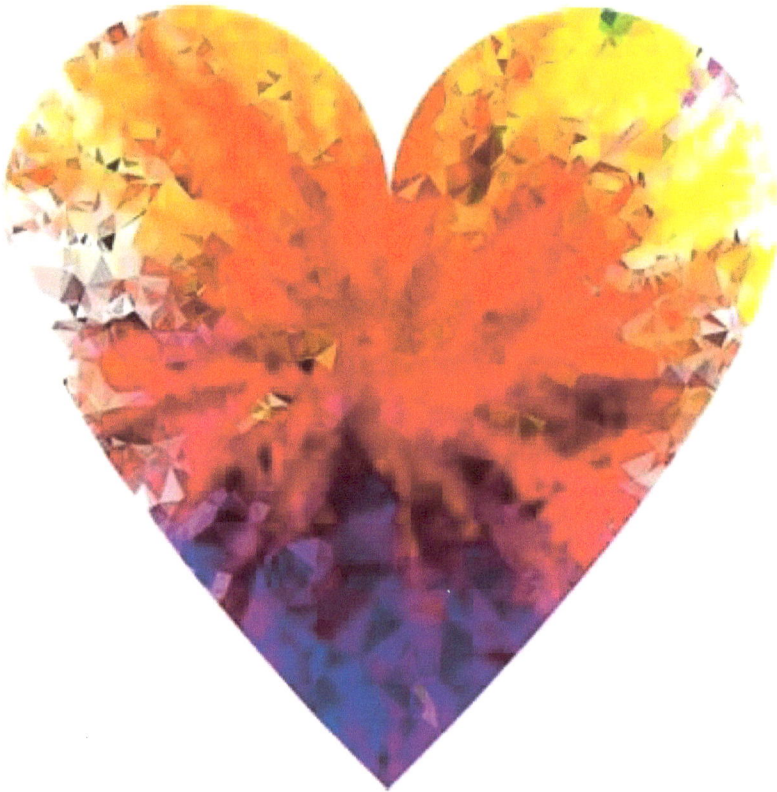

Fig. (7.1). Advocacy, the Heart of Nursing. Source: www.pixabay.com

"You really can change the world if you care enough." Marian Wright Edelman, American Activist for children

Nursing advocacy entails action on behalf of others. Advocacy was introduced in earlier Chapters and it is a threaded theme throughout this book because it is so central to what nurses do. The title of this Chapter is, *Nursing Advocacy: The Heart of Nursing*, and it is a fitting title because that is what many of us believe to be true (Fig. **7.1**). Chapter Seven begins with the assertion that advocacy is the heart of nursing. It is argued that the ethic of care and advocacy are closely related because they are both concerned with taking responsibility for what happens to us and others. The focus then turns to how advocacy can occur on behalf of an individual or a social cause and the three key actions that The CNA Code of Ethics Part II (2017) expects of nurses.

Whistle-blowing is a more drastic form of advocacy and it should only be undertaken as a last resort. Specific actions are strongly advised before deciding to be a whistle-blower. We are made aware that a nurse is unlikely to advocate for a person or group of people that they have a bias toward. Ensuring cultural safety and affirmative action is recommended as a means to end discrimination. There are some negative consequences associated with advocacy that includes being morally silenced. The Chapter ends with a Case in Point where student nurse chooses to be the voice for the client.

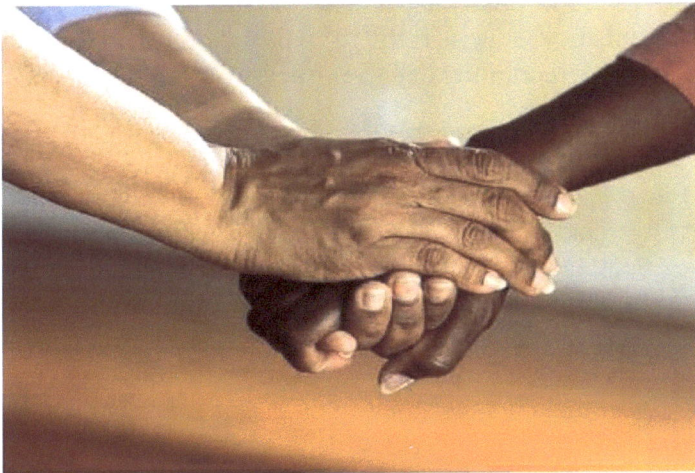

Fig. (7.2). Helping Hands. Source: www.pixabay.com

NURSING ADVOCACY & THE INDIVIDUAL

"What ever the tools or technologies, the job of the nurse will remain caregiver and advocate for the most sick and vulnerable members of our communities." Dr. Charles Tiffin, Professor of Human Science

One key role of nursing advocacy consists of being the voice for a specific individual or acting on their behalf (Fig. **7.2**). Clients sometimes have a tough time making their voices heard or asking for what they need. This happens when someone feels disempowered by the situation that they find themselves in. Individuals who have been admitted to hospital often relate to this feeling. Your clothes are removed; you are placed in a hospital gown where the back of the gown is often open; and you have to rely on complete strangers to care for you. Although we often claim that the client is the center of care when we are doing care planning, there is often a discrepancy between what the ideal goal is and what actually happens. Dewolf Bosek and Savage (2007) explains that due to their incapacitation and a sense of vulnerability, clients often feel disempowered and afraid to speak up on their own. That is why it is essential that the nurse be their voice (Dewolf Bosek & Savage, 2007).

Advocacy & Informed Consent

The CNA Code of Ethics (2017) Value C. Promoting and Protecting Informed Decision-making, expects that nurses will speak up and ensure that informed consent occurs and that the client's wishes are upheld. Recall that **informed consent** consists of ensuring that your client has a complete understanding of all of the treatment options available to them and any potential risks or benefits associated with each proposed treatment modality. As long as the client is mentally competent they have a right to make their own choices and to either follow or refuse the recommended treatment (CNA, 2017). In this manner informed consent honours a client's right to autonomy.

Paternalism & Advocacy

Sometimes a physician will want to decide what they believe is in the best interests of the client and may override what the client actually wants. This action is supported by the ethical principle of **paternalism**, also referred to as **parentalism**. However, as previously pointed out, paternalism is not a moral principle that nurses follow. When a doctor refuses to allow a mentally competent person to make informed choices about their care it is crucially important that the nurse speak up. However, when a nurse decides to be their client's voice and go against what the doctor may advise, they may face strong opposition because of the assumed power differential that exists between the two professions.

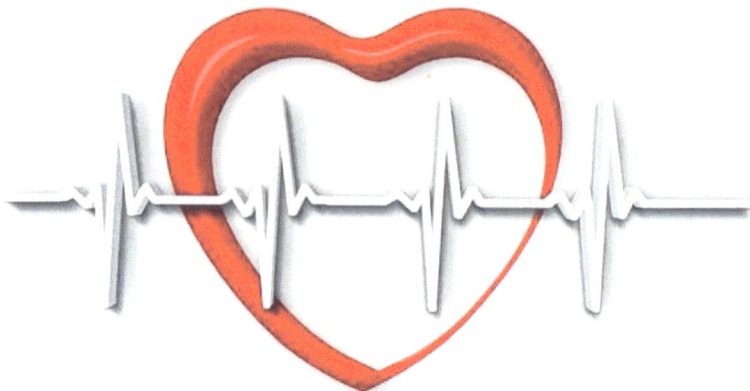

Fig. (7.3). Medicare. Source: www.pixabay.com

NURSING ADVOCACY & PROTECTING PUBLIC ACCESS TO HEALTH CARE

The CNA Code of Ethics Part II (2017) expects that nurses will work to protect the quality of public health care services and to preserve public access to health care for all (Fig. **7.3**). Nurses are specifically directed to take action to ensure that heath care delivery systems guarantee accessibility, universality and comprehensiveness of any necessary health services, to be provided at the right time and correct place (CNA, 2017). The type of care that nurses are mandated to protect include: health promotion, prevention of disease, diagnostics, as well as restorative and palliative care in hospitals, nursing homes and in the community (CNA, 2017).

Historical Underpinnings: Why Canada Has Publicly Funded Health Care

"I felt that no boy should have to depend either for his leg or his life upon the ability of his parents to raise enough money to bring a first-class surgeon to his bedside. And I think that out of this experience, not at the moment consciously, but through the years, that I came to believe that health services ought not to have a price tag on them, and that people should be able to get whatever health services they require irrespective of the individual's capacity to pay." Tommy Douglas, Canadian Politician & Forefather of Medicare

Medicare, which is publicly funded health care, has not always been available in Canada. In fact, it was not until July 1, 1962, that Medicare was first introduced in Saskatchewan as the first Government operated, single-payer medical insurance plan in North America (Brown & Taylor, 2012). The reason that Saskatchewan was the first province to embrace Medicare has a great deal to do with the Co-operative Commonwealth Federation (CCF) socialistic views led by Tommy Douglas. However, Medicare was not welcomed by all. The North American medical establishment and Canadian private insurance companies did everything they could to strop Medicare from spreading (Brown & Taylor, 2012). They were desperately afraid that Medicare would be popular and embraced by the public, and they were correct. Despite opposition, in 1966, universal health care was adopted in Canada with the passing of *The Medical Care Act*. This act was backed by all political parties: Tommy Douglas and the CCF, Progressive Conservatives lead by Diefenbaker, and by the Liberal Prime Minister, Lester Pearson (Samphir, 2015). Within ten years all of Canada was covered by public Medicare and very few politicians dared to oppose it (Brown & Taylor, 2012).

Health Care for all People

Samphir (2015) points out that, Universal access to health care is still an essential pillar of what it means to be Canadian. Yet, the same interest groups that tried to stop Medicare in Canada continue to try to destroy it today (Brown & Taylor, 2012). Many critics of our health care system site increased wait times for surgeries, not being able to find a family doctor, or long hours spent in the Emergency Room (ER) waiting to be treated, as reasons to privatize health care. Many of these criticisms are justified and there is room for improvement in how our health care is delivered. However, this does not mean that our system is no longer working. We need to be cognizant of the fact that everyone in this country can access basic health care without paying for it from their own pocket. In fact, tens of millions of Americans do not have access to affordable health care even though the United States is one of the richest countries in the world (Street, 2017). For instance, in comparison to Canadians, millions of Americans don't have medical coverage, especially the poor, and so many more lose their coverage just because they get sick or go without medical care because of a pre-existing medical condition (Alini, 2010). Reasons why it is not a very good idea to move toward a private health care system alongside our private system are clearly articulated in Box (**7:1**).

Box 7:1 WHY A MOVE TOWARD PRIVATE HEALTH CARE IS A BAD IDEA (adapted from The Supreme Court Ruling, 2005, of Chaoulli & Zeliotis *versus* Quebec & Canada, as cited in CNA, 2008).
* Those who seek private health insurance are people who can afford it and can qualify for it. They will be more advantaged members of society. They are differentiated from the general population, not by their health problems, which are found in every group in society, but by their income.
* While acknowledging the problem of shortage of providers, experience in all jurisdictions with two-tier health care systems (*e.g.*, the U.K., Australia, New Zealand and Israel) demonstrated a diversion of energy and commitment by physicians and surgeons from the public system to the more lucrative private option..
* Experts testified that there are no firm data whatsoever that a parallel private system would enhance potential for recruiting highly trained specialists
* Experience in other countries shows that an increase in private funding typically leads to a decrease in government funding.
* A service designed purely for members of society with less socio-economic power would probably lead to a decline in quality of services and a loss of political support.
* Evidence suggest that parallel private insurers prefer to siphon off high income patients (*e.g.* cream skimming) while shying away from patient populations that constitute higher risk. The public system is likely to wind up carrying the more complex high acuity end of the health care spectrum and consequently, increase rather than reduce demand in the public system for certain services.
* The existence of a private system in the United States has not eliminated waiting times. The availability, extent and timeliness of health care is rationed by private insurers, who may determine according to cost, not need, what is medically necessary health care and where and when it is to occur.

Sustainability of The Publicly Funded Canadian Health Care System & The Role of Nurses

"Registered nurses are deeply engaged in system transformation because they care about human health and about the delivery of responsible health care. More than caring, it is the professional and social responsibility of nurses to take a strong leadership stand on behalf of Canadians" (Canadian Nurses Association, 2012, p. 3).

Sustainability of the current Canadian health care system is dependent on the balance between the cultural, social and economic conditions that strive to meet the health care needs of individuals and populations (The Conference Board of Canada, 2019). Our health care system is as sustainable as we want it to be. Nurses, by their large numbers (>268,500) and their knowledge, are perfectly situated as advocates and change agents to take action to ensure that our health care is sustainable (CNA, 2012). According to The National Expert Commission, the best way to achieve sustainable health care is to address the social inequities and determinants of health (CNA, 2012). For example, we need to achieve and maintain better health outcomes through initiatives such as: better management of chronic diseases, embracing preventative and health promotional initiatives, adopt measures that decrease poverty and eliminate homelessness (CNA, 2012). All these initiatives reduce costs and improve upon the health of the population (The Conference Board of Canada, 2019). We will now proceed with a discussion of how nurses can specifically advocate for social justice which will improve the health of Canadians, especially the most vulnerable.

NURSING ADVOCACY & SOCIAL JUSTICE

"Until the great mass of people shall be filled with the sense of responsibility for each other's welfare, social justice can never be attained." Helen Keller, American Author, Political Activist, Lecturer, & first blind-deaf person to obtain a Bachelor of Science Degree

the CNA Code of Ethics (2017) expects nurses to advocate for social justice. **Social justice** emphasizes the relative position of specific groups in relationship to others in society and strives for increased equality. Social justice is supported by the **ethic of justice** and **the ethic of care** because they share the goal of creating a society with fewer inequalities. The ethic of care condemns exploitation or the hurting of others and calls on nurses to take action to stop and prevent all deliberate mistreatment of people (Gilligan, 1982).

Florence Nightingale, one of our beloved, historical nursing role models firmly believed in advocating for social reform. Box (**7:2**) Florence Nightingale who practiced as a nurse primarily in the nineteenth century, was outraged by the enormous difference in degree of wealth. Very few people were well off and the greater masses were extremely poor (McDonald, 2010). In fact, most people did not own property and did not enjoy very many comforts. Nearly a third of the population lived in absolute poverty (McDonald, 2010).

Box 7:2 The Florence Nightingale Pledge (as cited in DeWolf Bosek & Savage, 2007, p. 46)
I solemnly pledge myself before God and the presence of this assembly, to pass my life in purity. I will abstain from whatever is deleterious and mischievous and will not take or knowingly administer any harmful drug. I will do all in my power to maintain and elevate the standard of my profession and will hold in confidence all personal matters committed to my keeping and family affairs coming to my knowledge in the practice of my calling. With loyalty will I endeavor to aid the physician in his work and devote myself to the welfare of those committed to my care.

Poverty is a worldwide problem that has been growing instead of subsiding and has a negative impact on people's health (CNA, 2008, World Health Organization (WHO), 2018). The most impoverished people experience the poorest health (Public Health Agency of Canada (PHAC), 2004). According to WHO (2018), **social determinants of health** consist of the situations that people are born into, live in, work in, and age in. Social determinants of health are shaped by the distribution of money and resources at the global, national and local levels of government (WHO, 2018). They are further influenced by the following: conditions of early childhood; access to education; type of employment; working conditions; availability of adequate shelter and food; accessibility to enough income to sustain health and well-being; and the degree of social inclusion (WHO, 2018).

Unfortunately, social inequities and human misery are not only a historical fact, they still exist in Canada today. Although Canadians live longer and healthier lives than they did 25 to 50 years ago, there are disparities in health for many people. The relationship between socio-economic status and health outcomes is real. A higher social and economic status is associated with better health, yet it is estimated that one in seven Canadians live in poverty and just under 24% of Indigenous peoples live below the poverty line (Citizens for Public Justice, 2017). In this textbook, the term **Indigenous** is used as an inclusive and international term. It describes individuals and collectives who consider themselves as being related to and/or having historical continuity with "First Peoples," whose civilizations in many parts of the world, predate those of subsequent invading or colonizing populations (Allan & Smylie, 2015). For a summary of key demographics of persons living in poverty in Canada refer to Box (**7:3**).

Box 7:3 Key Demographics of People in Canada with High Poverty Rates (as adapted from Citizens for Public Justice, 2017).
Working-aged Adults - 14.7 %.
Single working aged Adults - 33.7 %
People with Disabilities aged 22 – 66 - 23 %
Indigenous peoples – 23.6 %
Children in Single Parent Families 43.4 %

Although Canada is one of the richest countries in the world one is six children live in poverty and the rate of childhood poverty for Indigenous children is twice that of other children. Over half of Indigenous peoples, whether they live on or off reserves, are poor and they are four times more likely to complain of hunger (CNA, 2010; Government of Canada, 2018). They are also more likely to live shorter and less healthy lives, be less productive for the nation and use more expensive health services (CNA, 2008). Twenty to 25 percent of Indigenous peoples have poor access to clean community water and sanitation services which poses additional risks to their health (CNA, 2010). The CNA (2008) quite poignantly pointed out that we cannot build or sustain a healthy nation in Canada if our Indigenous peoples are living in conditions of poverty.

The Real Cost of Homelessness

"The greatness of a nation can be judged by how it treats its weakest member." Mahatma Gandhi, Indian Civil Rights Activist.

Many policy makers and politicians complain about escalating costs associated with the delivery of health services in Canada. They may be unaware or unwilling to acknowledge the fact that social economic determinants of health are closely tied to health outcomes with the poor costing the healthcare system more in dollars (Public Health Agency of Canada (PHAC), 2004). Let's examine the real cost of homelessness in this country. Homelessness negatively affects the lives of people physically and mentally and greatly decreases their quality of life. In fact, large numbers of the homeless suffer from mental illness and addictions (Goering *et al.*, 2014). Furthermore, living in shelters requires tremendous energy just to survive (Goering *et al.*, 2014). Homelessness has more than doubled in certain parts of Canada in the past few decades, especially in high density areas, but it is prevalent in every area of the country. On any given night in Canada approximately 35,000 people sleep on the street and annually roughly 200,000 people are homeless (Canadian Public Health Association, (CPHA) 2015; Goering *et al.*, 2014). See (Fig. **7.4**).

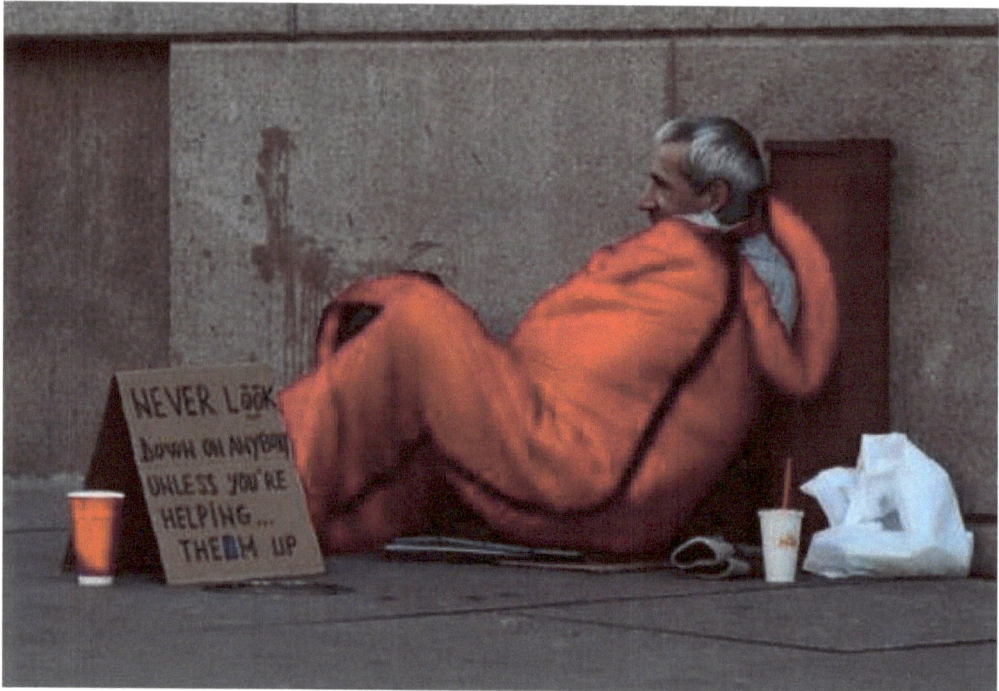

Fig. (7.4). Homeless man. Source: www.pixabay.com

The number of homeless continues to rise despite almost seven Billion dollars being spent on health care, the justice system and social services (Gaetz, Gulliver & Richter, 2014). Why has homelessness been increasing? Homelessness in Canada emerged as a significant problem in the 1990's due to the federal government's withdrawal of funding for affordable housing, declining wages, inflation and reduced funding for social services and pensions. Furthermore, this funding has not been restored by subsequent governments (Gaetz *et al.*, 2014).

One might argue that it is too expensive to provide housing and treatment for people who suffer from addictions, mental illness and homelessness when it is costing much more than we think to leave them on the street. The Canadian Institute for Health Information (CIHI) (2007) data indicate that mental health issues among the homeless population account for large numbers of Emergency Department visits (35%) and hospital stays (52%) when compared with the population as a whole. A study entitled, *Housing and Support for Adults with Severe Addictions and/or Mental Illness in British Columbia (BC)* revealed the actual cost per homeless person in BC. The research project was conducted by five academics from Simon Fraser University, the University of BC and the University of Calgary (Patterson, Somers, McIntosh, Shiell & Franklin, 2008).

The final report concluded that it costs the taxpayer $55,000 per homeless person or $644.3 million annually in health, corrections and social services. The study argued that if housing and support were offered to these people, it would cost the system much less – just $37,000 a year, and greatly improve the lives of those who are affected (Patterson *et al.*, 2008).

At Home /Chez Soi Study

A more recent study by the Mental Health Commission of Canada (MHCC) called, *At Home /Chez Soi* was conducted by the federal government where $110 million was spent over five years for a research project that focused on approaches for people with serious mental illness and homelessness (Goering *et al.*, 2014). Five cities were involved: Vancouver, Winnipeg, Toronto, Montreal and Moncton. More than 2,000 participants were followed over two years in a pragmatic, randomized controlled study to identify "what works, at what cost, for whom, and in which environments" (Goering *et al.*, 2014, p. 6). Two specific support services were introduced:

1. For persons with high needs, Assertive Community Treatment (ACT)
2. For those with moderate needs, Intensive Case Management (ICM)

A qualitative component was included in order to better interpret the quantitative results (Goering *et al.*, 2014). The study examined quality of life, community resources, recovery and employment opportunities. *Housing First* was employed which "supports people who are homeless, living with mental illness by providing permanent housing with wrap-around supports" (Goering *et al.*, 2014, p. 10). The results of the study revealed that mental health and substance use problems improved which was attributed to housing along with accessibility of available services, although individual results were quite diverse. Housing stability, quality of life and community functioning outcomes were also quite positive (Goering *et al.*, 2014). This study clearly demonstrated that we can improve the life of the homeless who are mentally ill or addicted[1].

CNA Code of Ethic Part II: Ethical Endeavours Related to Broad Societal Issues

"Never doubt that a small group of thoughtful, committed citizens can change the world. Indeed it is the only thing that ever has." Margaret Mead, American Cultural Anthropologist.

The CNA (2017) Code of Ethics Part II proposes that nurses have a professional and ethical responsibility to promote health equity through action on the social determinants of health. **Health equity** refers to reasonable access and opportunity for all people to meet their health care requirements (CNA, 2010). *The CNA (2018) Position Statement on Social Determinants of Health* advises a shift from a biomedical approach to a biopsychosocial model, because a biopsychosocial model more fully reflects social determinants of health. Reutter and Kuschner (2010) propose that nurses are well positioned to get involved in policy initiatives that will improve living and working conditions such as promoting: a living wage; affordable housing; quality and affordable child care services; early childhood education; and social inclusion (Reutter & Kuschner, 2010; CNA, 2018). Part II of The CNA Code of Ethics (2017) advises that nurses individually and collectively advocate for, and work toward, eliminating social inequities by the following means. Box (**7:4**).

Box 7:4 The CNA Code of Ethics Part II: Ethical Endeavours Related to Broad Societal Issues (CNA, 2017, pp. 18 - 19).
1. Advocating for publicly administered health systems that ensure accessibility, universality, portability and comprehensiveness in necessary health-care services.
2. Utilizing the principles of primary health care for the benefit of the public and persons receiving care.
3. Recognizing and working to address organizational, social, economic and political factors that influence health and well-being within the context of nurses' roles in the delivery of care.
4. Advocating for a full continuum of accessible health-care services at the right time, in the right place, by the right provider. This continuum includes health promotion, disease prevention and diagnostic, restorative, rehabilitative and palliative care services in hospital, nursing homes, home care and the community.
5. Recognizing the significance of social determinants of health and advocating for policies and programs that address them (*e.g.*, safe housing, supervised consumption sites).
6. Maintaining an awareness of major health concerns, such as poverty, inadequate shelter, food insecurity and violence, while working for social justice (individually and with others) and advocating for laws, policies and procedures that bring about equity.
7. Working with people and advocating for expanding the range of available health-care choices.
8. Collaborating with other health-care team members and professional organizations to advocate for changes to unethical health and social policies, legislation and regulations.
9. Recognizing that vulnerable groups in society are systematically disadvantaged (which leads to diminished health and well-being) and advocating to improve their quality of life while taking action to overcome barriers to health care.
10. Promoting the participation of persons considered incapable in consenting to care in the health-related discussions and decisions that affect them (*e.g.*, minors, persons with impaired mental function).
11. Call on all levels of government to acknowledge the current state of Indigenous health in Canada and to implement health-care rights and take actions with Indigenous peoples to improve their health services (Truth & Reconciliation Commission (TRC), 2015).
12. Supporting environmental preservation and restoration while advocating for initiatives that reduce environmentally harmful practices in order to promote health and well-being.

13. Advocating for the discussion of ethical issues among health-care team members, persons receiving care and students, encouraging ethical reflection and working to develop their own and others' awareness of ethics in practice.
14. Maintaining awareness of broader global health concerns, such as violations of human rights, war, world hunger, gender inequities and environmental changes, and working and advocating (individually and with others) to bring about change locally and globally.
15. Advocating for excellence in palliative and end-of-life care for palliative care options that are available to all – at home, in long-term care, acute care and hospice care.
16. Becoming well-informed about laws (*e.g.*, safe contraception, medical assistance in dying) and advocating for and working with others to create policies and processes that provide ethical guidance to all nurses.

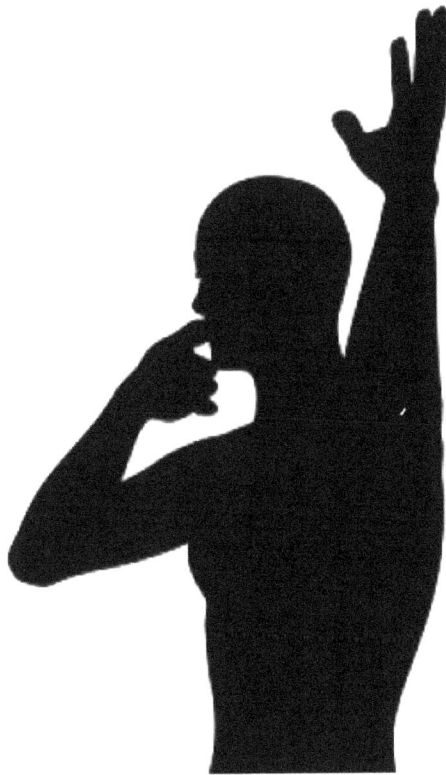

Fig. (7.5). Whistle-blowing. Source: www.pixabay.com

WHISTLE-BLOWING AS A LAST RESORT

Whistle-blowing is akin to blowing off a high-pitched whistle to draw attention to a situation (Fig. **7.5**) .The act of whistle blowing consists of reporting unethical or unsafe practice of a nurse or another health professional for incompetence, negligence or patient abuse (Burkhardt, Nathaniel & Walton, 2015; Oberle &

Bouchal, 2009). It is a drastic form of advocacy and must only be used as a last resort. In Box (**7:5**) nine specific actions are listed that a nurse should seriously consider before embarking on the act of whistle blowing.

Box 7:5 ACTIONS TO CONSIDER BEFORE WHISTLE-BLOWING (as adapted from Burkhardt et al., 2015).
1. Whistle-blowing should only be used when a person has unsuccessfully exhausted all other appropriate organizational channels to right the wrong. For example, the nurse must have already reported the problem, issue or event through proper channels in the organization.
2. The nurse who is considering whistle-blowing must be convinced or have evidence that the act of speaking out will likely result in positive or desired change.
3. There must be serious harm or potential harm to individuals or to the public.
4. Determine if you are ready, both personally and professionally, to act through personal reflection or consultation with others.
5. Consult with a member of your professional association or a lawyer for legal advice.
6. Collect evidence in the form of a paper trail where you record what you witnessed as compromised care. Pay attention to dates, times and outcomes. Keep a copy of all of the documentation, including electronic communication.
7. Remember when communicating by email that you do not make statements that may be attributed to you in the front page of a newspaper.
8. Build leadership skills and unity with your colleagues.
9. Develop a strong sense of ethical integrity in your nursing community. Find places to dialogue about issues of inequity or threats to others' integrity and care, as well as professionally safe venues for voicing nursing practice concerns.

The ensuring narrative is an example of when whistle-blowing became the only remaining action to ensure patient safety. Box (**7:6**).

HOW STEREOTYPICAL BIASES ACT AS AN IMPEDIMENT TO NURSING ADVOCACY

"I used to be afraid of people who suffer from mental illness. They scared me because I expected them to be violent. It wasn't until I did my mental health rotation in nursing, where I began to work closely with them, that I realized that they were just people like everyone else. I also learned that persons who suffer from a mental illness are more likely to be the victims of violence rather than the perpetrators." Douglas College Student Nurse.

If an individual nurse or group of nurses hold stereotypical biases toward marginalized populations, they will be unwilling or incapable of advocating on their behalf. There are many marginalized groups that nurses may hold a bias against: seniors, persons with a sexual orientation other than heterosexuality, people with religious beliefs that differ from one's own, street youth, sex trade workers, developmentally challenged persons, the addicted, the homeless, Indigenous peoples and those suffering from mental illness. For the purpose of brevity, we will primarily explore nurses' and other health care professionals' prejudicial biases toward Indigenous peoples and those suffering from mental illness.

Box 7:6 Narrative: When Whistle-Blowing Becomes Necessary
Samirah is an experienced emergency room (ER) nurse with an extensive critical care background. She recently changed jobs and works in a small community hospital. At this facility the Day Surgery Clinic operates alongside the ER and it is only staffed from 0700 – 1500 hours from Monday to Friday. After 1500 hours on weekdays, the ER nurses are expected to care for clients who are transferred from the Post-anesthesia Care Unit (PACU) to the Day Surgery area. The PACU is completely closed on weekends so when urgent surgery is performed patients are transferred directly to the Day Surgery area from the operating room (OR) without being recovered. Samirah strongly believes that this practice is unsafe and has made her views known to her supervisors. Oftentimes the ER gets quite busy so checking on post-operative patients in a timely manner is challenging. There have been many documented incidents when something untoward has occurred, like the time a patient fainted when she tried to get up to the bathroom on her own and a nurse did not discover her for over an hour. Administration has repeatedly refused to address the safety issues, citing increased costs for more staff. It is Saturday and another busy day in the ER. A 41-yea-old fresh post-operative patient, Mr. Brian, just underwent an urgent appendectomy, and has been transferred directly from the OR to the Day Surgery Clinic. Samirah is concerned so she stays with Mr. Brian for the first 40 minutes, places him on a cardiac monitor and sets the alarms. Mr. Brian's vital signs are fairly stable although he needs encouragement to take deep breaths and he keeps removing his oxygen mask. Samirah is called away to the trauma room to attend an urgent case. She pages the Nurse Supervisor and requests that someone come and watch Mr. Brian in her absence. She is informed that there is no nurse available. Samirah is working in the trauma room with another nurse and they are waiting for a physician to arrive. After a few minutes Samirah hears an alarm go off in the distance. She quickly realizes that the sound is coming from the Day Surgery area. She runs over to the unit to discover that Mr. Brian is unresponsive and making oral grunting noises. She looks up at the monitor and sees that he is in ventricular tachycardia. Samirah screams for help and pushes the emergency button. She proceeds to use the paddles from the crash cart to administer 300 joules of shock to the patient's chest but she must repeat this action three times before a normal sinus rhythm is restored. Mr. Brian regains consciousness once his heart rate is returned to normal. Samirah stays with her patient until Mr. Brian is transferred to a tertiary center for further tests and for constant surveillance in a Coronary Care Unit (CCU). That evening Samirah carefully documents all that has transpired and fills out a Patient Alert. She faxes the document to her nursing regulatory body and to a union representative. When Samirah returns to work after four days off she learns that the Day Surgery Clinic is closed until proper staffing levels can be arranged for evenings and weekends. Samirah's Manager expressed anger toward Samirah for the action she took, but Samirah knows that she did the right thing.

Biases Toward Indigenous Peoples

A study called *First Peoples, second class treatment: The role of racism in the health and well-being of Indigenous peoples in Canada,* was conducted by the Wellesley Institute (Allan & Smylie, 2015). The study results indicate that there is solid evidence of health disparities in people who are Indigenous when compared with those who are non-Indigenous. The research revealed that these disparities are rooted in colonial policies, like segregation and residential schools (Allan & Smylie, 2015). The study indicates that Indigenous peoples experience racism from health-care workers so frequently that they often strategize before they go the Emergency Room or they avoid seeking treatment all together. Such avoidance has resulted in delayed treatment for some, even those with cancer. For many others their presenting health complaints or concerns have been either ignored or dismissed solely because they are not Caucasian (Allan & Smylie, 2015). Stereotypical and hurtful attitudes include assuming all Indigenous persons abuse alcohol or drugs, that they are not worthy of the same care as others, and that they are wasting caregivers' time (Allan & Smylie, 2015).

Biases Toward Those Suffering from Mental Illness

Ross and Goldner (2009) conducted a comprehensive literature review of the stigma, negative attitudes and discrimination toward mental illness within the profession of nursing. Their findings are cause for concern, some of which are summarized in Box (**7:7**).

Nurses, Sigma, Negative Attitudes & Discrimination Toward the Mentally Ill (as adapted from Ross & Goldner, 2009).
* Surveys consistently revealed that patients who presented to hospital with mental illness, felt that they had been treated with a lack of dignity and caring.
* Stigma also appeared to be a barrier to caring treatment even when a patient's primary reason for admission was not related to their psychiatric illness.
* Even though nurses stated that they believed that mental health patients' care was an important component of holistic patient care, negative attitudes were still found to be evident towards these people and toward psychiatry in general.
* Large numbers of nurses appear to share the general population's stereotypical beliefs that persons who suffer from mental illness are dangerous, unpredictable, violent and bizarre.
* Many nurses self-identified that they lacked the skills to confidently and competently manage mental health patients' behavioural symptoms, and they linked this knowledge gap to their fear of the patients.
* Many general nurses hold beliefs that mental illness is caused by factors such as weakness or morals, character or will, laziness, malingering, and a lack of discipline and control.
* Serious gaps were noted in general nurses' clinical knowledge about suicide. Para-suicidal gesturing or self-harming was also viewed judgmentally by nurses.
* Nurses exhibited judgmental attitudes towards other nurses who suffer from mental illness and their negative opinions were not only directed at colleagues but self-directed as well.

Changing Negative Stigma with Cultural Safety & Affirmative Action

Cultural Safety & Indigenous Peoples

Cultural safety is one of several helpful strategies that can be implemented to help to change the negative stereotypes held by nurses and others in the health care setting, especially toward Indigenous Peoples. **Cultural safety** promotes respectful engagement and strives to address the power imbalances inherent in the health care system by cultivating an environment that is free of racism and discrimination (Allan & Smylie, 2015). For example, Allan & Smylie (2015) recommend cultural safety training for non-Indigenous health-care workers, that we employ more Indigenous health-care workers, and that we provide Sacred Spaces where traditional healing can be incorporated into care. Thorne (2018) as cited in De Souza (2019) quite poignantly and powerfully speaks to the importance of advocacy in relationship to cultural safety. Box (**7:8**).

Box 7:8 Nursing Advocacy & Cultural Safety (Thorne, 2018)
As an advocacy profession, we could collectively make such a wonderful contribution if we prioritized (cultural safety) as a major strategic direction. Nursing should be on the side of transformational change within our societies and our health-care systems. We ought to become as skilled at detecting an infringement of cultural safety as we are with infection control or careful monitoring of clinical signs. But achieving that level of skill in matters of cultural bias would require that we embark and nurture a shared recognition of why it matters. It would require an understanding that we all - not merely the designated advocates for whom this may be a special interest – have an essential role to play. And it would require that we begin to consider effective professional communication skills and working respectfully across difference as fundamental and essential attributes for which each and every member of the nursing profession ought to be held accountable.

Affirmative Action & Those Who Suffer from Mental Illness

Affirmative action is another strategy that can be implemented to help to change the negative stereotypes held by nurses, especially toward people suffering from mental illness. **Affirmative action** consists of an active effort to improve the employment or education of members of a known minority group (Merriam-Webster Dictionary, n.d.). Nurses need to become educated about what it is like to suffer from a mental illness in order to develop empathy and compassion. The evidence indicates that nurses who do become familiar with the lived experiences of people who are suffering from a mental illness and other minorities are more likely to develop positive attitudes toward them (Ross & Goldner, 2009). Familiarity can also occur through assertive action by the nursing profession to minimize the stigma and discrimination. It would a good idea for nurse leaders, including administrators and educators, to include a candid discussion of these issues in their education curriculum (Ross & Goldner, 2009). Box (**7:9**).

BOX 7:9 LEARNING ACTIVITY: CHANGING NEGATIVE STEREOTYPES
In addition to the already suggested strategies to end nurses' discrimination toward vulnerable populations, what other techniques can you suggest to positively change existing negative attitudes?.

Nursing Advocacy & The Risk of Being Morally Silenced

"If we want people to show up, to bring their whole selves including their unarmored, whole hearts – so that we can innovate, solve problems, and serve people – we have to be vigilant about creating a culture in which people feel safe, seen, heard, and respected." From Dr. Brene Brown's Book, *Dare to Lead: Daring Greatly & Rising Strong at Work*

The act of advocacy can sometimes negatively impact the nurse who dares to do what they know in their heart is right. A very real threat to the nurse advocate is that of being morally silenced by colleagues, other members of the health care team or administration. **Moral silence** occurs when the ability to voice your moral convictions is stifled (Bird, 2002). According to Bird (2002) moral silencing occurs in two keyways. The first is in the form of a personal attack upon the individual's integrity. The second is by instilling fear in the person who would like to speak up, but because they are afraid of losing their job or being punished in the work setting, they remain quiet. Subsequently, persons who cannot defend their ideals and feel pressured to be quiet often cave into the pressure. However, there are worse consequences, emotionally and psychologically to succumbing to the pressure of being morally silenced. To retreat and pull back will eventually lead to self-loathing, sadness and even depression which is anger turned inward. Other risks include developing **moral residue** which is deep feelings of guilt and remorse because you are unable to act on your personal moral beliefs. Therefore, I would encourage nurses to be as courageous as possible. However, before taking action, make sure that you get the support that you need from like-minded colleagues, your professional association (*e.g.*, the CNA) or your regulatory body. You are not meant to do this alone.

Questions Pertaining to the Case in Point:

1. How can a person be labelled with a mental disorder when they haven't even been properly assessed due to a language barrier?
2. Do you think this happens in practice and what can be done to prevent it from happening again?
3. If Inderpreet had not intervened and properly assessed Mrs. Gill, what do you think would have happened to her?

BOX 7:10 CASE IN POINT: WHEN A STUDENT NURSE CHOOSES TO BE THE VOICE FOR HER CLIENT

Inderpreet is a newly graduated Registered Psychiatric Nurse (RPN). She has just been hired to work in Adult Psychiatry at a local hospital. She arrived to work on Monday morning and learned in report that a 44 year-old South Asian woman, Mrs. Gill, had been admitted with depression five days ago, after a neighbor heard her crying excessively through the walls of her apartment. Mrs. Gill does not speak English, but no one had arranged for an interpreter to help with assessment. Inderpreet wondered how a definitive diagnosis could be made or appropriate treatment planned, without ever hearing Mrs. Gill's story. Inderpreet subsequently offered to interview Mrs. Gill in their native language of Punjabi. During the interview Mrs. Gill began to cry when she told Inderpreet that her only son was killed in a serious car accident 10 days ago and that she hasn't been herself since then. She admits that she has been crying and feeling alone but she is still eating and sleeping and she has made arrangements to return to India to be with her family. Mrs. Gill was in Canada to help her son while he attended University. She tells Inderpreet that she doesn't know why she is in hospital and that she is really worried about not being able to get out of hospital in time to make her scheduled trip back home. (Note: Mrs. Gill has no close relatives in Canada and her husband lives in India). After performing a full Mental Status Examination (MSE) [2] Inderpreet took the initiative to convey all that she learned to the whole mental health team. Mrs. Gills' diagnosis was changed to acute grief reaction and the plan of care altered accordingly. Mrs. Gill was discharged and referred to a support group in the Indo-Canadian community for help with her grief.

REFLECTING BACK

Summary of Key Points Covered in Chapter 7

- Nursing advocacy was defined as acting on behalf of others.
- Two key avenues for advocacy were presented, acting on behalf of an individual or in support of a larger cause.
- Nurses are expected to take the lead to preserve public access to health care for all people living in Canada.
- Social justice emphasizes the relative position of specific groups in relationship to others in society and strives for increased equality.
- Social justice is supported by the ethic of justice and ethic of care because they have the mutual goal of creating a society with fewer inequalities.
- Poverty is a world-wide problem that has been growing instead of subsiding and has a negative effect on people's lives.
- Homelessness is on the increase in Canada.
- The perception is that it is too expensive to provide housing and treatment for people who are homeless and suffer from addictions and or mental illness. Yet this is not supported by fact.
- Health equity refers to reasonable access and opportunity for all people to meet their health care requirements.
- Sixteen specific strategies were recommended by the CNA Code of Ethics Part II for nurses to employ, either individually or collectively, to end social inequities.

- Whistle blowing is a more drastic form of advocacy and should only be used as a last resort and when all other avenues of advocacy have been exhausted.
- Before participating in the act of whistle-blowing the nurse must have already reported the problem through the appropriate channels. They must be convinced or have evidence that the act of speaking out will likely result in the desired change. There must also be serious harm or potential harm to individuals or to the public.
- The literature provides evidence that nurses, and other health professionals, harbor stereotypical biases toward Indigenous peoples and the mentally ill.
- Cultural safety and taking affirmative action were recommended strategies to combat biases.
- The greatest threat to the nurse who dares to do what they know in their heart is right is that of being morally silenced. Nurses were encouraged to be as courageous as possible but to ensure that they are well supported.

SOMETHING TO PONDER

1. Currently some services in our Canadian health delivery are not funded. Should all health services be covered by the system? If not, what services would you exclude and why?
2. What can be done to ensure that people who live in remote communities have equitable access to health care?
3. If it costs more for people with severe addictions and/or mental illness to remain homeless than it does to provide them with housing and treatment, why isn't more being done and faster?
4. In addition to what was mentioned in this Chapter, what else do you think can be done to decrease the negative attitudes and discrimination toward Indigenous peoples and the mentally ill that exists within the profession of nursing?
5. Does the notion of being morally silenced for standing up for what you believe is right scare you? If yes, what do you think can be done to stop activity in the workplace that causes and/or perpetrates the act of moral silencing?

CLASSROOM GROUP EXERCISES

1. In a small group or as a class discuss whether you believe that health care is a right or a privilege?
2. Break into groups of four or five. Come up with an exhaustive list of persons or groups that need assistance in the form of nursing advocacy. Spend some time thinking seriously about how you might begin to help at least one marginalized population on your list, then create a plan.

ON YOUR OWN

1. Make a concerted effort to connect with like-minded people in your community in order to work toward improving the lives of those who are struggling. Remind yourself that no action is too small to be of help.

Recommended Readings

Fortier, J., & Douglas, J. (March 2012). Advocacy inside the maze. *Canadian Nurse*. Retrieved from: https://canadian-nurse.com/en/articles/issues/2012/march-2012/advocacy-inside-the-maze

Gaetz, S., Gulliver, T., & Richter, T. (2014). *The state of homelessness in Canada: 2014*. Toronto: The Homelessness Hub Press. Retrieved from: https://homelesshub. ca/sites/default/files/attachments/SOHC2014.pdf

Goering, P., Veldhuizen, S., Watson, A., Adair, C., Kopp, B., Latimer, I., Nelson, G., MacNaughton, E., Streiner, D., & Aubry, T. (2014). *At home/Chez Soi finalreport cross-site*. Alberta: Mental Health Commission of Canada (MHCC). Retrieved from: https://www.mentalhealthcommission.ca/English

Greenwood, M., de Leeuw, S., Lindsay, N. M., & Reading, C. (2015). *Determinants ofIndigenous peoples' health in Canada: Beyond the social*. Toronto: Canadian Scholar's Press.

Truth & Reconciliation Commission of Canada: Call to Action. (2017). Retrieved from: http://trc.ca/assets/pdf/Calls_to_Action_English2.pdf

Web Resources

Web Resource: YouTube Video: Health Care: U.S. *versus* Canada https://www. youtube.com/watch?v=iYOf6hXGx6M

Web Resource: The CNA Policy on Advocacy https://cna-aiic.ca/policy-advocacy

Web Resource: Class Activity: Social Advocacy Exercises by Melanie McFadyen https://community.macmillan.com/docs/DOC-9051-class-activity-social-advocacy-exercises

CONSENT FOR PUBLICATION

Not applicable.

CONFLICT OF INTEREST

The authors confirm that this chapter contents have no conflict of interest.

ACKNOWLEDGEMENTS

Declared none.

NOTES

[1] Note: For a complete report on the *At Home /Chez Soi* study, refer to the recommended reading list at the end of this Chapter.

[2] Note: A Mental Status Examination (MSE) is a standardized way of assessing a person's present mental capacity. The examiner seeks to gain an understanding of the following categories of information: general behaviour; appearance and attitude; characteristics of speech; emotional state; content of thought like special preoccupations; suicidal or homicidal ideation; hallucinations; delusions; orientation and memory (Trigoboff & Ren Kneisl, 2009).

REFERENCES

Affirmative action. (n.d.). *Merriam Webster Dictionary.*https://www.merriam-webster.com/dictionary/affirmative%20action

Allan, B & Smylie, J (2015) *First Peoples, second class treatment: The role of racism in the health and well-being of Indigenous peoples in Canada.*The Wellesley Institute, Toronto, Ontario.http://www.wellesleyinstitute.com/wp-content/uploads/2015/02/Summary-First-Peoples-Second-Class-Treatment-Final.pdf

Alini, E (2010) Everyone's a critic. *Macleans Magazine, 123,* 100-1.

Bird, FB (2002) *The muted conscience, moral silence and the practice of ethics in business.*Quorum Books, USA.

Brown, L & Taylor, D (2012) The birth of medicare: From Saskatchewan to Canada-wide coverage. *Can Dimens, 46*https://canadiandimension.com/articles/view/the-birth-of-medicare

Burkhardt, MA, Nathaniel, AK & Walton, NA (2015) *Ethics and issues in contemporary nursing* Nelson Education Limited, Toronto, Ontario.

Canadian Nurses Association (CNA) (2008) *Toward 2020: Visions for Nursing.*Author, Ottawa.

Canadian Nurses Association (CNA) (2010) *Social justice, a means to an end in itself* Author, Ottawa.

Canadian Nurses Association (CNA) (2012) *A nursing call to action: The health of our nation, the future of our health system.*Author, Ottawa.https://www.cna-aiic.ca/~/media/cna/files/en/nec_report_e.pdf

Canadian Nurses Association (CNA) (2017) *CNA Code of Ethics for Registered Nurses.*Author, Ottawa.

Canadian Nurses Association (CNA) (2018) *Social determinant of health position statement.* https://www.cna-aiic.ca/-/media/cna/page-content/pdf-en/social-determinants-of-health-position-statement_dec-2018.pdf?la=en&hash=CCD26634EF89E493DA64F60345A3AAB399089797

Canadian Public Health Association (CPHA) (2015) *Homelessness and public health* https://www.cpha.ca/homelessness-and-public-health

Citizens for Public Justice. (2019) *Poverty trends 2017.* Retrieved from: https://www.cpj.ca/poverty-trend--2017

De Souza, R (@DeSouzaRN). (April 21, 2019). Sally Thorne # Cultural Safety. RETWEET. Retrieved from: https://twitter.com/desouzarn?lang=en

DeWolf Bosek, M S & Savage, T A (2007) *The ethical component of nursing education: Integrating ethics into clinical experience.*Lippincott Williams & Wilkins., New York.

Gaetz, S, Gulliver, T & Richter, T (2014) *The state of homelessness in Canada.*The Homelessness Hub Press, Toronto.https://homelesshub.ca/sites/default/files/attachments/SOHC2014.pdf

Gilligan, C (1982) *In a different voice: Psychological theory and women's development.*MA: Harvard University Press, Cambridge.

Goering, P, Veldhuizen, S, Watson, A, Adair, C, Kopp, B, Latimer, I & Nelson, G (2014) *At home/Chez Soi final report cross-site.* Mental Health Commission of Canada (MHCC), Alberta. https://www. mentalhealthcommission.ca/English

Government of Canada (2018) *Social determinants of health and health inequalities* https://www. canada.ca/en/public-health/services/health-promotion/population-health/what-determines-health.html

McDonald, L (2010) *Florence Nightingale at first hand.*Wilfred Laurier, Canada.

Patterson, M, Somers, J M, McIntosh, K, Shiell, A & Franklin, C J (2008) *Housing and support for adults with severe addictions and/or mental illness in British Columbia.*Simon Fraser University, Burnaby, BC: Centre for Applied Research in Mental Health and Addictions (CARMHA).

Reutter, L & Kushner, KE (2010) 'Health equity through action on the social determinants of health': Taking up the challenge in nursing. *Nurs Inq,* 17, 269-80.
[http://dx.doi.org/10.1111/j.1440-1800.2010.00500.x] [PMID: 20712665]

Ross, CA & Goldner, EM (2009) Stigma, negative attitudes and discrimination towards mental illness within the nursing profession: A review of the literature. *J Psychiatr Ment Health Nurs,* 16, 558-67.
[http://dx.doi.org/10.1111/j.1365-2850.2009.01399.x] [PMID: 19594679]

Salzberg, S (2004) *Lovingkindness: The revolutionary art of happiness.* London: Shambala.

Samphir, H (2017) Resist the silent war on Canadian Medicare. *Canadian Dimension* https://canadiandimension.com/articles/view/resist-the-silent-war-on-canadian-medicare

Street, P (2017) The empire has no clothes. *Canadian Dimension* https://canadiandimension.com/articles/view/the-empire-has-no-clothes

The Conference Board of Canada. *Principles of sustainable health care* https://www.conferenceboard.ca/CASHC/principles.aspx?AspxAutoDetectCookieSupport=1

Trigoboff, E & Ren Kneisl, C (2009) Assessing.*Contemporary psychiatric-mental health nursing* Pearson Prentice Hall, New Jersey 215-34.

Truth and Reconciliation Commission of Canada (TRC) (2015) *Honouring the truth, reconciling for the future Summary of the final report of the Truth and Reconciliation c Commission* http://www.chaireconditionautochtone.fss.ulaval.ca/documents/pdf/Honouring-the-truth- reconciling-for-the-future.pdf

Watson, J (2008) *Nursing: The philosophy of caring (Revised edition).*University Press of Colorado, Boulder, Colorado.

World Health Organization (WHO) (2018) *Social determinants of health.*Retrieved. https://www.who.int/social_determinants/en/

In an Age of Technological Advancements: Ensuring that Caring Remains in Practice

Abstract: Chapter Eight explores how technological advances enhance healthcare delivery but also create new challenges for nurses. Caring as technology refers to the meaning of health care delivery in relationship to technology. Many benefits of technology in health care include, expediency of care delivery, improving the working conditions of nurses, safer learning opportunities for student nurses, and decreased overall costs for health care. There are also some draw backs such as, a decrease in direct communication, a negative impact on relational practice, an increased risk of privacy violations and the loss of nursing jobs. It was pointed out that, in modern health practices the nurturing aspects of caring for the ill or aged is increasingly viewed by some institutional bodies as less important than other more mechanistic aspects of service. Modern advances of science have also somewhat blurred the boundaries of when life begins and when it ends. Nursing the dying person can be difficult for nurses. No matter how many future changes occur the challenge to the profession of nursing is not to lose the capacity to care. Mindfulness was recommended as a tool to help nurses to connect with their clients in a caring way. In the Case in Point a distraught family member shares her story of how it felt to be left in the dark about the imminent death of her loved one.

Keywords: Affirmation, Caring as technology, Futility, Morbidity, Mortality, Mindful listening, Robots, Simulation, Virtual reality.

LEARNING GUIDE

After Completing this Chapter, the Reader Should be Able to

- Define caring as technology.
- Be aware that although technological advances have improved many aspects of health care delivery it has also created new challenges.
- Understand how modern advances of science have also somewhat blurred the boundaries of when life begins and when it ends.
- Recognize that nursing the dying person can often be difficult for nurses.
- Appreciate that no matter how many future changes occur the challenge to the profession of nursing is not to lose the capacity to care.

- Explain the value of mindful listening and how to use it to connect with clients in a caring way.
- Apply what was learned to the Case in Point: When the family feels that they have been left in the dark.

"It is ironic that nursing education and practice require so much knowledge and skill to do the job, but very little effort is directed toward developing how to 'Be' while doing the real work of the job." Jean Watson, American Nurse, Author, Professor & Care Theorist

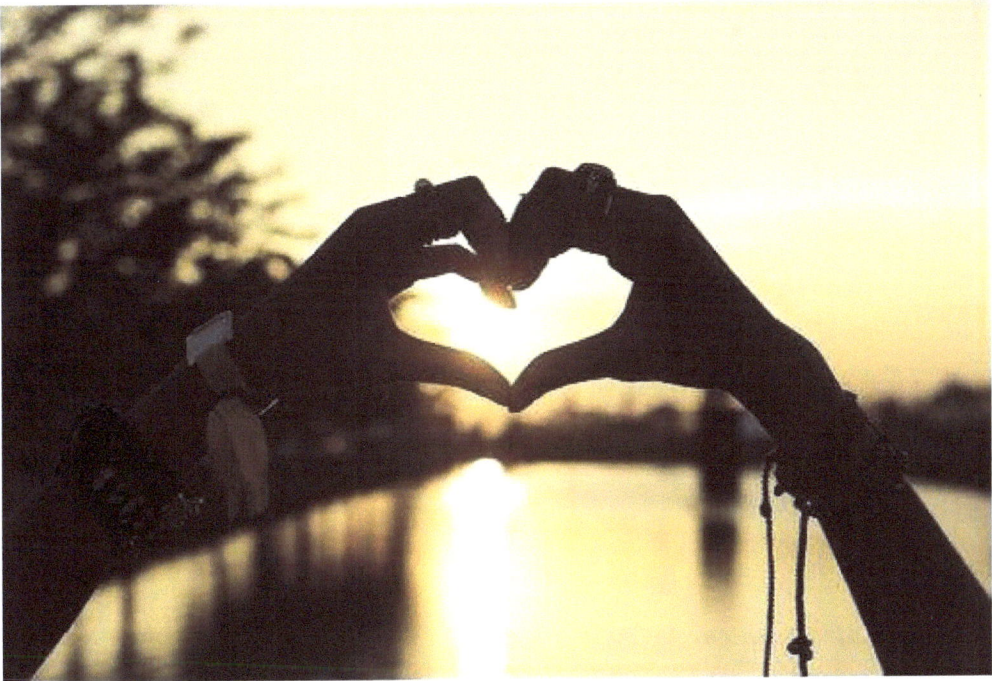

Fig. (8.1). Caring. Source: www.pixabay.com

Caring as technology refers to caring in relationship to technology and such things as virtual reality, machines that support life and robots. Chapter Eight points out that, although technological advances can enhance healthcare delivery, it can also create new challenges for nurses. In modern health practices the nurturing aspects of caring for the ill or aged is increasingly viewed by some institutional bodies as less important than other more mechanistic aspects of service. Furthermore, advances of science have somewhat blurred the boundaries of when life begins and when it ends. Subsequently, nursing the dying person can often be difficult for nurses. No matter how many changes occur in the future, the challenge to the profession of nursing is not to lose the capacity to care. A way to focus on the needs of our clients in a caring way is through the art of mindful listening. The Case in Point shares a heart wrenching story as told by a family member, who felt devastated that they were not informed that their loved one was dying. Nurses are challenged to explore ways in which this situation could have been handled in a more compassionate manner.

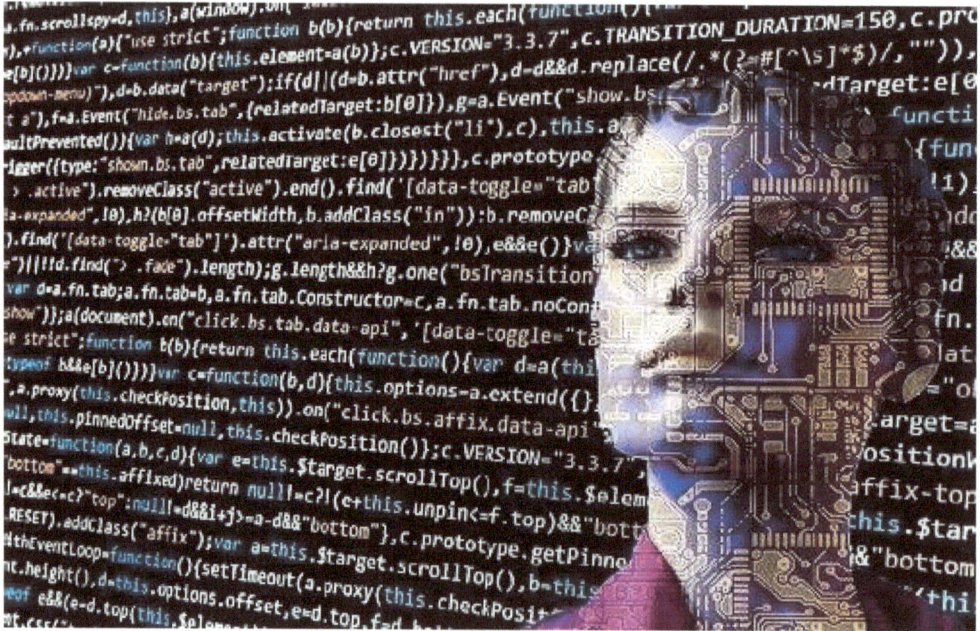

Fig. (8.2). Artificial Intelligence & Robotics. Source: www.pixabay.com

TECHNOLOGICAL ADVANCES IN HEALTHCARE: HOW IT IS CHANGING THE WAY THAT WE NURSE

The Benefits

There are many benefits to making use of technological advancements in health care such as, the ability to instantly access electronic records; global positioning systems' (GPS) tracking of medical equipment; and enhanced access to diagnostic tests in real time (Gionet, 2017; Elrick, 2017). Work is made easier for nurses by the use of electronic lifts to move clients, and by robots who can do a great deal of the manual labor formerly only performed by nurses (Wirkus, 2017). Costs for health care delivery are decreased because less nurses are needed to do the work, and nurses' salaries are one of the biggest expenditures of providing direct client care (Rouleau, Gagnon & Cote, 2015).

Nursing informatics in the form of laboratory simulation has become prevalent in schools of nursing and has enhanced student learning while reducing the risk of injury to patients. For example, simulation allows students to learn in real time and to make errors without harming an actual patient (Gionet, 2017). Similarly, student nurses' access virtual reality case studies by computer that very accurately depict situations that can occur in the hospital setting (Rouleau *et al.*, 2015). The artificial intelligence associated with virtual reality is even able to track the level of learning and knowledge gaps of the individual accessing the program.

The Disadvantages

Even though there are many advantages to the use of technology in practice, there are also some drawbacks. Technology is very much jeopardizing the way in which nurses have traditionally provided care to their clients. For example, Elrick (2017) points out that, direct communication between caregivers suffers. There is a decrease in nurse to client and nurse to family contact, especially as the use of robots for direct patient care increases (SreeRaja, 2018). This decrease in direct contact impacts relational practice and a nurse's connection to those in their care. Privacy violations are often threatened because of easy computer access and security breaches. Nurses are also in danger of losing some of their jobs, especially when robots can replace them at a reduced cost (SreeRaja, 2018).

When Care is Deemed Less Crucial Than Efficiency

"The dominant approach separates fact from value and meaning, separates subject from object, focuses on value free intellectual, factual, technical education and pedagogies to the exclusion of the intentional, the relational, the intersubjectivity, the care contextual, the evolving, growing human consciousness." Olivia Bevis & Jean Watson, Authors of *Toward a Caring Curriculum: A New Pedagogy for Nursing.*

In Current times caring practice is being viewed as less crucial by some nurses than efficiency, and that can negatively impact the relationship between nurse and client (Ray, 2016). For example, many nurses see a clear relationship between morality and practice when they are personally attending to patients with direct hands-on care that previously constituted much of nursing, but when engaged in complicated technological care, they find it difficult to recognize or feel the moral sense in that care (Ray, 2016). This is especially true in technical activities that require giving more attention to technique than to the patient (Watson, 2008; Barnard & Locsin, 2007). When nursing students seem to be more concerned with knowing the routine of the ward and getting things done than they are with client needs, I become concerned. Ward, Cody, Schaal and Hojat, (2012) point out that, over emphasizing technology, scientific knowledge and computers as a priority, in conjunction with de-emphasizing the art of caring, can contribute to student nurses becoming good technicians but not caring compassionate ones.

Caring for the Ill or Aged is Viewed as Less Important

There is also some evidence to indicate that in modern health practices the nurturing aspect of caring for the ill or aged is increasingly viewed by institutional bodies as less important than other more mechanistic aspects of service (Ray, 2016). In fact, robots are now being used globally in nursing care (Carter-Templeton, Frasier, Wu & Wyatt, 2018). They are being utilized to combat loneliness in the elderly population and with those suffering from dementia (SreeRaja, 2018). However, Harrington (2018) stresses that robots are not always able to perform nursing tasks in the same caring way that humans do. There is also lack of research being conducted to assess how the lonely and aged feel about being cared for by a machine rather than a human being (Carter-Templeton *et al.*, 2018; Harrington, 2018). The question is posed, should robots be allowed to replace nurses? Box (**8:1**).

BOX 8:1 LEARNING ACTIVITY: SHOULD ROBOTS REPLACE NURSES? (as adapted from SreeRaja, 2018; Carter-Templeton *et al.,* 2018; Harrington, 2018)
Robots are being utilized to control loneliness in the elderly population and with those suffering from dementia. There is also lack of research being conducted to assess how the lonely and aged feel about being cared for by a machine rather than a human being. 1. Discuss whether robots should be allowed to replace nurses. Why or why not? 2. Which activities are permissible for robots to take over and which ones should only be conducted by humans?   1. Discuss whether robots should be allowed to replace nurses. Why or why not?   2. Which activities are permissible for robots to take over and which ones should only be conducted by humans?

HOW MODERN SCIENCE SOMETIMES BLURS THE BOUNDARIES BETWEEN LIFE & DEATH

Caring for Premature Babies

Modern advances of science have somewhat blurred the boundaries of when life begins and when it ends (Burkhardt, Nathaniel & Walton, 2015). Newborn infants can now survive at earlier gestational stages. In the not so distant past this would not have been possible. Yet in the past few decades the survival of premature and low-birth newborns has improved significantly due to technological and therapeutic advances (Keatings & Smith, 2016). Infants as young as < 24 weeks of gestation can be kept alive but not without the potential for complications (Green, Darbyshire, Adams, & Jackson, 2014). Congenital heart disease, genetic anomalies and neonatal bowel obstruction are but a few of the long list of potential difficulties (Keatings & Smith, 2016). Even though infant mortality rates have decreased, infant morbidity has increased. **Mortality** consists of the relative frequency of deaths in a specific population. **Morbidity** refers to the types of health challenges in a particular group. The highest morbidity for these premature newborns is directly correlated with the amount of time spent in the Neonatal Intensive Care Unit (NICU) (Keatings & Smith, 2016) (Fig. **8.3**). For instance, the number of extremely premature infants in the NICU is going up and Neonatal nurses are finding the experience very challenging (Green *et al.*, 2014).

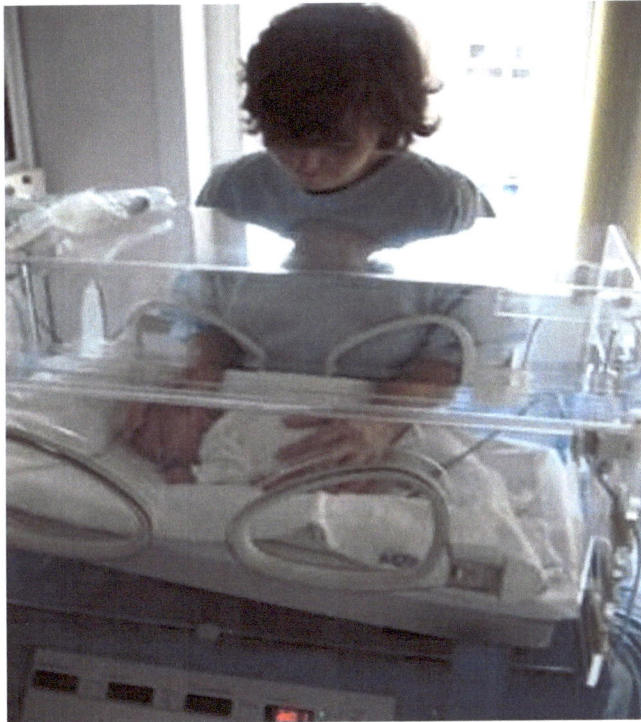

Fig. (8.3). Premature Baby. Source: www.pixabay.com

Futility & Trying to Save them All

The moral anguish that is associated with caring for the dying newborn is seldom reported due to the health care team giving up too soon. Rather, what is portrayed as most disturbing is the overuse of technology to try and save a life that can't be saved (Green *et al.*, 2014). Many of the Neonatal nurses who care for extremely premature newborns find some of the interventions to be futile, although they are not always open about it (Green *et al.*, 2016). **Futility** is concerned with carrying out treatment that is destined to fail to sustain life or is instigated when the prognosis for recovery is hopeless. Two examples of futility in health practice include, the overuse of technology to try and save a premature baby when it is evident that the child's life cannot be saved and performing CPR on someone suffering from the end stages of a terminal illness.

However, some research findings indicate that there is a benefit associated with carrying out futile efforts when death of an infant or other type of patients is forthcoming. For instance, those efforts may help the new parents or other family members with a bit more time to process the fact that their loved one is dying (Mohammed & Peter, 2009).

When a Cure is No Longer Possible: Caring for the Terminally Ill

The notion of death as a real possibility is not only troubling for the client and their family, it is also difficult for many care givers. Death may be viewed by some health professionals as something to be avoided because it is distressful (Kuhl, 2003). Subsequently, caregivers may sometimes avoid spending time with the terminally ill person, exactly when the patient is petrified with fear and so badly in need of personal attention. Clients may even feel abandoned by their doctor (Kuhl, 2003). The neglect does not necessarily surface in the form of not attending to the person's physical necessities, but usually takes on the form of subtly negating the client's emotional and spiritual needs (Siegel, 1989; Kuhl, 2003). Yet, as health care providers, one of the greatest gifts you can give others in these trying circumstances is your presence and care. The following story demonstrates the stark reality that often the nurse is the only person left to deal with the emotional anguish of a family who has just experienced the death of a loved one. Box (**8:2**).

BOX 8:2 Narrative: When a Nurse is Left to Deal with the Family's Anguish
After a trying repeat occurrence at work, Annie decided to resign from her valued critical care position to work on another unit and she had her reasons. Twice in one week the cardiac surgeon urgently transferred a client from the operating Room (OR) to the Critical Care Unit (CCU) unit because the surgery was unsuccessful, and death was forthcoming. After several requests for the cardiac surgeon to remain in the CCU so he could speak with the family, he refused. When Annie questioned him as to why he was in so much of a hurry to leave, his reply was, *"I have other lives to save and no patient dies under my direct care."* Annie was left to deal with both families' emotional anguish and outbursts

Why Caregivers Disconnect with the Dying

Discomfort with death and dying is not the only reason why caregivers may emotionally abandon their clients. Kuhl (2003) points out that most doctors do not intend to neglect their patient's emotional distress. They actually want to help. They sometimes shy away from emotionally connecting with patients because of a lack of communication skills, the doctor's own psychological issues, demands on their time, or a sense that they have somehow failed their patient by not making them well (Kuhl, 2003; Siegel, 1993). Doctors are not the only ones who have trouble dealing with the dying patient. Nurses also experience difficulty dealing with death. The following story as told by a physician, surgeon and well-known author, conveys this stark and poignant reality. Box (**8:3**).

BOX 8:3 Narrative: When Nurses Avoid Dealing with a Patient's Death (Siegel, 1993, pp. 210 – 211)

It's amazing how seldom members of the hospital staff visit patients who are close to death. If you shut the door, no one comes in. I was at a meeting when I received a call from Muriel, a young woman also unable to breathe and near death from extensive cancer. She told me, *"You say dying is easy. I looked up at the sky and said, I'm ready, and nothing happened."* So, I explained, *"It's because you're too agitated. I can't get there until five o'clock, but then I'll come and help you."* When I came in, she was filled with fear and anger, and been given no sedation. I tried to tell her that it is hard to die angry and fearful. You have to let go. Then I asked for some morphine, enough to calm her and ease her pain. Because of Muriel's youth, this was a frightening scene for the nurses. They had to be thinking, this could be one of us in that bed. Only a brave medical student was there besides me and the patient's family. After the morphine took effect, her breathing became easier and we had a wonderful couple of hours, filled with love and laughter. She literally came alive again. By seven o'clock Muriel looked so much better that I thought maybe she was changing her mind. I asked her, *"Do you mind if I go get some dinner?"* She said no. I came back in half an hour, and she had died. The nurses had announced that she had died, but when I walked into the room, Muriel's eyes were still open, the intravenous pump was still running and everything else was connected, as though she were still alive. The nurses had difficulty dealing with her death.

COMING TO TERMS WITH DEATH & DYING IN OUR PRACTICE

"Rainbows are relatively rare occurrences since, in order to see one, both precipitation and sunshine must share the same space in the sky at the same time. To this day, the sight of one still astonishes me." Michael Levine, Author

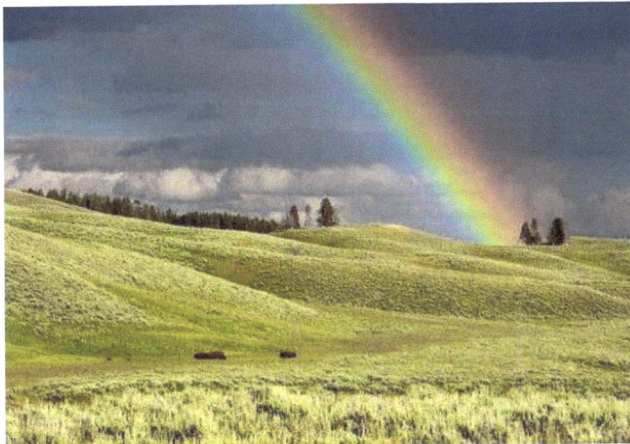

Fig. (8.4). Rainbow. Source: www.pixabay.com

The Circle of Life

Dealing with death and dying is a part of what nurses do but that does not mean it is easy. Yet, we can only help others through grief and loss associated with death, if we ourselves are able to make peace with the concept of taking care of the dying person. One way to cope with death is to learn to view death as an integral part of life. When we try to understand both the frailty and wonder of all of life, we are more likely to come to terms with the possibility that we are part of something else other than what exists in the physical realm (Watson, 2008). Some refer to this entity as God, the life force, the circle of life or universal energy. It does not matter what you call it, or if you prefer not to believe in anything outside of physical reality. What matters is that you are able to deal sufficiently with death so that you do not abandon or avoid caring for the dying client or their loved ones in their time of need.

Understand that Every Life Has Meaning

Miller-Tiedeman (1999), advises that we think of each and every person as having unique gifts and a purpose for their life and that their life has meaning. She tells us to remember that we have a unique purpose for coming into this world and that when we die we leave an imprint of what we have created behind, which includes how we have served others. Miller-Tiedeman believes that in this way we will be better equipped to deal with the loss of life that is so very much a part of our work as nurses. Salzberg (2004) so poignantly points out that, even if we do not know what to do or say to make things better for those who are experiencing loss or are about to pass away, we cannot fail if our intention is to be fully present, and to act with lovingkindness, empathy and care.

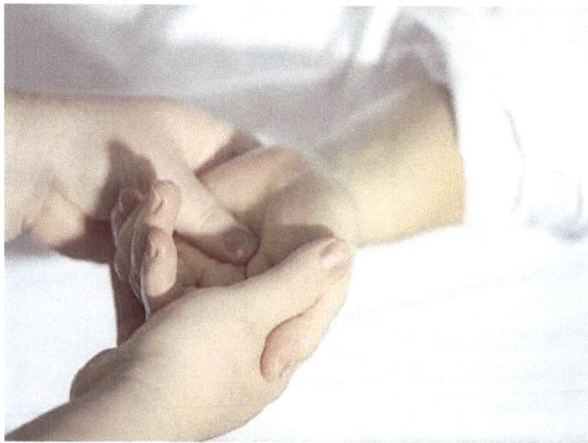

Fig. (8.5). Our capacity to Care. Source: www.pixabay.com

HOW NOT TO LOSE OUR CAPACITY TO CARE: THE GIFT OF MINDFUL LISTENING

"A great attraction of care ethics, I think is its refusal to encode or construct a catalog of principles and rules. One who cares must meet the cared for just as he or she is, as a whole human being with individual needs and interests. At most it directs us to attend, to listen, to respond as positively as possible." Nel Noddings, American Feminist, Educationalist & Philosopher.

No matter how many changes occur in the future, the challenge to the profession of nursing is not to lose the capacity to care. It is our ability to connect with our clients, to listen to their concerns, to allow them to tell their story and to share what they fear the most, that makes nursing rewarding. The person who is living through the experience is as important as the treatment, prognosis or outcome. Therefore, despite our frenzied schedules, computer work, and excessive demands on our time, it is still feasible to prioritize the needs of our clients (Shafir, 2008). A way to focus on the needs of suffering clients is through the art of mindful listening. Mindful listening is caring at its best because it puts the goal of human connection and understanding above everything else (Walker, 2010). **Mindful listening** refers to actively listening to what is being said and to the overall theme of what is shared. It is concerned with holding time still and listening from the heart (Shafir, 2008; Schmidt, 2002). Why is mindful listening important? Mayerhoff (1971) explains that when we want to genuinely demonstrate that we care for a person we must know many things. We need to know who the person is, what their strengths and weaknesses are, what do they really need in this very moment, in order to know how best to help them. We must not be tempted to end the silence and offer advice because we are uncomfortable. This sort of reactive action closes the door to trust. We must conscientiously remind ourselves that this encounter is not about us, but about our client.

If done with genuine care and concern, the result of mindful listening may be transformative. It can sometimes result in a conversation that is especially memorable and even life changing (Shafir, 2008). Walker (2010) points out that every time a client trusts her enough to share something personal about their life story, she tells them, *"It's a privilege to know this about you"* (p. 43). What often occurs after she says this is that the client acknowledges that they feel valued and truly cared for. Box (**8:4**) summarizes how to be effective at mindful listening. Box (**8:5**) contains a powerful affirmation that can be used at the onset of a new to help you stay focused on what matters most.

BOX 8:4 HOW TO BE EFFECTIVE AT MINDFUL LISTENING (as adapted from Walker, 2010; Shafir, 2008)
1. Make it your intention to be a warm and safe place.
2. Remind yourself that everyone has limitations and vulnerabilities.
3. Be willing to listen without expectations and without judging.
4. Be fully present and in the moment.
5. Pay 100% attention to what the person is trying to tell you.
6. Listen for the whole message. Concentrate as much on what has not been said as what has been said.
7. Become aware of the hidden messages in the metaphors and themes.
8. Make the person who is speaking feel valued and respected.
9. If necessary, say nothing because often it is the silence that allows the other person to process what they are feeling.

BOX 8:5 AN AFFIRMATION TO BEGIN YOUR WORKDAY (Shafir, 2008, p. 230)
First, let me consider the mystery of what is about to occur. Let me remember that my patient is a unique human being and that my interaction, to the extent that it's genuine, will be unprecedented. Let me remember that each moment is brimming with possibilities, that by listening mindfully, I may be able to see more deeply, by letting myself be touched by their experience, I will convey to the patient that I care.

BOX 8:6 CASE IN POINT: WHEN THE FAMILY FEELS THAT THEY HAVE BEEN LEFT IN THE DARK
Our beloved Aunt Viola was 84 years of age and quite a feisty lady. I was her next of kin and on a beautiful Spring morning, I received a call that Viola had been admitted to the Emergency Room (ER) because of trouble breathing. At first, I was told that Viola would be coming home real soon. The second phone call relayed a different message, that Viola would be admitted to hospital instead. That was when I decided to go to the hospital to be with my Aunt. Viola was admitted to the ER because there were no hospital beds. The nurse told me that Viola's official diagnosis was pneumonia. At first glance, Viola seemed to me to be doing okay, but I wasn't a health professional, so I could not judge how sick she was. After spending several hours with Viola I went home late that evening with the intention of returning to the hospital the next day. Apparently sometime during the night Viola got off her stretcher to go to the bathroom and fell and broke her arm. No one called me during the night to notify me of this accident. When I returned to the ER the next morning I noticed that Viola's arm was injured, wrapped in bandages and elevated on a pillow. The nurse promptly informed me that Viola needed surgery to repair her badly broken arm but she did not qualify for a general anesthetic because she had a bad heart. That was the first time I heard of Viola having a heart condition. No one explained what was going on, but I also didn't ask a lot of questions, maybe because I didn't know what to ask. The nurse also informed me that Viola had an advance directive that she would not get CPR if she died suddenly. I thought it was strange that she would tell me that. Nevertheless, I called the whole family to come and see Viola, because heart problems sounded serious to me. Although she seemed to be in good spirits, Viola was now visibly short of breath and had continuous Oxygen running. Maybe that was a clue. Information was relayed to us by one of the doctors that my Aunt had suffered a heart attack. They gave Viola some Morphine for her pain and a drug called Lasix to help take the fluid away from her lungs so she could breathe better. No one told us that Viola was dying so we acted like she would be okay. Perhaps we were in denial. The nurses kept coming back into the room to give Viola more

Morphine through the intravenous. They didn't explain why she needed more Morphine. I assumed it was for her arm pain. Once Viola seemed settled we all left for a bit to get some coffee. When we returned, Viola was lying on her stretcher and unresponsive. When I touched her she did not move and I noticed that she was no longer breathing. No one was in the room with her, not even a nurse. She was all alone. I felt so guilty about her dying without any of us there with her. No one said much to us. I still blame myself somehow.[1]

Question Pertaining to the Case in Point:

1. Recognizing the fact that the story as told, is through the eyes of a distraught family member, with no health care providers' input, is it still conceivable that the communication lines were not really clear? Regardless of the unknown details, what can be learned from this story? Is there anything that could have been done differently by the staff to help the family?

REFLECTING BACK

Summary of Key Points Covered in Chapter 8

- Caring as technology was defined as caring in relationship to technology and such things as virtual reality, machines that support life and robots.
- Although technological advances can enhance healthcare delivery it can also create new challenges for nurses.
- In modern health practices the nurturing aspects of caring for the ill or aged is increasingly viewed by some institutional bodies as less important than other more mechanistic aspects of service.
- Modern advances of science have somewhat blurred the boundaries of when life begins and when it ends.
- Even though we have been able to reduce the mortality rates of premature infants, infant morbidity has increased.
- Futility is concerned with carrying out treatment that is destined to fail to sustain life or instigated when the prognosis for recovery is hopeless. Two examples were given, the overuse of technology to try and save a premature baby when it is evident that the child's life cannot be saved and performing CPR on someone suffering from the end stages of a terminal illness.
- The notion of impending death as a real possibility is not only troubling for the client it is also difficult for many care givers.
- It is important for nurses to learn how to deal with death so that they will not abandon or avoid caring for the dying client or their loved ones in their time of need.
- No matter how many changes occur in the future the challenge to the profession of nursing is not to lose the capacity to care.
- A way to focus on the needs of our clients in trying times is through the art of mindful listening.

• Mindful listening refers to actively listening to what is being said and to the overall theme of what is shared.

SOMETHING TO PONDER

1. Are there types of new treatments based on scientific advances that you believe pose some controversy ethically? This would be a good topic for a classroom discussion or debate. Remember that no argument is one sided and to listen to all points of view.

CLASSROOM GROUP EXERCISE

1. Do a brain storming session on a White board in class to explore the following notion. Mindfulness was one suggestion to help to keep caring in the practice of nursing. What other actions or ideas can facilitate the enhancement of caring in our profession?

ON YOUR OWN

1. Reflect on what believe nurses need to support them when they are readily confronted with human suffering.
2. How can Nursing Regulatory Bodies, Nursing Associations or Health Boards better support nurses?

NOTES

[1] Note: The Case in Point was told by a family member who admits that she often cries when she thinks about her Aunt Viola. As always, many details have been either left out or altered, in order to ensure the anonymity of all of the persons who were involved.

CONSENT FOR PUBLICATION

Not applicable.

CONFLICT OF INTEREST

The authors confirm that this chapter contents have no conflict of interest.

ACKNOWLEDGEMENTS

Declared none.

REFERENCES

Barnard, A & Loscin, R (2007) *Technology & nursing: Practice, concepts and issues.*Palgrave MacMillan, Hampshire, United Kingdom.

Burkhardt, MA, Nathaniel, AK & Walton, NA (2015) Ethics and issues in contemporary nursing. Second Canadian Edition Nelson Education Limited., Toronto, Ontario.

Carter-Templeton, H, Frazier, RM, Wu, L & H Wyatt, T (2018) Robotics in nursing: A bibliometric analysis. *J Nurs Scholarsh,* 50, 582-9.
[PMID: 29920944]

Chopra, D (2005) *Peace is the way.*Three Rivers Press, USA.

Colwell, B (2010) Cancer: A practical guide for general practitioners. *The Canadian Journal of Diagnoses.* 27 (8), 45-47.

Elrick, L (2017) Technology in nursing: How electronics are changing the field. *Rasmussen College.*https://www.rasmussen.edu/degrees/nursing/blog/technology-in-nursing/

Gionet, K (2017) *Nurses of the future must embrace high-tech.*The Conversation. Retrieved from: http://theconversation.com/nurses-of-the-future-must-embrace-high-tech-86042

Green, J, Darbyshire, P, Adams, A & Jackson, D (2015) Looking like a proper baby: Nurses' experiences of caring for extremely premature infants. *J Clin Nurs,* 24, 81-9.
[http://dx.doi.org/10.1111/jocn.12608] [PMID: 24810931]

Harrington, L (2018) Nurse Robots. *AACN Adv Crit Care,* 29, 107-10.
[PMID: 29875105]

Keatings, M & Smith, OB (2016) *Ethical & legal issues in Canadian nursing (Kindle ed).*c Canada: Saunders.

Kuhl, D (2003) *What dying people want: Practical wisdom for the end of life.*Anchor Canada, Canada.

Mayerhoff, M (1971) *On caring.*Harper & Row, New York.

Miller-Tiedeman, A (1999) *Learning, practicing, and living the new careering.*Taylor & Francis Group, USA.

Mohammed, S & Peters, E (2009) Rituals, death and the moral practices of medical futility. *Nursing Ethics* 292-302.

Ray, MA (2016) Transcultural caring dynamics in nursing and health care, 2nd ed. F.A. Davis Company, Philadelphia.

Rouleau, G, Gagnon, M & Cote, J (2015) Impacts of information and communication technologies on nursing care: An overview of systematic reviews (protocol). *BioMed Central: The Open Access Publisher* https://www.ncbi.nlm.nih.gov/pmc/articles/PMC4449960/
[http://dx.doi.org/10.1186/s13643-015-0062-y]

Salzberg, S (2004) *Lovingkindness: The revolutionary art of happiness.* London: Shambhala.

Schmidt, J J (2002) *Intentional helping: A philosophy for proficient caring relationships..* Columbus, Ohio: Merrill Prentice Hall.

Shafir, RZ (2008) Mindful listening for better outcomes. In: Hicks, S.F., Bien, T., (Eds.), *Mindfulness and the therapeutic relationship.*The Guildford Press, New York. pp. 219-230.

Siegal, B (1989) *Peace, love & healing, body mind communication & the path to self-healing: An exploration..* New York: Harper & Row Publishers.

Siegal, B (1993) *How to live between office visits: Guide to life, love and health.* New York: Harper Collins Books.

SreeRaja, KR (2018) Robotic nursing in health care delivery. *International Journal of Nursing Education. 10*

(3), 148 – 151.

Walker, V (2010) *The art of comforting: What to say and do for people in distress.*Penguin Group, New York.

Ward, J, Cody, J, Schaal, M & Hojat, M (2012) The empathy enigma: an empirical study of decline in empathy among undergraduate nursing students. *J Prof Nurs,* 28, 34-40.
[PMID: 22261603]

Watson, J (2008) *Nursing: The philosophy of caring (Revised edition).*

Wirkus, M (2017) *A look at new nursing technologies & trends NurseZone* Retrieved from https://www.americanmobile.com/nursezone/new-graduates/look-at-new-nursing-technologies-and-trends/

CHAPTER 9

Embracing Diversity: Toward a Morally Inclusive Practice

Abstract: The goal of Chapter nine is to assist nurses to engage in a morally inclusive practice. A morally inclusive practice celebrates what people have in common as well as their differences. Diversity reflects variations in belief systems and ways of living and permeates everything that we do. Nurses are advised to diligently avoid stereotyping, which is expecting all people from a particular group to respond in a certain way based on perceived ideas. Systemic racism reinforces unfair inequalities among ethnic or racial groups and is a serious problem in health care. Education is the key to changing this culture. It is pointed out how Colonialism and Canadian residential schools resulted in historical trauma to Indigenous peoples that still negatively impacts large numbers of people. The Truth & Reconciliation Commission of Canada (TRCC) (2015) made a specific recommendation that Canadian medical and nursing schools include a mandatory course covering Aboriginal health issues. Applying the principles of trauma-informed care (TIC), cultural safety and cultural humility are recommended to help nurses be empathetic. Bullying is identified as a negative but harsh reality in nursing. Witnesses of bullying are asked to intervene to end bullying behaviours. A proposed Code of Conduct to encourage inclusion in nursing is recommended. The Chapter ends with a Case in Point: The Sinclair Case: Ignored to Death.

Keywords: Bullying, Culture, Cultural competence, Cultural awareness, Cultural sensitivity, Cultural safety, Colonialism, Cultural humility, Civility, Diversity, Ethnicity, Emotional intelligence, Inclusive practice, Incivility, Indigenous peoples, Racialized ethnicity, Residential Schools, Resiliency, Relationship-based care, Systemic racism, The Truth & Reconciliation Commission of Canada, The United Nations Declaration on the Rights and Freedom of Indigenous Peoples, Trauma-informed care, Trauma-sensitive, Trauma-responsiveness.

LEARNING GUIDE

After Completing this Chapter, the Reader Should be Able to

- Describe what is meant by a morally inclusive practice.
- Define diversity.

- Understand the differences between ethnicity, stereotyping, racialized ethnicity and systemic racism.
- Reflect on the important reasons why all nurses should avoid stereotypical biases and acts of systemic racism. Recognize that Colonialism and Canadian residential schools resulted in historical trauma that still negatively impact large numbers of Indigenous peoples.
- Gain a working understanding of what trauma-informed care (TIC) entails and how to implement its principles into practice.
- Appreciate that cultural safety and cultural humility are skills that helps nurses to be empathetic.
- Develop an appreciation of all the components associated with cultural competence and how to incorporate them into practice.
- Be motivated as nurses to take the lead in implementing cultural safety and cultural humility in the work-place.
- Realize that bullying is a negative but real aspect of the nursing culture.
- Become aware of ways that nurses can act individually or as a group to counteract workplace bullying.
- Understand the specific actions as proposed by Code of Conduct to encourage inclusivity in nursing.
- Apply what was learned to the Case in Point: The Sinclair Case, Where Racism Contributed to Death.
- Appreciate the importance of making cultural safety training a requirement for all health care professions.

Chapter Nine inspires nurses to whole-heartedly embrace diversity. Although diversity reflects variations in belief systems and ways of living, the current discussion deals primarily with the ethnic and cultural aspects of diversity. The current discussion deals primarily with the ethnic and cultural aspects of diversity. Chapter 10 will specifically cover the important topic of gender and sexual orientation. Chapter 11 will focus on the role of religion and spirituality in nursing. The intention of all three Chapters is to assist nurses to celebrate what we share with all people, including individuals and groups that are different from our own.

Nurses are advised to diligently avoid stereotyping. Systemic racism reinforces unfair inequalities among ethnic or racial groups and is a serious problem in health care. It is also crucial for nurses to understand how past trauma negatively affects many individuals and groups of people in our society. Applying the principles of trauma-informed care (TIC), cultural safety and cultural humility are suggested ways to help nurses to be empathetic.

Bullying is identified as a negative but harsh reality of the culture of nursing.

Witnesses of bullying are asked to intervene to end bullying behaviour. Specific actions are suggested by a proposed Code of Conduct to encourage inclusion in nursing. The Chapter ends with a Case in Point: The Sinclair Case: Ignored to Death.

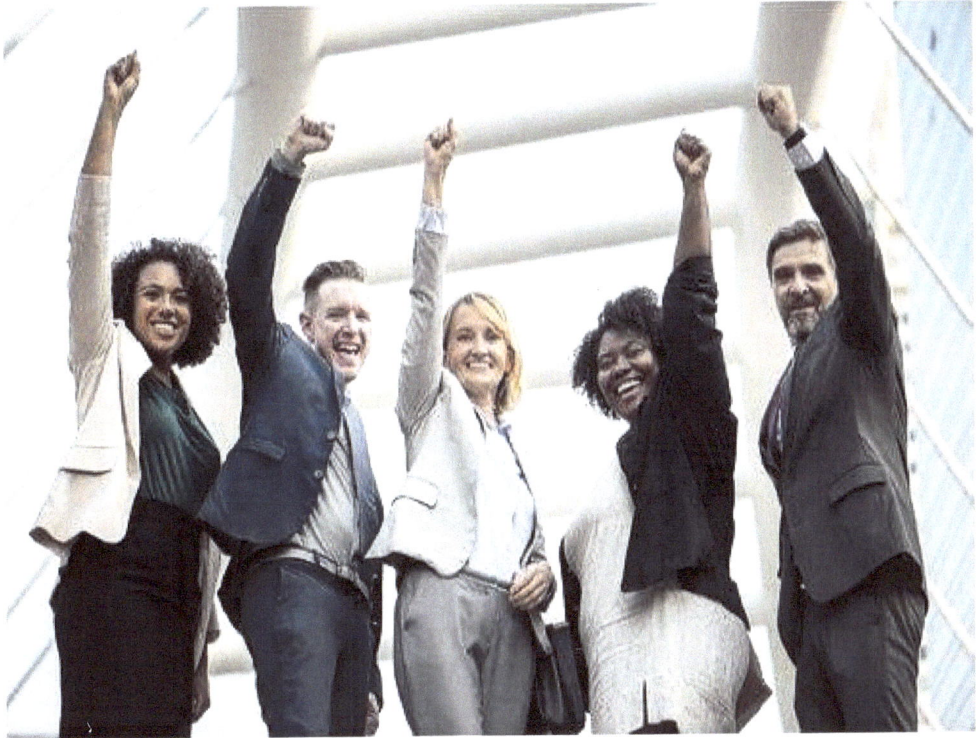

Fig. (9.1). Coming Together & Honoring Diversity. Source: www.pixabay.com

THE VAST LANDSCAPE OF DIVERSITY

The primary goal of this Chapter is to help nurses to engage in a morally inclusive practice (Fig. **9.1**). A **morally inclusive practice** celebrates what people have in common as well as their differences and involves the action of whole heartedly embracing diversity (Coehlo, & Manoogian, 2010). **Diversity** is a concept that reflects variations in belief systems and ways of living. It includes, but is not limited to ethnicity, culture, gender, sexual orientation, age, religious and spiritual beliefs, socioeconomic position and health status (Burkhardt, Watson & Nathaniel, 2015; Coehlo & Manoogian, 2010; Galanti, 2004). We have more in common than we think. By accepting a variety of lifestyles, nurses are better able to move away from fearing our differences and instead develop an appreciation of the strengths that come from the unity contained within diversity (Burkhardt,

Nathaniel & Walton, 2015).

Ethnicity, Stereotyping, Racialized Ethnicity & Systemic Racism

Ethnicity & Stereotyping

Ethnicity in the broadest sense refers to a group of people who share a common and distinctive culture, religion and language, often from a specific country or part of the world. People will frequently refer to their ethnicity as their association with their family of origin (*e.g.*, Italian, Chinese, Spanish, Mexican, German or Indigenous). An important characteristic of an effective caregiver, especially when it comes to caring for people who are different from us, is the act of suspending judgment (Ray, 2016). Nurses are advised to diligently avoid **stereotyping**, which is expecting all people from a particular group to respond in a certain way based on perceived ideas (Burkhardt *et al.*, 2015). Stereotypical bias is in no way limited to ethnicity and can be aimed at any of the following groups of individuals: adolescents, the aged, prisoners, people with physical or mental disabilities, the poor, the homeless, mentally ill, drug users, Indigenous peoples and others. The following story demonstrates how a Caucasian nurse experienced stereotypical bias for the first time. Box (**9:1**).

I work as a nurse. I am usually quite pale white in color, I guess because my family is from Scotland, but I have brown hair and black eyes. I had just returned from a trip to Mexico. I was nicely tanned and it was my first day back at work. That day, one of my assigned clients was an elderly gentleman who had undergone prostrate surgery and was quite miserable. I assumed that he was upset about his health challenges and I did my very best not to judge him and acted with kindness, like when I went to the hospital library to get him something to read. At the end of my shift my client stated that he was really pleased that I was so nice to him and apologized for being such a grouch. He explained that as a rule he disliked and mistrusted *"brown people"* but that I must be different because I seemed like a good nurse. I guess I had a rather puzzled look on my face, because he responded with, *"I hope I have not offended you."* I just stood there stunned with disbelief and speechless. For the first time in my life I got a glimpse of what it must feel like to be discriminated against because of skin color.

Racialized Ethnicity & Systemic Racism

"The most enduring stereotypical images about Indigenous peoples is a being prone to alcohol and substance use. The image of the 'drunken Indian' continues to be one of the most harmful stereotypes operating in healthcare settings." Brenda L. Gunn, Metis Law Professor & Member of The Sinclair Working Group

The act of stereotyping resembles the notion of racialized ethnicity, but rather than referring to any group, racialized ethnicity is primarily aimed at issues of race. **Race** refers to a group of individuals that are connected by ancestral origin and certain biological differences, such as skin pigmentation. **Racialized ethnicity** refers to the problems faced by people who are automatically associated with a particular ethnic background and are assumed to follow the characteristics of that ethnic group, even when that may, or may not be, the case (Burkhardt *et al.*, 2015). A problem occurs in health care delivery when a nurse, by thought or action, pigeonholes people into one specific group (Galanti, 2004). Nowhere is this problem more evident than in the biases that are directed to Indigenous peoples through acts of systemic racism (Allan & Smylie, 2015).

Systemic racism is a serious problem in health care and is also called structural or institutional racism. It consists of actions, practices and policies that either maintain, perpetrate or reinforce unfair inequalities among ethnic or racial groups (First Nations Health Authority (FNHA) n.d.). Boyer (2017) points out that systemic racism toward Indigenous peoples within the Canadian Health Care System is widespread. Its prevalence is high in central Canada. Box (**9:2**) identifies some harsh examples of systemic racism toward Indigenous peoples that exists today.

BOX 9:2 SYSTEMIC RACISM TOWARD INDIGENOUS PEOPLES (as adapted from FNHA, 2016; Boyer, 2017; Allan & Smylie, 2015; Gunn, 2017)
* Indigenous Peoples often report feeling the effects of direct stress from interactions with health care professionals that are perceived as discriminatory in nature.
* Some report experiencing denial of access to healthcare resources, even when available, based on racism.
* Indigenous women in Central Canada often feel pressured by doctors and other health professionals to be sterilized just following giving birth.
* Indigenous men are often ignored in the Emergency Room (ER) leading to at least one case of an avoidable death. For example, the Sinclair case where a 45-year-old First Nations man died of a treatable bladder infection after being ignored for 34 hours in the ER.
* 42 Percent of Aboriginal People in Canada Reported Experiencing Racism since 2017 and 74 Percent of that racism was perpetrated by non-Indigenous People.
* Studies demonstrate that Indigenous peoples experience racism from health care workers so often that they routinely make advance plans on how to best deal with it before they even arrive to the Emergency Room (ER), or they avoid getting care altogether.
* Recent research reveals that racism against aboriginal people in health care is prevalent and a major factor in inferior health among native people in Canada.

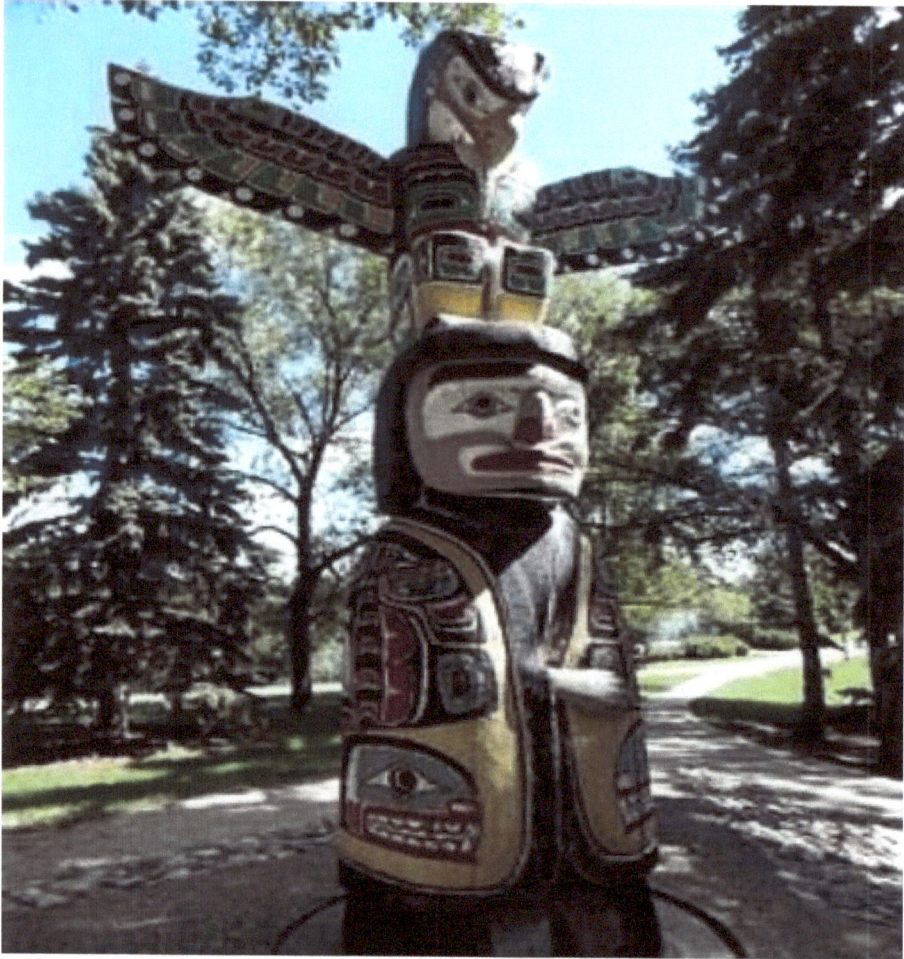

Fig. (9.2). First Nations Totem Pole. Source: www.pixabay.com

INDIGENOUS PEOPLES, COLONIALISM & RESIDENTIAL SCHOOLS: THE IMPACT OF HISTORICAL TRAUMA

Indigenous peoples refers to persons who consider themselves as being related to or having historical continuity with "First Peoples," whose civilizations in what is now known as Canada, the United States, the Americas, the Pacific Islands, New Zealand, Australia, Asia, and Africa predate those of subsequent invading or colonizing populations (Allan & Smylie, 2015, p. 3) (Fig. **9.2**). In Canada they consist of First Nations, Inuit and Metis (Roberts, 2016). The quote that follows is from the Truth & Reconciliation Commission of Canada (TRCC) (2015). It clearly summarizes the terrible historical trauma and "cultural genocide" inflicted upon Indigenous Peoples in Canada. Box (**9:3**).

BOX 9:3 SUMMARY OF HISTORICAL TRAUMA INFLICTED UPON INDIGENOUS PEOPLES IN CANADA (Truth & Reconciliation Commission of Canada (TRCC), 2015, p. 1).

For over century, the central goals of Canada's Aboriginal policy were to eliminate Aboriginal governments; ignore Aboriginal rights; terminate the Treaties; and through a process of assimilation cause Aboriginal peoples to cease to exist as distinct legal, social, cultural, religious, and racial entities in Canada. The Establishment of residential schools were a central element of this policy, which can best be described as "cultural genocide."

The History that Underlies the Trauma

In this section I endeavour to further clarify some of the background behind the terrible and inexcusable trauma and atrocities inflicted upon Indigenous peoples in Canada. There have been historical structures that have negatively impacted the physical and emotional health of Indigenous peoples in Canada. One such factor was colonization, conquest and attempted assimilation into the dominant society that drastically altered every aspect of the lives of Indigenous groups (Reading, 2015). What occurred historically is that European settlers decided that Indigenous ways of living were wrong and unacceptable. Prior to the Europeans landing in North America it is estimated that there were eighteen million Indigenous peoples who spoke more than 2,200 languages. They were a society that flourished as hunter gatherers, who lived primarily and respectfully off the land, and relied on the help of extended family to raise their children (Roberts, 2016). They enjoyed good health and wellness, ate traditional foods and were able to perform spiritual and emotional healing practices (FNHA, 2016).

After invasion of the Europeans and Colonization, the way of life for Indigenous Peoples was greatly changed through the establishment of legal treaties that made sure that Indian bands and tribes were relegated to living on reserves. In the late 1800s residential schools were established by Christian Missionaries (Roberts, 2016). The purpose of the residential schools was to assimilate the native children through education, cultural degradation and teaching the children to be ashamed of their native heritage (Roberts, 2016). Parents were required by law to send their children to residential schools where Indigenous customs and language were forbidden and children were severely punished physically and emotionally and sexual abuse was paramount (Reading, 2015). Education was substandard and children often went hungry. The last residential schools did not close in Canada until the 1990s and the experience still negatively impacts many Aboriginal men and women today (Roberts, 2016; Reading, 2015). Unfortunately, even today, substantive power imbalances remain between non-Indigenous and Indigenous people and that power differential is prevalent in the delivery of health care services (Boyle, 2017). Education and training are key to changing systemic racism that still exists in health care today.

The Truth & Reconciliation Commission of Canada & Recommendations for Future Curriculum

The Truth & Reconciliation Commission of Canada (TRCC) (2015) made specific recommendations that apply to Nursing Education curriculum. Part 24 from the *Calls to Action*, recommends that Canadian medical and nursing schools make it mandatory for all students to take a course covering Aboriginal health issues. It strongly suggests that the content of the course include the history and legacy of residential schools, Aboriginal rights, and Indigenous teachings and practices.

The Truth & Reconciliation Commission of Canada is not alone in recommending that nurses be better educated in Indigenous issues. Bearskin (2016) insists that all Canadian schools of nursing redesign their curriculum to include mandatory education in Indigenous health, teachings, customs and practices, and that all nurses become familiar with, *The United Nations Declaration on the Rights of Indigenous Peoples* (United Nations, 2006). Bearskin recommends that nurses use the knowledge from *The United Nations Declaration on the Rights of Indigenous Peoples* to inform their workplace decisions and the development of health care policies. Bearskin urges nurses to be prepared to ask difficult questions such as, *Is the Policy grounded in the UN declaration? Will it improve access to health care or will it create more barriers?* (Bearskin, 2016). It is also highly recommended that any course that is developed for health care professionals should also comprise of skills-based training in intercultural competency, conflict resolution, anti-racism and *The Canadian Charter of Rights and Freedoms.* (TRCC, 2015). Box (**9:4**) quotes the Charter on equality.

BOX 9:4 EQUALITY BEFORE AND UNDER LAW AND EQUAL PROTECTION AND BENEFIT OF LAW/ Affirmative action programs (Department of Justice, 1982)
Equality 15. (1) Every individual is equal before and under the law and has the right to equal protection and equal benefit of the law without discrimination based on race, national or ethnic origin, color, religion, sex, age or mental or physical disability.

The Importance of Health Professionals Becoming Trauma Sensitive

After a brief overview of the historical and current trauma experienced by Indigenous peoples, it is important for nurses to become trauma sensitive. To be **trauma sensitive** entails understanding that trauma is prevalent in our society and impacts many of the individual clients that we interact with and care for in health settings. It also affects large groups of people (Gerber, 2019). Individuals who have experienced adverse childhood experiences of trauma later develop a high propensity for developing mental illness and are prone to addictions and other self-destructive behaviours (Gerber, 2019). It is, therefore, crucially important for caregivers who are caring for persons with past trauma, to develop an understanding of how to best create an environment that promotes healing and recovery.

The Widespread Impact of Trauma

The impact of trauma is extensive. It is essential that health professionals to comprehend that individual traumatic experiences not only affect the person who has experienced them, they can also have ripple effects in other relationships. For example, learned, fear-based, ineffective and fearful ways of coping that are somewhat reactive in nature, can have varying degrees of negative impact on individuals, their families and a community, and can be passed on across generations (Berger & Quiros, 2016). Furthermore, traumatic experiences are not limited to those that happen to the individual person. Systemic events such as war, colonization, racism, genocide and other forms of violence happen to whole populations and affects their ability, or lack of ability, to cope with life's stressors (Gerber, 2019).

A Culture of Caregiver Judgement

Unfortunately, some caregivers harbour judgments toward specific vulnerable populations who have been traumatized. For example, the literature provides evidence that nurses, and other health professionals often possess stereotypical biases toward Indigenous people, the mentally ill, the addicted and other vulnerable groups (Ross & Goldner, 2009; Allan & Smylie, 2015; Hanson & Lang, 2016). Attitudes of practitioner bias and judgment have been known to interfere with establishing trust between the caregiver and client.

Behaviours Associated with Trauma

Behaviours commonly noted by those who have experienced trauma include, but are not limited to: a basic mistrust of anyone in an authoritarian role, a propensity for anger and angry outbursts, disinterest, disobedience, defiance, withdrawal in relationships, reoccurring behaviours of violence toward self or others, difficulties with school or work attendance, high rates of unemployment and all sorts of addictive behaviours (Berger & Quiros, 2016; Gerber, 2019) (Fig. **9.3**). The following excerpt from Dr. Peter Levine, a well-known international researcher in somatic reactions to trauma, paints a picture of how people react to a threat or impending injury. Box (**9:5**).

Box 9:5 THE SEQUELA OF THE TRAUMA RESPONSE (Dr. Peter Levine, International Trauma Response Researcher & Author of several books including, *Waking the Tiger: Healing Trauma*)

In response to threat and injury, animals, including humans, execute biologically based non-conscious action patterns that prepare them to meet the threat and defend themselves. The very structure of trauma including activation, dissociation and freezing are based on the evolution of survival behaviours. When threatened or injured, all animals draw from a library of possible responses. We orient, dodge, duck, stiffen, brace, retract, fight, flee, freeze, collapse, etc. All these coordinated responses are somatically based – they are things that the body does to protect and defend itself. It is when these orientating and defending responses are overwhelmed that we see trauma.

Fig. (9.3). The Negative impact of Trauma. Source: www.pixabay.com

Trauma-Responsiveness

Awareness of the facts that trauma is pervasive and prevalent in society is the first step for health care providers to change any preconceived negative assumptions about persons who have been traumatized. The second step is for practitioners to learn how to act with **trauma-responsiveness** which consists of acting with understanding when confronted with somewhat reactive behaviours associated with past trauma. Trauma responsiveness consists of creating settings that are safe and welcoming environments that cultivate opportunities for healing to take place. Although, it is beyond the scope of this current book to explore TIC in depth, it is highly recommended that nurses become educated in what TIC consists of and how to implement its principles into practice.

Trauma-informed Care (TIC)

Trauma-informed care (TIC) is strength based and is founded on the premise of sincere responsiveness to the full impact of trauma. Although, it is beyond the scope of this current book to explore trauma-informed care (TIC) in depth, it is highly recommended that nurses become educated in what TIC consists of and how to implement its principles into practice. With TIC, healing is facilitated through practicing non-judgment and acceptance, increasing a sense of connectedness and through empowerment (Hanson & Lang, 2016). The definition of TIC also includes the many co-occurring disorders associated with trauma and does not force the client to reveal their specific trauma history in order to receive help (Hanson & Lang, 2016).

Key Principles of Trauma Informed Care: Safety & Trust, Empowerment & Resiliency

Although the exact labels may differ somewhat, there are generally key principles associated with trauma-informed care such as: cultivating safety & trust, empowerment & building resiliency (Fig. **9.4**).

Safety & Trust

When people are survivors of trauma they often experience a violation of safety and trust. Subsequently, any steps toward healing must begin by creating safety (Gerber, 2019). Therefore, TIC accentuates the importance of physical, psychological and emotional safety for survivors of trauma as well as their care givers (Hopper, Bassuk & Olivet, 2009).

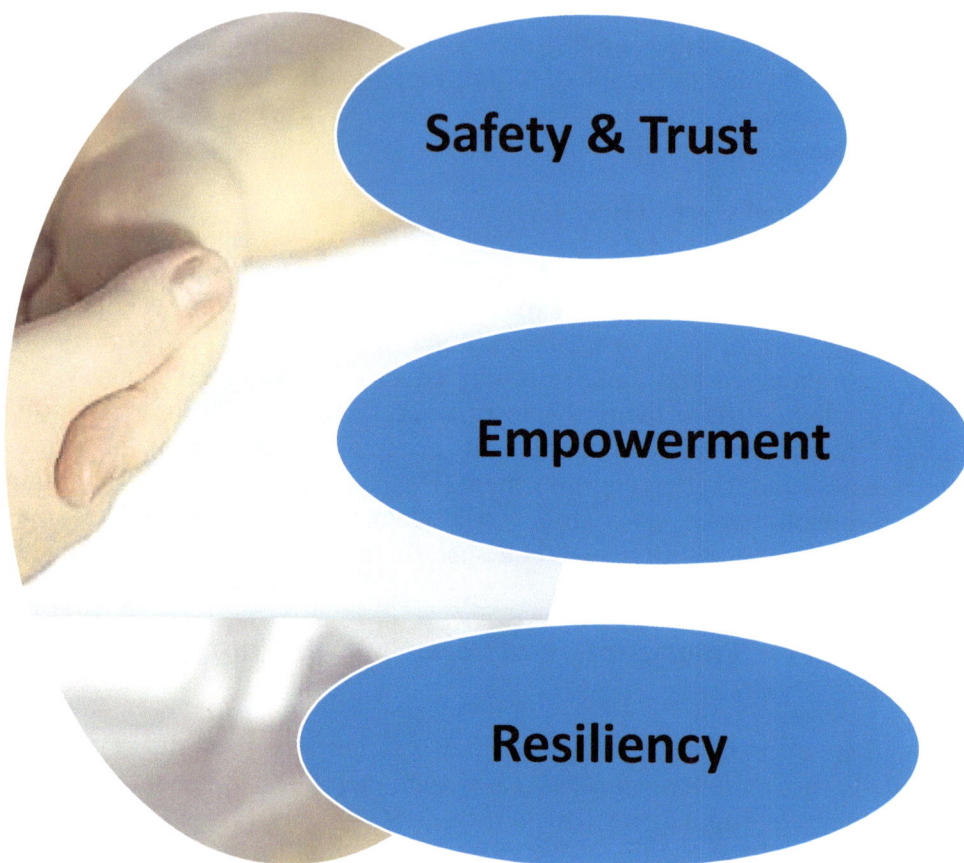

Fig. (9.4). Three Key Principles of TIC. Source: K. Stephany

Empowerment

Empowerment begins with acknowledging that the trauma has happened, along with a willingness to listen to what the person has to say. Since they have often felt a loss of control, TIC creates opportunities for survivors of trauma to re-build a sense of control by allowing them to make their own choices (Gerber, 2019' Berger & Quiros, 2016; Hopper *et al.,* 2009).

Resiliency

Resiliency, which is the ability to gain strength from adversity, can be created by helping traumatized clients to understand that because they have survived the trauma, they have developed new capabilities and strengths of character. One of those strengths is the capacity to empathize and feel compassion for others who also have suffered (Hooper *et al.*, 2009: Berger & Quiros, 2016). As previously pointed out, this discussion of TIC has been very brief. Please refer to the recommended reading list or reference list for additional resources.

CULTURAL COMPETENCE: PRACTICING IN EMPATHETIC & HELPFUL WAYS

Cultural Awareness & Cultural Sensitivity

Cultural competence is a skill that helps nurses to deal with cultural issues in practice in understanding, empathetic and helpful ways. There are several key aspects to incorporating cultural competence into nursing: cultural awareness, cultural sensitivity, cultural safety, relationship-based care and cultural humility (Burkhardt *et al.*, 2015; FNHA, 2016). **Cultural awareness** consists of the action of wanting to know what values, beliefs and behaviours are important to people who are from cultures other than our own (Burkhardt *et al.*, 2015). **Cultural sensitivity** goes beyond cultural awareness and seeks to incorporate a client's cultural beliefs directly into nursing practice (Burkhardt *et al.*, 2015).

Cultural Safety, Relationship-based Care & Cultural Humility

Cultural safety helps change the negative stereotypes held by nurses and others in the health care setting. Cultural safety promotes respectful engagement by addressing the power imbalances inherent in the health care system and is accomplished through cultivating a safe environment that is free of racism and discrimination (Allan & Smylie, 2015).

Cultural safety also includes care providers purposefully seeking to understand what health and wellness means to the clients they are caring for. For example, The First Nations view of health and wellbeing is holistic and includes the spiritual, emotional, physical and social (FNIIA, 2016; Gunn, 2017). For Indigenous Peoples good health outcomes need to include traditional medicines and foods (Gunn, 2017). Indigenous peoples also believe that good health and wellness begins with each individual and expands outward to embrace broader cultural, social, economic and environmental elements of health and wellness (FNHA, 2016).

Cultural safety is best cultivated in conjunction with relationship-based care (First Nations Health Authority (FNHA), 2016a). **Relationship-based care** creates a healing environment through purposeful acts of compassion offered by health care professionals to the persons that they are assigned to care for and about (FNHA, 2016). It consists of the caregiver being fully present; empowering others to be themselves, helping them to feel good about their heritage, and allowing them to tell their stories without feeling judged (Bearskin, 2016).

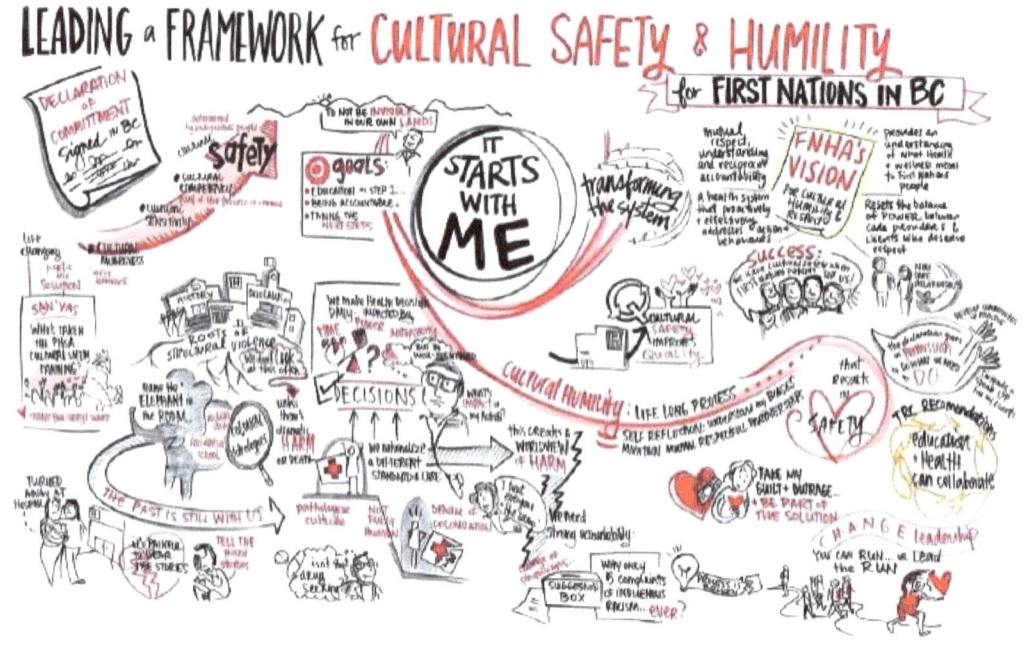

Fig. (9.5). First Nations Health Authority Poster on Cultural Humility. Source: www.fnha.ca/culturalhumility

Cultural humility is closely aligned with cultural safety and involves a commitment by the care practitioner to sincerely seek to fully understand what another person has experienced (FNHA, 2016). It is about a willingness to begin by becoming aware of your own inherent biases. Therefore, cultural humility involves caregiver self-reflection in order to uncover personal and systemic biases and to genuinely replace them with respectful behaviours that enhance dignity (FNHA, 2016).

WHEN THE CULTURE OF NURSING TAKES AN UGLY TURN: NURSES AS BULLIES

Modern Views of Culture

When a person thinks of the term culture, they usually depict images of beliefs, values, knowledge and behaviours of an identified ethnic group (Galanti, 2004). However, more recent definitions of culture portray the concept more broadly. **Culture** is defined as the beliefs, values, behaviours, customs and way of living of any group of individuals (Burkhardt *et al*, 2015; Ray, 2016). In fact, culture is fluid and ever evolving and permeates everything we do. Unique cultural expressions can occur from many groups, including nursing.

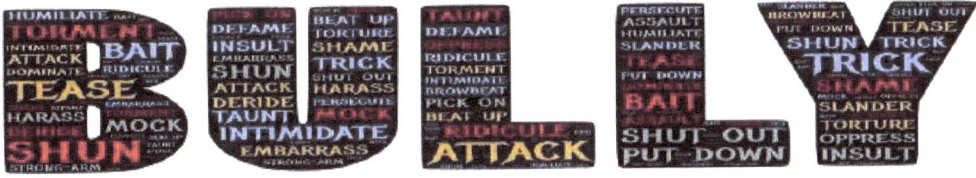

Fig. (**9.6**). Bullying. Source: www.pixabay.com

Nursing Culture & Bullying

"Nurses are really vicious to each other. It's not one hospital. It's not one type of nurse. It's the new nurse, it's the nurse who transferred from another floor, it's the ICU nurses feeling superior to the med-surg nurses – its endless." Dr. Cheryl Dellasega, RN, PhD, Professor of Women's Studies, Researcher & Author.

Nurses belong to their own culture but not all aspects of nursing social interaction are positive. **Civility** in nursing is behaviour that is tantamount with respectful, gracious, polite and courteous conduct (Meires, 2018). **Incivility**, is the opposite to civility and consists of activity that is intentionally rude, intimidating and hostile toward others. One specific and harmful form of incivility is bullying. Bullying has many names: vertical, lateral or horizontal violence; nurse to nurse hostility; workplace intimidation and negative behaviour (Stokowski, 2010). Although it does not matter what you call it, it is important to identify the characteristics of this type of aggression.

Bullying is workplace violence (Stokowski, 2010). It consists of repeated, unreasonable and purposeful cruel actions of either individuals or groups that is directed toward a person or group of employees. The goal of bullying is to intimidate, belittle and cause harm. Therefore, it creates a risk to the health and safety of the target (Stokowski, 2010) (Fig. **9.6**). Bullying is also an abuse of power that is intended to inflict physical or emotional harm and injury (Dellasega, 2009). A nurse bully is someone who routinely intimidates or causes harm to another nurse that they believe to be vulnerable or beneath their level of competence (Meires, 2018). There are real tangible costs to bullying. For instance, bullying creates a toxic work environment, can pose safety risks to patients and interferes with teamwork and communication (Stokowski, 2010; Dellasaga, 2009).

How Often Does Bullying Occur in Nursing?

We do not know for sure how often bullying in nursing occurs, or what the exact numbers are for a variety of reasons. For instance, there is a wide variation in the definition of bullying, individual perceptions of what constitutes bullying differs, and some nurses are too intimidated to call it bullying when they suspect that it is occurring (Stokowski, 201). However, some studies have revealed a documented prevalence rate somewhere between 17% – 85% (Edmonson, Bolick & Lee, 2017; Castronovo, Pullizzi & Evans, 2016). These same studies point out that bullying affects nurses of all ages and stages, although new nurses seem to be targeted more often than others (Edmonson *et al.,* 2017; Castronovo *et al.,* 2016). Dellasega (2009) believes that everyone has experienced bullying in one of three ways sometime in their nursing career: as the bully, as the victim, or as the by-stander. So, what does bullying look like? Box (**9:6**) lists some specific examples of acts of intimidation, but by no means includes all forms or types of bullying actions.

BOX 9:6 EXAMPLES OF BULLYING BEHAVIOURS (as adapted from: Stokowski, 2010; Dellasega, 2009; Meires, 2018)
1. Giving a co-worker the "cold treatment" (*e.g.*, refusing to speak to the person).
2. Unwarranted criticism.
3. Blaming the other nurse without any evidence of wrongdoing.
4. Acting in an intimidating fashion toward the other person.
5. Gossiping or spreading rumors, which may include telling lies to tarnish their reputation.
6. Assigning them a more difficult workload when compared to other nurses.
7. Withholding crucial information about a client they are assigned to care for, on purpose to get them into trouble.
8. Treating someone differently from the others (*e.g.*, social isolation).
9. Being condescending or patronizing.
10. Eye rolling when the other person speaks.
11. Shouting at the other person.

Why Does Bullying Occur?

Why do some nurses resort to bullying others? Bullies, typically, are insecure, angry, frustrated with their work or home life, unhappy, stressed or unable to handle the demands in their life (Meires, 2018). Some bullies may also be immature and may lack **emotional intelligence,** which is the ability to think about the consequences of your choices before acting (Meires, 2018; Stokowski, 2010). Others argue that high stress work areas such as Critical Care Units, Emergency Rooms and other high specialty units create conditions that incite lateral violence because the work environment is extremely demanding (Meires, 2018).

It has also been argued that because relational aggression is often preferred by women over physical aggression, and that the profession of nursing is still primarily occupied by women, that nurse to nurse aggression is an inevitable part of this culture (Archer & Cote, 2005; Pugh, 2006). Dellasega (2009) is convinced that because nurses are in a subservient position to medical staff they are often subjected to vertical insults and being pushed around. Therefore, they in turn exert lateral violence on their fellow nurses. Although these theories may explain the behaviour, they do not condone it.

Who is Doing the Bullying, Where is it Happening & Who is Targeted?

Perpetrators of the abuse are most often those in supervisory positions or those who believe that they are more skilled than ordinary nurses (Dellasaga, 2009). For example, a study conducted by Vessey *et al.* (2009) revealed the following breakdown of the type of nurse who was mainly the perpetrator of the abuse: Senior nurses (24%), Charge Nurses (17%), and Nurse Managers (14%). The types of units where the maltreatment generally occurred, divided into percentages, from the most to least common include: Medical Surgical Units 23%, Critical Care Units 18%, Emergency Rooms 12%, Perioperative Areas 9%, and Obstetrics Units 7% (Vessey *et al.,* 2009). What is disturbing to note, is that evidence indicates that bullying behaviours may even start in nursing school (Stokowski, 2010).

Who is most often the target of the bullying? Stokowski (2010) found that a new graduate or new hire is targeted first. Next in line are those who have been promoted. When someone is promoted some of the other nurses who have been overlooked, feel jealous. The same occurs for nurses who receive special attention by the medical staff (Stokowski, 2010).

What Can be Done to Combat Bullying in Nursing?

The CNA Code of Ethics (2017) clearly advises that nurses make a conscious effort to treat each other with respect, which includes fellow nurses, students and other health professionals. The CNA also points out that it is important to understand the power differences between all these individuals. However, being mandated to act with respect is not enough. Nurses need to do their part, both individually and collectively to end the bullying behaviour. So what can be done to end bullying in nursing? I believe that every nurse that is a witness to any form of aggression toward another, has an ethical obligation to act. If you look the other way you become part of the problem instead of the solution (Fig. **9.6**). Let's examine some of the ways in which that end can be accomplished.

Meires (2018) proposes that if the bullying behaviour is pointed out in a diplomatic manner that may be enough. She uses the example of having coffee with the person and telling them how their behaviour impacted them or someone else. However, Meires is aware that this simple strategy may not work with everyone. If the bully's bad behaviour continues then the perpetrator may need to be reported to a supervisor. However, if the supervisor is the bully, then you may need to look up what your institution's policies and procedures are concerning incivility in the workplace (Merires, 2018).

Murray (2009) recommends that nurses take an approach that involves looking out for each other, which includes supporting the victim of the abuse during and after it occurs and filing an incident report. You can also intervene as an individual by asking the victim to help you with your assignment to get them away from the situation, speak up on their behalf or just stand beside them so they feel supported (Dellasaga, 2009).

There is also a more collective way to intervene and there is power in numbers. For instance, Dellasaga (2009) points out that bystanders usually outnumber both bullies and the victims combined, and if the witnesses to the abuse unite, they can foster change. One suggestion is to intervene as a group right when the bullying occurs by calling their behaviour out. Bullies are usually insecure and will often back off when directly confronted, especially if confronted by more than one person at a time (Stokowski, 2010). The learning activity in Box (**9:7**) features an inspiring you tube video with ideas on how to eradicate a culture of lateral violence in nursing and replace it with civility.

BOX 9:7 LEARNING ACTIVITY: WORKING TOWARD A CULTURE OF CIVILITY IN NURSING
1. Watch the following you tube video by Kathleen Bartholomew called, *Lessons from Nursing the World* at: https://www.youtube.com/watch?v=Qh4HW3yx00w
2. After watching the video, have an open discussion of the recommended strategies put forward by Kathleen Bartholomew to help to eradicate a culture of lateral violence between nurses.

A CODE OF CONDUCT TO FOSTER INCLUSIVENESS & DIVERSITY IN NURSING

"We can't solve problems by using the same kind of thinking we used when we created them." Albert Einstein, German-born Theoretical Physicist.

Schmidt, MacWilliams & Neal-Boylan (2016) point out that there is an escalation of concerns within the profession of nursing about the lack of diversity and an increase in exclusionary behaviours. Types of exclusivity actions include: isolation of persons or groups who are different, incivility, bullying and workplace violence (Schmidt *et al.*, 2016) (Fig. **9.7**). Extensive review of the literature reveals that there are no specific nursing codes of conduct that specifically deal with inclusion (Schmidt *et al.*, 2016). Therefore, the authors developed a comprehensive nursing code of conduct for inclusion that builds on existing nursing codes of ethics. They ensured that what they developed would be applicable to nursing students, nurses in practice and nurses in educational settings (Schmidt *et al.*, 2016). Highlights of this code of conduct include: that it addresses exclusionary behaviours in the profession; holds every nurse in every setting accountable for their actions; can be used as a foundation for measurement; and promotes diversity and co-operation (Schmidt *et al.*, 2016). The code directives are applicable in three different ways, nursing interactions with patients, and with colleagues, and directed to the profession at large. However, only those key features of the code of conduct that pertains specifically to nurse/patient relationships are included in Box (**9:8**).

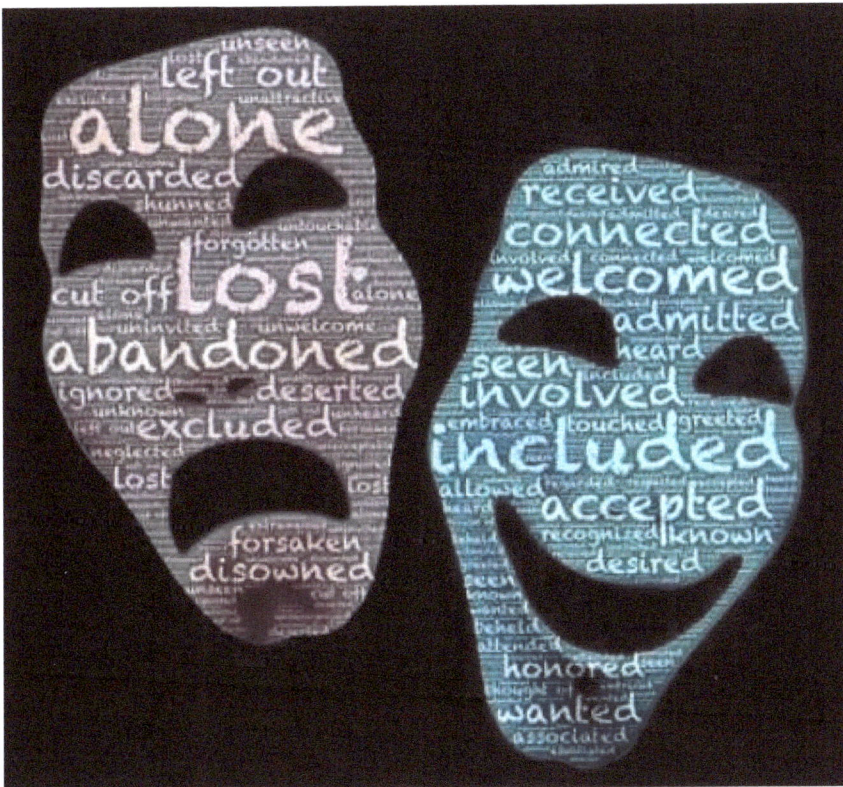

Fig. (9.7). Exclusivity Behaviors *versus* Inclusiveness. Source: www.pixabay.com

BOX 9:8 A PROPOSED CODE OF CONDUCT FOR INCLUSION AND DIVERSITY (as adapted from Schmidt *et al.*, 2016, pp. 104 – 105)
As it Pertains to Nurse/Patients Relationships

1. Treat everyone impartially without regard to age, ethnicity, gender, sexual orientation, disability, nationality, language, economic status, religious or spiritual beliefs, geographical status or political beliefs. Avoid all forms of stereotyping, discrimination and prejudice (AACN, 2008 as cited in Schmidt *et al.*, 2016).
2. Ensure that you value the worth of others & practice patient centered care (ANA, 2015b; Nursing Council of New Zealand, 2012 as cited in Schmidt *et al.*, 2016).
3. Listen actively and avoid interrupting or imposing your own opinions.
4. Elicit and acknowledge feedback from others (*e.g.*, express a willingness to learn from others).
5. Communicate in an open, compassionate, and positive manner (*e.g.*, transparent and kind communication, avoid negative tones).
6. Acknowledge and respect different beliefs, values and practices (*e.g.*, holistic care, agreeing to disagree) (ANA, 2015b; Nursing Council of New Zealand, 2012 as cited in Schmidt *et al.*, 2016).
7. Provide honest, accurate, and understandable information to others (Nursing Council of New Zealand, 2012 as cited in Schmidt *et al.*, 2016).
8. Involve others as partners in decision-making and support the rights of others to make choices for themselves.
9. Advocate for others when they are unable to advocate for themselves or in instances of prejudice or discrimination (Nursing Midwifery Board of Australia, 2013 as cited in Schmidt *et al., 2016*).
10. Attend to the needs of others in a compassionate and safe manner.
11. Follow-up on commitments made to others (ANA, 2015b as cited in Schmidt *et al.*, 2016).
12. Correct one's own actions or make changes in behavior when needed.
13. Engage in reflection and self-critique. Consider consequences to others before acting.
14. Collaborate with patients/families to resolve complaints or conflicts in an honest and respectful manner (Nursing Council of New Zealand, 2012 as cited in Schmidt *et al.*, 2016).
15. Avoid aggressive behavior toward patients/families, including mental, physical, and verbal abuse (*e.g.*, nonthreatening communications, absence of passive-aggressive behaviors).
16. Keep personal information confidential unless permitted to share (ICN, 2012 as cited in Schmidt *et al.*, 2016).
17. Protect privacy during patient care.

Every nurse should be held responsible for ensuring that they utilize inclusive behaviours in practice and there is evidence that pledges have proven to be effective in business cultures. Therefore, Schmidt *et al.* (2016) highly recommend that all nurses use a pledge for inclusion like the one in Box (**9:9**).

BOX 9:9 Pledge for Nurses:A Commitment to Inclusion (as adapted from Schmidt *et al.*, 2016, p. 106)

As a professional nurse, I commit to inclusive behaviours with my patients, students, colleagues, the profession, and society as a whole. The values underlying these behaviors are dignity, autonomy, altruism, justice, and integrity. I believe that I can achieve professional integrity by acting in a legal, ethical, and fair manner and through self-regulation. I therefore promise to abide by the Nursing Code of Ethics and the behaviors outlined in the Code of Conduct.

BOX 9:10 CASE IN POINT:THE SINCLAIR CASE: IGNORED TO DEATH (as adapted from Gunn, 2017).

Brian Sinclair was a 45-year-old Indigenous man from Central Canada. He died in September of 2008 in the Emergency Room (ER) of Winnipeg's Health Science Centre (HSC), which is one of the most comprehensive hospitals in Manitoba. Prior to presenting to the ER, Mr. Sinclair sought care from a family physician at a primary care clinic who then sent him by taxis to the ER which was only a few blocks away from the clinic. After 34 hours of being ignored, unattended to and uncared-for, Mr. Sinclair died of complications of a treatable bladder infection. Five years after his death an Inquest occurred. The goal of Phase I of the Inquest was to examine the circumstances under which Mr. Sinclair's death occurred. Phase II was mandated to determine what could have been done to prevent similar deaths in the future. In Phase I many witnesses testified that staff at the HSC made assumptions about Mr. Sinclair, such as, that he was intoxicated and homeless. Nurses testified that they did not notice that Mr. Sinclair was seated in a wheelchair in the waiting room of the ER. However, hospital video cameras showed many nurses walking right by him, but not one attended to him. Many of the ER staff testified that racism did not affect the care that they provided because they treat everyone the same. In January 2014 the presiding judge at the Inquest ruled that issues of race, racism, poverty, disability and substance use were beyond the scope of the Inquest. Subsequently, Part II, which was charged with identifying how to prevent a similar death in the future, was completely ignored. What this ruling meant, was that there would not be an examination of the role that social exclusion and classism may have played in the inadequate care that was provided to Mr. Sinclair while he resided in the ER. As a result of the neglect of the Inquest to address these crucial issues, *The Sinclair Group* was formed which consisted of Indigenous leaders, physicians, nurses, health advocates, legal experts, academics and health researchers. *The Sinclair Group* determined, that contrary to the Inquest testimony of the nurses, wait times were not the cause of Brian Sinclair's death. Mr. Sinclair died of racism. He required a simple procedure and antibiotics to treat a bladder infection which never occurred. Preconceived negative stereotypical notions of Indigenous Peoples, embedded in the health care system permitted the hospital staff to ignore Mr. Sinclair to death. Security, clerical, nurses and medical staff all ignored him throughout several shift changes resulting in his demise.

Question Pertaining to the Case in Point & Recommendation:

1. What biases do you suspect were inherent in some of the nurses who were assigned to care for Mr. Sinclair? Do you think that those same biases still exist today and how can we make real progress in changing them?

Recommendation: In order to overcome systemic racism within health care, it is highly recommended that all health care professionals take cultural safety training. Ideally the training would include some of the following themes.

a. Education on terminology, diversity colonialization, residential schools and Indian hospitals would need to be included (Gunn, 2017).
b. A review of how culture and stereotypical biases negatively impact the treatment received by Indigenous Peoples who interface with the health care system.
c. Strategies for cultivating empathetic communication and relationship skills (Gunn, 2017)

REFLECTING BACK

Summary of Key Points Covered in Chapter 9

- Nurses are encouraged to engage in a morally inclusive practice that celebrates what people have in common as well as their differences.
- Nurses are also expected to whole heartedly embrace diversity.
- Diversity reflects variations in belief systems and ways of living and includes many things such as: ethnicity, culture, gender, sexual orientation, age, religious and spiritual beliefs, socioeconomic position and health status.
- Ethnicity in the broadest sense refers to a group of people who share a common and distinctive culture, religion and language, often from a specific country or part of the world.
- Nurses are advised to diligently avoid stereotyping, which is expecting all people from a particular group to respond in a certain way based on perceived ideas.
- Systemic racism is a serious problem in health care. It consists of actions, practices and policies that either maintain, perpetuate or reinforce unfair inequalities among ethnic or racial groups.
- Systemic racism is evident in the biases that are directed to Indigenous peoples.
- Indigenous peoples refer to persons who consider themselves as being related to or having historical continuity with "First Peoples," whose civilizations predate those of subsequent invading or colonizing populations.
- There is a history of a series of inflicted trauma that occurred to Indigenous Peoples in Canada for over a century.
- The Truth & Reconciliation Commission of Canada (2015) recommends that Canadian medical and nursing schools make it mandatory for all students to take a course covering Aboriginal health issues.
- Unfortunately, a culture of caregiver judgement exists where some health professionals harbour judgments toward specific vulnerable populations who have been traumatized.
- It is important for nurses to become trauma sensitive, which is understanding that trauma is prevalent in our society and that it has negative impacts on individual health and relationships.

- Nurses are also expected to learn how to be trauma-responsive which consists of acting with understanding when confronted with somewhat reactive behaviours associated with past trauma.
- Trauma Informed Care (TIC) is a recommended strategy that is strength based and founded on the premise of sincere responsiveness to the full impact of trauma.
- Cultural competence is a skill that helps nurses to deal with cultural issues in practice in understanding, empathetic and helpful ways.
- There are several key aspects to incorporating cultural competence into nursing: cultural awareness, cultural sensitivity, cultural safety, relationship-based care and cultural humility.
- Bullying is workplace violence. It consists of repeated, unreasonable and purposeful cruel actions of either individuals or groups that is directed toward a person or group of employees.
- Bullying is a negative but harsh reality of the culture of nursing. Witnesses of bullying are asked to intervene either individually or collectively to end the bullying behaviour.
- Due to an escalation of concerns within the profession of nursing about the lack of diversity and an increase in exclusionary behaviours, a comprehensive nursing code of conduct for inclusion was recommended.

SOMETHING TO PONDER

1. Have you seen any evidence that some health professionals demonstrate biases and judgements toward some people or groups who have experienced trauma?
2. If caregivers judge traumatized clients, how will that impede care?

CLASSROOM GROUP EXERCISES

1. Break into groups of four. Discuss specific ways that nurses, individually and as a group, can advance cultural safety within the delivery of health care services.
2. As a White Board exercise brainstorm to develop strategies, as individuals or as a group of professionals to change negative stereotypes?

ON YOUR OWN

1. Reflect and journal in order to increase self-awareness of any potential inherent biases you may have toward people of other cultures.
   a. What culture, if any, do you primarily identify with?
   b. What beliefs about other differing cultures do you hold strongly to?
   c. What is your view of Indigenous cultures?

    d. Where do your ideas or assumptions come from?

    e. Are you able to identify any inherent biases that can be categorized as stereotypical or as systemic racism?

    f. What specific actions can you take to change your negative attitudes into ones that are positive and inclusive?

Recommended Readings

Dellasega,C.(2011).*When nurses hurt nurses:Recognizing and overcoming the cycle of bullying.* Indianapolis,USA:The Honor Society of Nursing:Sigma Theta Tau International.

Gerber,M.R.(2019).*Trauma informed healthcare approaches:A guide for primary care.* Switzerland:Springer Nature.

Truth & Reconciliation Commission of Canada (TRCC) (2015). *Honouring the truth,* reconciling the future: Summary of the final report of the Truth & Reconciliation *Commission of Canada.* Retrieved from: http://publications.gc.ca/collections/collection_2015/trc/IR4-7-2015-eng.pdf

United Nations (2006). *United Nations declaration on the rights of Indigenous peoples.* Retrieved from: https://www.un.org/esa/socdev/unpfii/documents/DRIPS _en.pdf

Web Resources:

Web Resource:*The Indigenous Cultural Competency Training (ICC) Program,* by the Provincial Health Services Authority (PHSA) in BC. http://www.sanyas.ca/

Web Resource:How to Recognize & Prevent Bullying in Nursing https://www. nurse.com/blog/2017/08/23/how-to-recognize-and-prevent-bullying-in-nursing/

CONSENT FOR PUBLICATION

Not applicable.

CONFLICT OF INTEREST

The authors confirm that this chapter contents have no conflict of interest.

ACKNOWLEDGEMENTS

Declared none.

REFERENCES

Allan, B & Smylie, J (2015) *First Peoples, second class treatment: The role of racism in the health and well-being of Indigenous peoples in Canada.*The Wellesley Institute, Toronto, Ontario. http://www.welles leyinstitute.com/wp-content/uploads/2015/02/Summary-First-Peoples-Second-Class-Treatment-Final.pdf

Archer, J & Cote, S (2005) Sex differences in aggressive behaviour. In: Tremblay, R.E., Hartup, R.E., (Eds.), *Developmental origins of aggression* Guildford Press, New York 425-30.

Bearskin, RLB (2016) *Through the lens of truth and reconciliation: Next steps Canadian Nurse Retrieved from:*https://www.canadian-nurse.com/en/articles/issues/2016/march-2016/through-the-lens-of-trth-and-reconciliation-next-steps

Berger, R & Quiros, L (2016) Best practices for training trauma-informed practitioners: Supervisors voice. *Traumatology,* 22, 145-54.
[http://dx.doi.org/10.1037/trm0000076]

Boyer, Y Healing racism in Canadian health care. *Canadian Medical Association Journal (CMAJ),* 189, 1408-9.https://www.ncbi.nlm.nih.gov/pmc/articles/PMC5698028/
[http://dx.doi.org/10.1503/cmaj.171234]

Burkhardt, MA, Nathaniel, AK & Walton, NA (2015) Ethics and issues in contemporary nursing. Second Canadian Edition Nelson Education Limited., Toronto, Ontario.

Castronovo, MA, Pullizzi, A & Evans, S (2016) proposed solution. *Nurs Outlook,* 64, 208-14.
[http://dx.doi.org/10.1016/j.outlook.2015.11.008] [PMID: 26732552]

Canadian Nurses Association (CNA). (2017)*CNA Code of Ethics for Registered Nurses.*(Revised Edition). Ottawa: Author.

Coehlo, DP & Manoogian, M (2010). Culturally sensitive nursing care of families. In J. R. Kaakinen, V. Gedaly-Duff, D. P. Coehlo & S. M. H. Hanson (Eds.). *Family health care nursing: Theory, practice and research*, 4th ed. Philadelphia: F. A. Davis Company, pp. 151 – 174.

Kaakinen, JR, Gedaly-Duff, V, Coehlo, DP, Hanson, SMH *Family health care nursing: Theory, practice and research* F. A. Davis Company, Philadelphia 151-74.

Dellasega, CA (2009) Bullying among nurses. *Am J Nurs,* 109, 52-8.
[http://dx.doi.org/10.1097/01.NAJ.0000344039.11651.08] [PMID: 19112267]

Department of Justice (1982) *The Canadian Charter of Rights and Freedoms.*Retrieved.http://pub lications.gc.ca/collections/Collection/CH37-4-3-2002E.pdf

Edmonson, C, Bolick, B & Lee, J (2017) A moral imperative for nurse leaders: Addressing incivility and bullying in health care. *Nurse Lead,* 15, 40-4.
[http://dx.doi.org/10.1016/j.mnl.2016.07.012]

First Nations Health Authority (FNHA) (2016) *Creating a climate for change: Cultural safety and humility in health services delivery for First Nations and Aboriginal Peoples in British Columbia (BC).*Author. Retrieved from,
BC.
http://www.fnha.ca/Documents/FNHA-Creating-a-Climate-For-Change-Cultural-Humility-Resource-Booklet .pdf

First Nations Health Authority (FNHA) (2016) *Cultural safety and humility: Key Drivers and ideas for change.*Retrieved
from.
http://www.fnha.ca/Documents/FNHA-Cultural-Safety-and-Humility-Key-Drivers-and-Ideas-for-Change.pdf

Galanti, G (2004) Caring for clients from different cultures. 3rd ed University of Pennsylvania Press, Philadelphia.

Gerber, M R (2019) *Trauma informed healthcare approaches: A guide for primary care.* Switzerland: Springer Nature.

[http://dx.doi.org/10.1007/978-3-030-04342-1]

Gunn, B L (2017) Ignored to death: Systemic racism in the Canadian Healthcare system. *Expert Mechanism on the Rights of Indigenous Peoples (EMRIP)* Retrieved from: https://www.ohchr.org/Documents/Issues /IPeoples/EMRIP/Health/UniversityManitobca.pdf

Hanson, RF & Lang, J (2016) A critical look at trauma-informed care among agencies and systems serving maltreated youth and their families. *Sage Publications,* 21, 95-100.https://journals.sagepub.com/doi/abs /10.1177/1077559516635274

Hopper, EK, Bassuik, EL & Olivet, J (2009) Shelter from the storm: Trauma-Informed care in homelessness services settings. *Open Health Serv Policy J,* 2, 131-51.http://www.traumacenter.org/products/pdf_files /shelter_from_storm.pdf

Meires, J (2018) Workplace incivility, the essentials: Here's what you need to know about bullying in nursing. *Urol Nurs,* 38, 95-7.

Murray, J S (2009) *Workplace bullying in nursing: A problem that cannot be ignored Pearson*

Provincial Health Authority Services (PHAS) in British Columbia (2015) *Indigenous cultural safety training*http://www.sanyas.ca/

Reading, C (2015) Structural determinants of Aboriginal Peoples' health.*Determinants of Indigenous peoples' health in Canada: Beyond the social* Canadian Scholar's Press, Toronto 3-15.

Roberts, RA Aboriginal health.*Community health nursing: A Canadian perspective, 4th ed.* Toronto: Pearson Education Canada, pp. 401 – 414.

Ross, CA & Goldner, EM (2009) Stigma, negative attitudes and discrimination towards mental illness within the nursing profession: a review of the literature. *J Psychiatr Ment Health Nurs,* 16, 558-67. [http://dx.doi.org/10.1111/j.1365-2850.2009.01399.x] [PMID: 19594679]

Schmidt, B J, MacWilliams, B R & Neal0Boylan, L (2016) Becoming inclusive: A code of Conduct for inclusion and diversity. *Journal of Professional Nursing,* 33, 102-7.

Stokowski, L A (2010) *A matter of respect and dignity: Bullying in the nursing profession USA: Medscape Retrieved from:.*https://pdfs.semanticscholar.org/673d/4c5fc45f73a0 c86f1e60e5a85a0079c44c29.pdf

Ray, M (2016) Transcultural caring dynamic in nursing and health care, 2nd ed. Philadelphia, PA: F. A. Davis Company.

Truth & Reconciliation Commission of Canada (TRCC) (2015) *Honouring the truth, reconciling the future: Summary of the final report of the Truth & Reconciliation Commission of Canada.*http://publications.gc.ca/collections/collection_2015/trc/IR4-7-2015-eng.pdf

United Nations (2006) *United Nations declaration on the rights of Indigenous peoples* Retrieved from https://www.un.org/esa/socdev/unpfii/documents/DRIPS_en.pdf

Vessey, JA, Demarco, RF, Gaffney, DA & Budin, WC (2009) Bullying of staff registered nurses in the workplace: a preliminary study for developing personal and organizational strategies for the transformation of hostile to healthy workplace environments. *J Prof Nurs,* 25, 299-306. [http://dx.doi.org/10.1016/j.profnurs.2009.01.022] [PMID: 19751935]

Watson, J (2008) *Nursing: The philosophy of caring (Revised edition).*Boulder, Colorado: University Press of Colorado..

CHAPTER 10

Ethics, Gender & Sexual Orientation: Moving Beyond Tolerance to Acceptance

Abstract: Chapter ten deals with the somewhat sensitive subject matter of ethics, gender and sexual orientation. Nurses are encouraged to move beyond tolerance and to accept and respect life choices that differ from their own. The issue of gender style and ethical decision-making is reviewed. It is pointed out that male ways of approaching moral decision-making may be different from females but not inferior to them. The reasons why Canadian nurses are still primarily women is explored. Nurses are obligated to have a working knowledge of the varying forms of sexual and gender orientation and they are not allowed to discriminate against any individual for any reason. It is pointed out that members who identify as lesbian, gay, bi-sexual, transgender, queer or questioning their sexual identity, or 2 spirit (LGBTQ2S) are often victims of both acute and chronic trauma. They are often not well understood or treated by members of the health community. Nurses are advised to become familiar with treatment guidelines in order to more effectively manage gender assessments. A strategy to foster compassion is recommended. The Chapter ends with a Case in Point: When Coming Out Seems to Cost too much.

Keywords: 2-spirit, Asexuality, Bisexuality, Ethic of justice, Ethic of care, Gender orientation, Gay, Gender non-conforming, Heterosexuality, Homosexuality, Heterosexism, Lesbian, Non-binary, Queer, Questioning their sexual identity, Transgender.

LEARNING GUIDE

After Completing this Chapter, the Reader Should be Able to

* Explain the differences between tolerance and acceptance.

* Appreciate that ethic of care theorist, Gilligan (1982) viewed male ways of approaching moral decision-making as different from females but not inferior to them.

* Explain key reasons why the profession of nursing is still primarily occupied by women.

* Be informed of some of the various forms of sexual and gender orientation.

* Understand that persons who identify as lesbian, gay, bi-sexual, transgender and queer or questioning their sexual identity and 2 Spirt (LGBTQ2S), are often victims of both acute and chronic trauma.

* Realize that members of the LGBTQ2S group are frequently not well understood or treated well by members of the health community.

* Become familiar with treatment guidelines that foster inclusiveness in order to more effectively manage gender assessments.

* Learn to adopt a strategy to develop compassion.

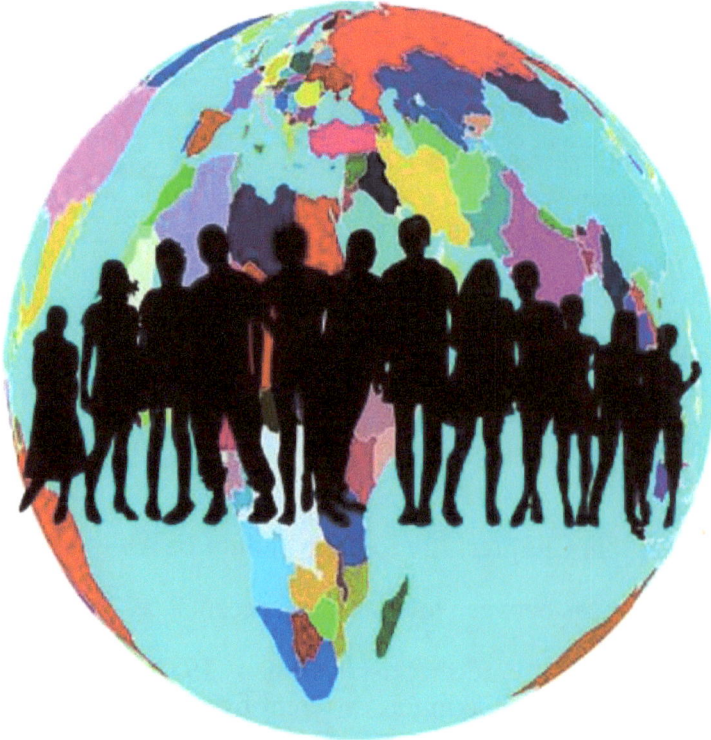

Fig. (10.1). Gender Diversity. Source: www.pixabay.com

GENDER ISSUES IN NURSING

"A healthy, vital society is not one in which we all agree. It is one in which those who disagree can do so with honor and respect for other people's opinions and an appreciation of shared humanity." Marianne Williamson.

The primary goal of the previous Chapter was to inspire nurses to engage in a morally inclusive practice that embraces diversity. The current Chapter is written as an extension of that dialogue and deals with the somewhat sensitive subject matter of ethics, gender and sexual orientation (Fig. **10.1**). The goal is to encourage nurses to move beyond tolerance and to accept and respect life choices that differ from their own. Box **(10:1).** The issue of gender style and ethical decision-making is reviewed. It is pointed out that male ways of approaching moral decision-making may be different from females but not inferior to them. The reasons why Canadian nurses are still primarily women is explored. Nurses are obligated to have a working knowledge of the varying forms of sexual and gender orientation and they are not allowed to discriminate against any individual for any reason. It is pointed out that members who identify as lesbian, gay, bi-sexual, transgender, queer or questioning their sexual identity, or 2 spirit (LGBTQ2S) are often victims of both acute and chronic trauma. They are often not well understood or treated by members of the health community. Nurses are advised to become familiar with treatment guidelines in order to more effectively manage gender assessments. A specific exercise to foster compassion is also recommended. The Chapter ends with a Case in Point: When Coming Out Seems to Cost too much.

BOX 10:1 MOVING BEYOND TOLERANCE (Source: K. Stephany)
Acceptance goes beyond tolerance and although it may not involve agreeing with a person's choices or orientation, it acknowledges that they are valid.

Re-Visiting the Issue of Gender & Ethical Decision-Making

The traditional manner of dealing with ethical issues originated historically with male philosophers and was referred to as an ethic of justice. The **ethic of justice** is objective, rule orientated and based on the idea of fairness (Smolkin, Bourgeois and Findler, 2010). The ethic of care theorist, Gilligan (1982), in her original research, found that when it came to ethical decision-making in nursing, the ethic of justice on its own was insufficient. Her conclusions were based on the fact that the profession of nursing is mostly occupied by women and data that revealed that females, in general, appear to differ from males in what they viewed as most important. Gilligan concluded that, as a group, women tend to focus more on caring, relationships, connectedness and responsibility, which is the essence of the **ethic of care**, and less on algorithms for making decisions. Gilligan was trying to stress that being aware and sensing the needs of others is just as important as applying rules to decision-making (Smolkin *et al.*, 2010; Noddings, 1984). What needs to be emphasized is that although Gilligan viewed male ways of approaching moral decision-making as different from females, she did not consider them to be inferior. Gilligan's primary goal was to emphasize the importance of both perspectives working together. As Botes (2010) stresses, although the ethic of justice and the ethic of care represent polar opposites, if only one of these perspectives is exclusively used in ethical decision-making, then some ethical dilemmas would be unresolved. What is proposed as the best way to attain balance in making moral choices in health care is to ensure that the fair and reasonable treatment of everyone occurs (the ethic of justice), while also guaranteeing that all people are treated in an all-inclusive, contextual and need based manner (the ethic of care) (Botes, 2010). Box **(10:2).** However, Gilligan did believe that nurses should rely a bit more heavily upon the ethic of care when dealing with moral issues because the essence of caring practice is foundational and an intractable part of nursing (Gilligan, 1982; Watson, 2008).

BOX 10:2 BALANCE IN ETHICAL DECISION-MAKING INCLUDES THE ETHIC OF JUSTICE & THE ETHIC OF CARE (as adapted from Botes, 2010)

What is proposed as the best way to attain balance in making ethical decisions in health care is to ensure that the fair and reasonable treatment of everyone occurs (the ethic of justice), while also guaranteeing that all people are treated in an all-inclusive, contextual and need based manner (the ethic of care).

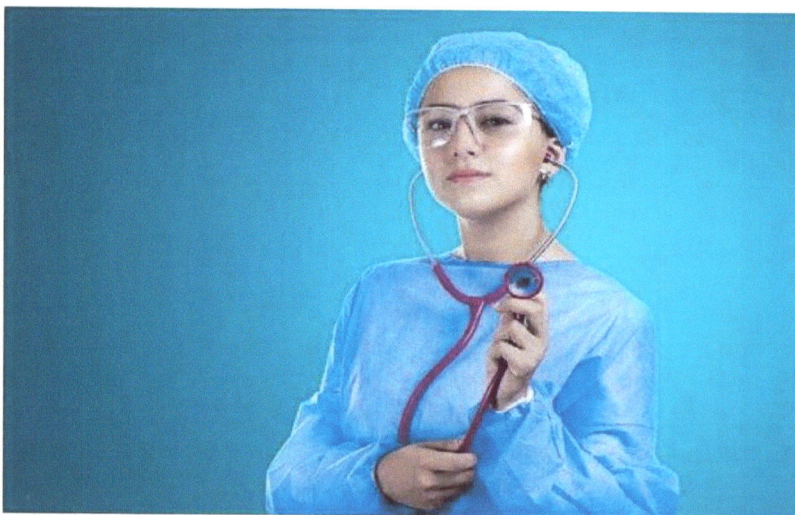

Fig. **(10.2).** Female Nurse. Source: www.pixabay.com

Canadian Nurses are Still Primarily Women: A Historical Perspective

Nursing workforces in both the USA and Canada are still primarily female. In the USA 90% of nurses are female and 10% male (Long, 2018). In Canada the statistics are quite similar with 92% female and 8% male (CNA, 2017) (Fig. **10.2**). Why is nursing still primarily a female dominated profession? The problem of women dominating the profession originates from the time of Florence

Nightingale in the 19th Century. Florence Nightingale believed that there was no room for men in the profession of nursing except, perhaps, on occasions when their physical strength may have proved beneficial (Skretkowicz, 2010). Nevertheless, long before the time of Florence Nightingale, there was a tradition of men as nurses. For example, documentation of men doing the work of caring for the sick goes back as far as 1600 years before Christ (BC) and well into the 2nd Century Common Era (CE) (Kenny, 2008). In the middle ages religious orders employed both males and females to care for the sick. However, during the Crusades, the same monastic orders ensured that their own hospitals were largely run by men because the role was thought to be too dangerous for women (Kelly, 2008). We will now examine a few key reasons why nursing still mostly consists of women followed by a story told by a male nursing student who experienced stereotypical discrimination because of his career choice. Box **(10:3)** & Box **(10:4)**.

BOX 10:3 WHY NURSES ARE STILL PRIMARILY WOMEN (as adapted from Burkhardt, Nathaniel & Walton, 2015; Vera-Jones, 2008).
1. Societal stereotyping of the profession as being best suited for women.
2. Nursing roles and tasks being viewed by the public in general as mostly women's work.
3. Nursing being traditionally associated with a religious call to serve (*e.g.*, nurses as ministering angels).
4. The unsubstantiated assumption that female nurses possess more caring qualities than male nurses do.
5. The perception that all traditional female dominated career choices as lacking in pay parity when compared to male dominated jobs.
6. Males who enter the professional of nursing being automatically viewed as having more feminine *versus* masculine attributes.
7. A fear by heterosexual males of being automatically assumed to be gay.
8. Males being seen as suitable for only very specific areas of nursing (*e.g.*, psychiatry, operating room, and critical care) and excluded from more traditional nursing settings.

BOX 10:4 Narrative: A Male Student Nurse Experiences Discrimination
My name is Jim and I am a student nurse. I was glad that we took time in class to talk about gender issues in nursing. Our group was asked to come up with reasons why we think the profession of nursing was still mostly occupied by women. The other members of my group asked me to share my story. I think that many men are afraid of becoming a nurse because they don't want to be seen as a sissy. I am a big guy. I work out and lift weights to keep in shape for soccer. When I told my soccer buddies that I was becoming a nurse they started to tease me, at first just a little and then it got out of hand, so much so, that I quit playing. They called me a fag and some other nasty stuff. It was so annoying. The worst thing is that for the first time I got a sense of what it must be like to have people hate you because of what they think your sexual orientation is. I am not gay and I have a wife and three children. But it shouldn't matter whether I am gay or not. If I was gay and did professional wrestling for a living they would probably think I was straight. Because I am a man and student nurse, they assume the opposite.

The Rise of Men in Nursing

The good news is that the number of males in nursing is increasing, in fact the numbers have more than tripled since the 1970s (Fig. **10.3**). The financial recession of 2008 also saw a spike of men entering the profession and is slowly increasing since then. Some of the reasons why men now choose nursing as a career include: opportunities for gainful employment due to a shortage of nurses, increased salaries, some flexibility in work schedules, and expanding job prospects (Long, 2018). In order to be better informed about the experiences of men in nursing Long (2018) conducted interviews with three types of male nurses, a male student nurse, a male Emergency Room (ER) nurse and a high-level male nursing executive. Some of the questions posed and their responses are described below.

BOX 10:5 THE EXPERIENCES OF MEN IN NURSING (Long, 2018, p. 8)
What is the biggest challenge of being a man in nursing? **Nursing Student:** The stigma from a female dominated industry, and the idea that I may not have what it takes or not be smart enough to accomplish what women have done extremely well since the beginning of nursing. **ER Nurse:** I wanted to work in the ER as a nurse after I had been a paramedic for many years. I wanted more challenging skills and that was nursing. **Nurse Executive:** I liked the potential for flexibility and opportunity in the medical field without having to go through years of medical school. How is nursing different due to more men now in nursing? **Nursing Student:** I feel that nursing needs men just as the workforce needs women. Diversity isn't such a bad thing when it remains unbiased. **ER Nurse:** Men add different insights and ways of thinking in emergency situations and in medicine and when combined with the way women think, the team is stronger. I'll always be grateful for working with such talented and smart women in nursing. They've taught me a lot. **Nurse Executive:** Men add a new dimension to the field of nursing because we think differently and that can be helpful in discussing new ways of doing things. What advice do you have for men in nursing? **Nursing Student:** Some older female nurses will dismiss you based on your gender. Keep that in mind and focus on what you need to accomplish. Remember that you're not there to please other nurses, you're there to care for people (not patients, people). **ER Nurse:** Come join the party because we need more men in nursing. It's a great profession and you get to work with a lot of great women. **Nurse Executive:** Don't be afraid of being around so many smart and beautiful women.

ACCEPTING SEXUAL & GENDER ORIENTATIONS THAT DIFFER FROM YOUR OWN

"We simply assume that the way we see things is the way they should be. And our attitudes and behaviors grow out of these assumptions." Stephen Covey, American Educator, Author & Keynote Speaker.

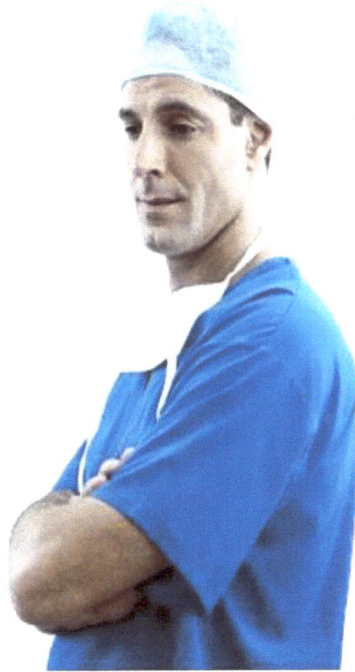

Fig. (10.3). Male Nurse. Source: www.pixabay.com

Sexual Orientation

Sexual orientation can be used to refer to sexual identity, sexual behavior or both. Although progress has been made over the course of the last 40 years, much is still needed to deal more progressively with acts of overt or covert prejudice against individuals because of sexual preference. Nurses are given clear directives by the CNA Code of Ethics (2017a) that they must not discriminate against any individual for any reason. An attitude of **heterosexism** is prohibited, which is the stereotypical bias that assumes that the most preferred and only accepted form of sexual practice is heterosexuality (Kavanagh, 1996). The following is a brief description from Merriam-Webster Dictionary (n.d.) of some of the different sexual orientations that nurses need to be aware of. It is by no means exhaustive.

Heterosexuality: a person attracted to individuals of the opposite sex.

Homosexuality, also referred to as the terms, Lesbian and Gay, is an individual attracted to persons of the same sex.

Bisexuality: a person attracted to both sexes.

Asexuality: the individual is devoid of sexual attraction.

Gender Orientation

Aside from sexual orientation there is gender orientation. While related culturally, sexual and gender orientations are separate phenomena and do not necessarily influence each other. When someone doesn't conform to their original biological gender in some way, they may use the umbrella term "Transgender." **Transgender** can be defined as identifying with a gender that differs from the one which corresponds to the person's sex at birth (Planned Parenthood, n.d.). The way in which transgender persons may describe their identities may differ from person to person. For example, they may refer to themselves in any of the following ways: trans, trans*, trans and gender diverse, trans and gender-no--conforming, and 2 spirit (Lane, 2019). Therefore, it is extremely important to approach persons who identify as different with a sincere desire to refer to them in the term that they prefer (Planned Parenthood, n.d.). For further clarification and understanding, note that **gender non-conforming** is used to refer to persons who do not conform to cultural or social expectations of what is usually associated with their gender (Planned Parenthood, n.d.). **Non-binary** refers to those who do not identify as exclusively masculine or feminine because gender is seen as a spectrum (Lane, 2019). In Canadian culture the term **2-spirit** refers to Indigenous persons who identify as trans, gender diverse or gender-non-conforming. Therefore, the politically correct abbreviation for members from this community is LGBTQ2S.

Box 10:6 LEARNING ACTIVITY: AN EXERCISE IN EMPATHY (as adapted from the Organization for Youth Education about Homophobia, 2003)
1. Break into groups of two. In complete silence, think of the three most fun things that you did this past weekend. Take at least 2 minutes to gather your thoughts. Once you've had a chance to come up with your three favorites things, begin conversing with the individual sitting across from you, without EVER mentioning those three things. Try to maintain a conversation for at least five minutes.
2. Debrief: How did it feel when you could not share what stood out for you as most important, even when you wanted to? Was it easy to maintain a conversation for a full five minutes? Consider how difficult it is for someone who identifies as LGBTQ2S to not be able share their experiences with other people because they fear being judged or worse. Imagine what it would be like to come out. Some people have a difficult time understanding why someone would choose to come out at all. Hopefully this exercise will help you to feel empathy for those who are afraid to be themselves for fear of being judged or rejected.

Trauma & Members of the LGBTQ Community

It is important for nurses to become aware that individuals who identify as LGBTQ2S are often victims of both acute and chronic trauma (National Coalition of Anti-violence Programs, 2014). The most common types of trauma are comprised of hate violence which includes discrimination, domestic abuse and sexual assault (Kudler, Presley & Savage, 2015). When it comes to violence and harassment, members who identify as LGBTQ2S are 2 ½ times more likely to face hate crimes when compared to any other group. Transgender persons are 1.9 times more likely to be targets of physical violence and 3.9 times more likely to be discriminated against by intimate partners (Kudler *et al.*, 2015). Members of the LGBTQ2S group also have a high rate of anxiety, mental illness and suicide. The rates of suicide are quite troubling. For transgender or gender non-conforming individuals the suicide rate is 41% (Kudler *et al.*, 2015). Suicide rates for lesbian, gay or bisexual individuals is 20%; and for the overall LGBTQ2S community it is 4.6% (Kudler *et al.*, 2015). Lane (2019) points out that for trans, gender-diverse and non-binary people suicide risk becomes higher when access to medical gender transition is delayed or restricted.

Trauma Informed Care

Since many members of the LGBTQ2S group are exposed to trauma, it is imperative that nurses incorporate Trauma-informed care (TIC) into their practice when caring for members of this population. As we learned in Chapter Nine, **trauma-informed care** (TIC) is strength based and involves a sincere responsiveness to the full impact of trauma. Healing occurs through non-judgment, the establishment of safety and trust, acknowledging that the trauma has occurred, fostering connectedness, and through empowerment (Hanson & Lang, 2016). Best practices in caring for LGBTQ2S persons who have been traumatized advises that as a caregiver, you do not have to know everything about their experience to be supportive. You need to aim to be respectful, a good listener, to be willing to empathize with their suffering and to be supportive. If you want to know what helps or what they need in terms of care, ask them to tell you (Cornelius & Carrick, 2015; Kudler *et al.*, 2015).

HEALTH CARE, KNOWLEDGE DEFICITS & NEGATIVE ATTITUDES TOWARD LGBTQ2S

"A belief system is nothing more that a thought you've thought over and over again." Dr. Wayne Dyer, American Self-help Author & Motivational Speaker.

Knowledge Deficits Exist

Nurses have an ethical responsibility to be knowledgeable and sensitive to the health care needs of all marginalized or vulnerable groups, which includes those who identify as LGBTQ2S (Cornelius & Carrick, 2015). However, even though 10% of the people in the United States and Canada declare that they are part of the LGBTQ2S group, many health care professionals, including nurses, have insufficient skills in how to best care for them (Fig. **10.4**). The following caregiver knowledge deficits lead to poorer health outcomes for members of this population: unfamiliarity with specific types of presenting health complaints associated with being LGBTQ2S; a lack of understanding or curiosity about the person's fears or their concerns; and a complete unawareness of trauma history, co-occurring mental illness or suicide risk (National Coalition of Anti-violence Programs, 2014).

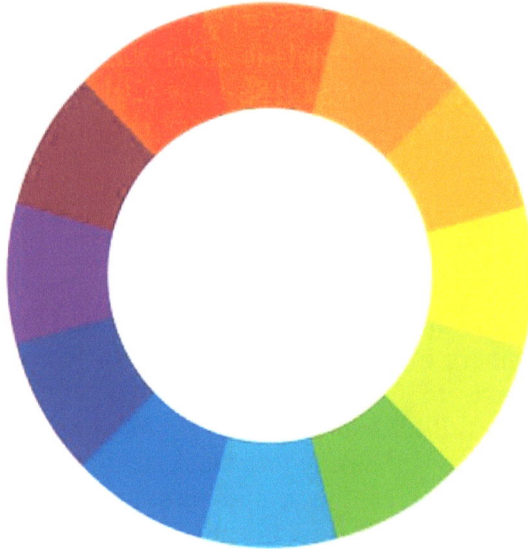

Fig. (10.4). Color Circle Symbol for LGBTQ2S. Source: www.pixabay.com

Disrespectful Attitudes

Knowledge deficits are not the only impediment to persons who identify as LGBTQ2S receiving comprehensive health care. Disrespectful attitudes and inherent biases pose additional barriers. For example, members of the LGBTQ2S community are frequently not treated very respectfully by nurses. How bad are the barriers to health care and discrimination for this group? Research into transgender and non-conforming persons reveal alarming statistics on the seriousness of the barriers to adequate health care. Nineteen percent of persons who identify as LGBTQ2S were refused medical care due to their reported gender status; 28% conveyed that they had been harassed; 50% reported that their caregivers lacked knowledge about their health care needs and 28% did not seek medical care when they needed it because of discrimination (Grant, Mottet & Tanis, 2010 as cited in Cornelius & Carrick 2015).

Education is Needed to Foster Inclusiveness

Due to the existence of gaps in knowledge and the inherent biases that exist, nurses are advised to become familiar with treatment guidelines that foster inclusiveness, and to be more respectfully conducting gender assessments of persons who identify as LGBTQ2S. Studies confirm that student nurses have inadequate knowledge of LGBTQ2S health concerns and often report being uncomfortable when caring for these clients, and they also need additional education specific to this population (Cornelius & Carrick, 2015). It is advisable that the curriculum in schools of nursing ensure that student nurses are taught how to develop LGBTQ2S care plans that include health assessment questions about sexual orientation and preferences, as well as other culturally and gender specific care (Cornelius & Carrick, 2015; Lang, 2019). Learning to employ respectful use of language is also important, as is the implementation of clinical record systems that are more LGBTQ2S inclusive (Lang, 2019).

LEARNING HOW TO ESTEEM THE VIEWS OF OTHERS THAT DIFFER FROM YOUR OWN

"If you change the way you look at things, the things that you look at change."

Dr. Wayne Dyer, American Self-help Author & Motivational Speaker.

A person does not need to agree with another individual's sexual choices, views or gender orientation to respect the person. Ideally, a nurse should always strive to value views that differ from their own. However, often it is fear and a lack of understanding that causes persons to reject others or their way of living. Salzberg (2004) points out that we tend to respond with numbness or complete terror if our hearts are restricted when we are unwilling to accept other ways of living that differ from our own. However, the journey to changing judgment and fear into acceptance and care, begins with a willingness to want to understand. Subsequently, we need to make it our intention to try to imagine the world as the other views it (Salzberg, 2004).

Chopra (2005) advises that we can begin to build bridges when we see others as a part of us rather than as us *versus* them. No one is your enemy. Any person that we disagree with, whether it is a belief system or life choice, is just another human being with a difference of opinion. They are still human just like us and they are worthy of respectful consideration. To help foster tolerance, acceptance and compassion, contemplate doing the following exercise, *Developing Concern for Others,* by the Dalai Lama. Box **(10:7)**.

Question Pertaining to the Case in Point

1. Do you agree with the student's perspective that teaching tolerance and acceptance is futile? Why or why not?

2. If teaching tolerance and acceptance is not the best way to change strong biases, what else can be done?

BOX 10:7 Developing Concern for Others by the Dalai Lama (Hopkins, 2002, p. 93)

1. Develop a disciplined attitude of true other concern, in which you cherish others more than yourself.
2. Care about others always.
3. If you cannot help than do no harm.
4. Remind yourself daily, that true heartfelt caring does no harm to anyone, temporarily or in the long run.
5. Practice compassion, which is identifying with the suffering of another, for it is a priceless jewel.

BOX 10:8 CASE IN POINT: WHEN COMING OUT SEEMS TO COST TOO MUCH

Note: The following story is derived from an email that was sent to a nursing instructor.

I want to thank-you for your lecture on the importance of nurses not judging others concerning their sexual orientation. But I have some stuff to share with you so you can better understand what it is really like to live a life where you must hide who you really are. It is all good and fine for you to try and teach tolerance, but can it be taught to nurses who learned to hate certain people when they were growing up? Student nurses sometimes agree with their instructor so they can pass the course, but inside they feel differently and outside the classroom they act differently too. I know because I have seen it all before. Some of my former classmates have been really mean to students who openly admit that they have different sexual preferences than the status quo. I am not straight but no one would know it. I carefully hide my sexual orientation by the way that I dress and act. I pretend that I am not who I am because if the truth came out my life as I know it would end. My family openly preaches that they hate gay people, even though I think that my father has some homosexual tendencies. But if I ever come out they will disown me and that would be the end of me. I don't know what the answer is, but I don't think you can teach people to be open-minded when they are not. Sorry for being so down and pessimistic. I hope that someday I will feel different.

REFLECTING BACK

Summary of Key Points Covered in Chapter 10

* It was proposed that ethical decision-making in nursing is best made from both an ethic of justice and ethic of care perspective. However, it is highly recommended by Gilligan (1982) that nurses should rely a bit more heavily upon the ethic of care.

* The profession of nursing is still primarily comprised of women. For example, in both the USA and Canada greater that 90% of the nursing workforce is staffed by women.

* Some reasons why Canadian nurses as still women include that, the profession is thought to be best suited for women and women's work; nursing has been associated as a religious calling; female caring is viewed as superior to male caring; the perception of a lack pay parity; males automatically assumed as

feminine in nature or gay; and men seen as only suitable for specific areas of nursing.

* The good news is that the number of males in nursing is on the rise, in fact the numbers have more than tripled since the 1970s and keep growing.

* Unfortunately, those who identify as lesbian, gay, bi-sexual, transgender, queer or questioning their sexual identity, and 2 spirit (LGBTQ2S) are frequently not well understood or treated well by members of the health community.

* Nurses are advised to become familiar with treatment guidelines that foster inclusiveness and to obtain better experience in managing gender assessments.

* We were also made aware that members of the LGBTQ2S community are often victims of both acute and chronic trauma. Subsequently nurses are strongly advised to utilize the tools associated with trauma-informed practice when caring for these clients.

* Nurses need to learn to value and respect views that differ from their own. Subsequently, the following exercises was recommended to foster compassion, *Developing Concern for Others* by the Dalai Lama.

SOMETHING TO PONDER

1. Debate the merits *versus* the downside of relying on both the ethic of justice and the ethic of care when dealing with moral decision-making in nursing practice.

2. Given the fact that nurses in Canada are still largely female, what can be done to recruit more men into the profession?

CLASSROOM GROUP EXERCISE

1. Do a White Board brain-storming session. In addition to what was suggested in the Chapter, identify alternative strategies that can be used to develop genuine understanding and concern for others who are different than us?

ON YOUR OWN

1. Journal about your own biases concerning sexual or gender orientation. Write about your preconceived views and intentionally challenge them. Remember to remind yourself that a belief is simply something that you assume to be true. It does not necessarily reflect reality.

2. If you experience fear or judgment toward a specific person or group, consider

performing the strategy suggested by the Dalai Lama.

CONSENT FOR PUBLICATION

Not applicable.

CONFLICT OF INTEREST

The authors confirm that this chapter contents have no conflict of interest.

ACKNOWLEDGEMENTS

Declared none.

REFERENCES

Botes, A (2000) A comparison between the ethics of justice and the ethics of care. *J Adv Nurs,* 32, 1071-5. [http://dx.doi.org/10.1046/j.1365-2648.2000.01576.x] [PMID: 11114990]

Burkhardt, MA, Nathaniel, AK & Walton, NA (2015) Ethics and issues in contemporary nursing. Second Canadian EditionNelson Education Limited, Toronto, Ontario.

Canadian Nurses Association. (2017). *Registered nurse profile (including nurse practitioners) in Canada.* Retrieved from: https://www.cna-aiic.ca/en/nursing-practice/the-practice-of-nursing/health-human-resources/nursing-statistics/canada

Chopra, D (2005) *Peace is the way.*Three Rivers Press, USA.

Cornelius, JB & Carrick, J (2015) A survey of nursing students' knowledge of and attitudes toward LGBT health care concerns. *Nurs Educ Perspect,* 36, 176-178. [http://dx.doi.org/10.5480/13-1223]

Gilligan, C (1982) *In a different voice: Psychological theory and women's development.*

Hanson, RF & Lang, J (2016) *A critical look at trauma-informed care among agencies and systems serving maltreated youth and their families*https://journals.sagepub.com/doi/abs/10.1177/1077559516635274 [http://dx.doi.org/10.1177/1077559516635274]

Hopkins, J (2002). *How to practice: The way to a meaningful life (his holiness the Dalai Lama).*Atria Books, Toronto.

Kavanagh, K (1996) Social and cultural dimensions of health and health care. In (Eds.) *Conceptual foundations of nursing practice*   Mosby, USA 285-308.

Kenny, PE (2008) Men in nursing – A history of caring and contribution to the profession (Part I). *Pa Nurse,* 63, 3-5. [Retrieved from]. https://0-web-b-ebscohost-com.orca.douglascollege.ca/ehost/pdfviewer/pdfviewer?vid=11&sid=da480039-83a0-43a7-b3db-58fec1c9bd3e%40pdc-v-sessmgr05

Kudler, B, Presley, C & Savage, M (2015) Trauma-Informed care: Addressing mental health risk factors. *Advancing Excellence in Transgender Care* Retrieved from: http://www.lgbthealtheducation.org /wp-content/uploads/Trauma-Informed-Care.pdf

Lane, R (2019) Developing inclusive primary care for trans, gender-diverse and nonbinary people. *Canadian Medical Association Journal (CMAJ),* 61, 14-6. [http://dx.doi.org/10.1503/cmaj.190011] [PMID: 30665974]

Long, T (2018) The rise of men in nursing. *Nevada RN Information,* 27, 8. Retrieved from: https://0-web-b-ebscohost-com.orca.douglascollege.ca/ehost/pdfviewer/pdfviewer?vid=7&sid=a3d4fe1e-6918-45c2-aba8-010e4532282d%40sessionmgr102

Merriam-Webster Dictionary. (n.d.). Retrieved from: https://www.merriam-webster.com/

McCormick, A, Scheyd, K & Terrazas, S (April 17, 2018). Trauma-Informed care and LGTBTQ youth: Considerations for advancing practice with youth with trauma experiences. *Families in Society: The Journal of Contemporary Social Services.* Retrieved from: https://journals.sagepub.com/doi/10.1177/1044389418768550

National Coalition of Anti-violence Programs (NCAP). (2014). Lesbian, Gay, Bisexual, Transgender, Queer, and HIV-Affected: Hate Violence (2014 Release Edition). Retrieved from: https://avp.org/wp-content/uploads/2017/04/2013_ncavp_hvreport_final.pdf

Noddings, N (1984) *Caring: A feminine approach to ethics and moral education.*University of California Press, Berkeley.

Organization for Youth Education about Homophobia. (2003). Workshop presentation manual. Langley, BC: Author. Planned Parenthood (n.d.). What are the appropriate labels for transgender people? Retrieved from: https://www.plannedparenthood.org/learn/sexual-orientation-gender/trans-and-gender-nonconfo-ming-identities/transgender-identity-terms-and-labels

Salzberg, S (2004) *Lovingkindness: The revolutionary art of happiness.*Shambala, London.

Skretkowicz, V (2010). *Florence Nightingale's notes on nursing and notes on nursing for the laboring classes: Commemorative edition with historical commentary.*Springer, New York.

Smolkin, D, Bourgeois, W & Findler, P (2010) *Debating health care ethics.*McGraw-Hill Ryerson, Canada.

Vere-Jones, E (2008) Why are there so few men in nursing? *Nurs Times,* 104, 18-9. [PMID: 18411991]

Watson, J (2008) Nursing: The philosophy of caring (Revised edition). Boulder, Colorado: University Press of Colorado.

The Role of Religion & Spirituality in Nursing: Respecting What the Client Believes

Abstract: The aim of Chapter eleven is to encourage nurses to work with their client's religious and spiritual values and not to discriminate when they differ from their own. The desire to believe in God or something beyond the physical is deemed universal. Theology, religion and spirituality are an integral part of the search for something more and what most religious and spiritual beliefs share is the notion that there is more to life than physical existence. The profession of nursing has a long and enduring history of a close association with spirituality and nursing has often been referred to as a mission or calling. It is argued that religious practices are still valid for present day nursing. The Canadian Nurses Association (CNA) supports this stand and recognizes parish nursing as valid. The ethic of care can be viewed as a means to spiritual connection because, like religion, spirituality values the relationship between people and all that exists in life. Nurses are also strongly encouraged to consider implementing transcultural caring guidelines for spirituality into their practice. The Chapter ends with a Case in Point: When a practicing Christian is assigned to care for an Atheist.

Keywords: Atheism, Ethic of care, Parish nurse, Religion, Spirituality, Theology.

LEARNING GUIDE

After Completing this Chapter, the Reader Should be Able to

* Be reminded that although nurses have the right to follow their own personal set of values, they cannot force their religious beliefs onto their clients.

* Become aware that although theology, religion and spirituality share many things in common, they are not exactly the same.

* Explain how the subject of spirituality is still relevant for nursing and how it is linked to the ethic of care.

* Draw a connection between spirituality and the ethic of care.

* Learn how to honour clients' religious and/or spiritual beliefs.

* Consider implementing transcultural caring guidelines for spirituality into practice.

* Apply what was learned to the Case in Point: When a Practicing Christian Nurse is Assigned to Care for an Atheist.

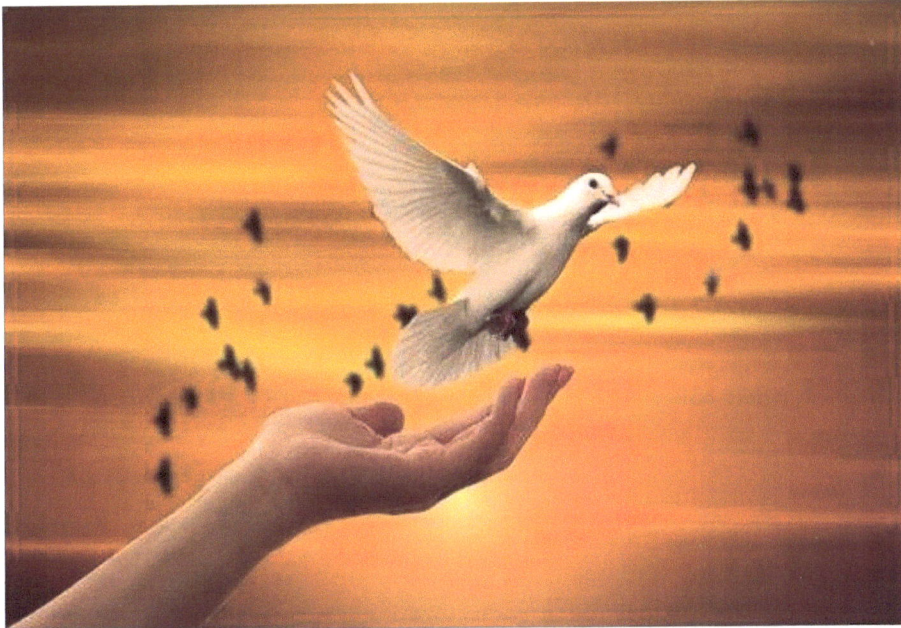

Fig. (11.1). The Dove & Symbol for Spirituality. Source: www.pixabay.com

RELIGION & SPIRITUALITY IN NURSING

"Regardless of whether one is conscious of one's own philosophy and value system, it is affecting the encounters, relationships, and moments we have with our self and others." Jean Watson, American Nurse, Author, Professor & Care Theorist.

The importance of embracing diversity was first formally introduced in Chapter Nine, expanded upon in Chapter Ten and continues in Chapter Eleven. In Chapter Four the values clarification process was introduced. Identifying what matters to nurses and clients and respecting the differences was declared to be the purpose of values clarification. It was also advised that, although nurses have the right to follow their own personal set of values, they cannot force what they believe onto their clients. This moral directive stands for all personal values including those that pertain to religion and spirituality. Subsequently, the goal of this Chapter is to encourage nurses to respect their client's religious and spiritual values and not discriminate when their views differ from their own.

The desire to believe in God or something beyond the physical is deemed universal. What most religious and spiritual beliefs share is the notion that there is more to life than physical existence. The profession of nursing has a long and enduring history of a close association with spirituality and nursing has often been referred to as a mission or calling. It is argued that religious practices are still valid for present day nursing. The Canadian Nurses Association (CNA) supports this stand and recognizes parish nursing as valid. It is strongly suggested that nurses consider implementing transcultural caring guidelines for spirituality into their practice. The Chapter ends with a Case in Point: When a practicing Christian is assigned to care for an Atheist.

Theology, Religion & Spirituality: How are they Similar & Different?

"Though we may differ greatly in how, who and what we worship, the basic code of behavior is common to all. It is this common denominator which binds us together in humanity and has helped us to continue to grow and survive." Leo Buscaglia, Psychologist, Author and Teacher

The longing to identify with something beyond the physical in life is one of the most significant quests of the human condition. Historically, the desire to come to understand God, to believe and have faith in something beyond our physical, no matter what you name it, is universal (Moorhouse, 2008). Theology, religion and spirituality are integral parts of the search for something more. However, even though they have much in common there are some distinct differences between them (Fig. **11.2**).

Theology is the study of the transcendent and supernatural, often referred to as God and includes the study of all religions and topics relevant to spirituality (Ray, 2016). **Religion** goes beyond studying the super-natural and at the heart of every **religion** is the worship of a greater power or a being outside of the individual person, such as God or deity. It also involves the following of sacred texts or a book of laws and rules and emphasizes prayer, service, and earning your place in the afterlife (Watson, 2008; Burkhardt, Nathaniel & Walton, 2015; Stanford, 2010). Religion has traditionally brought a sense of comfort to people living in times of great turmoil and fear. It is believed by some that religion has the purpose of creating order from chaos and gives humanity a code and rules to live by (Levine, 2003).

While theology involves studying the supernatural and religion focuses on the worship of something outside of ourselves such as God, **spirituality** concentrates more on the energy within the individual and the connection with an animating energy force that permeates every aspect of life (Ray, 2016; Watson, 2008). The use of silence, meditation, mindfulness and solitude are deemed important aspects of spirituality (Ray, 2016; Miller-Tiedeman, 1999). Despite their differences, there is considerable overlap between theology, religion and spirituality. Theology studies both religion and spiritual beliefs and many religions also practice activity normally associated with spirituality. Both the religious and spiritual life consist of a journey of the soul reaching out to a universal source for guidance and sustenance.

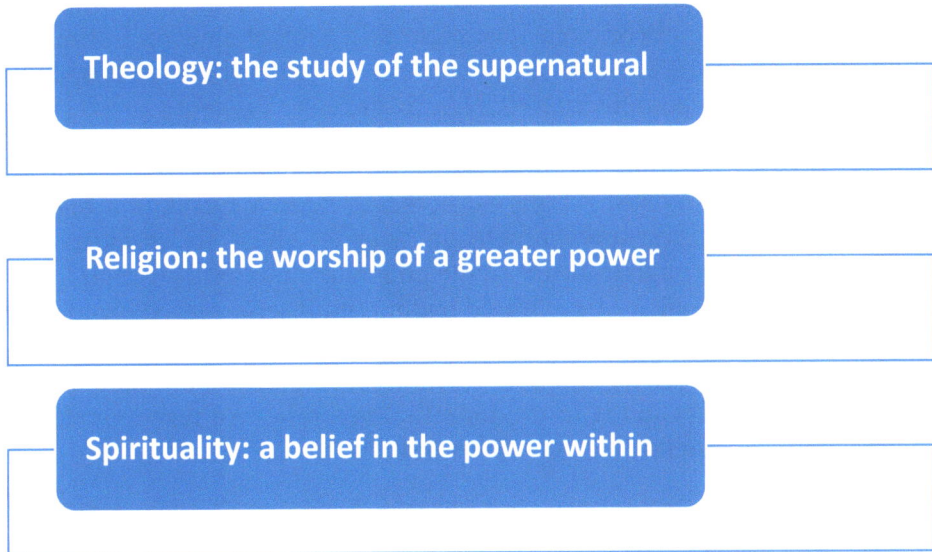

Theology: the study of the supernatural

Religion: the worship of a greater power

Spirituality: a belief in the power within

Fig. (11.2). Theology, Religion & Spirituality. Source: K. Stephany.

Spirituality & Nursing: Is it Still Important Today?

Religion and spirituality are universal human experiences that transcend culture, although they may be colored and shaped by cultural experiences (Burkhardt *et al.*, 2015). Even though the various religious faiths differ somewhat in how, who and what they worship, they agree that there is more to life than physical existence (Buscaglia, 1982). Box **(11:1).**

BOX 11:1 WHAT ALL RELIGIONS HAVE IN COMMON (Buscaglia, 1982)
Even though the various religious faiths differ somewhat in how, who and what they worship, they agree that there is more to life than physical existence

The profession of nurse has a long and enduring history of a close association with spirituality and nursing has often been referred to as a religious mission or a call to serve. (Burkhardt *et al.*, 2015). In fact, the word "nurse" is derived from Greek which means nurturing of the human spirit (Seidi, 1993). Florence

Nightingale believed that nurses help people to be in the right spiritual condition so that nature can work together with their soul state to help heal them (MacDonald, 2010).

The CNA (2017) Code of Ethics advises that nurses respect religious and spiritual choice in the same way that they do any other form of diversity. The CNA (2011)*Position Statement on Spirituality, Health and Nursing Practice*, asserts that recognition of a client's spirituality is an integral dimension of holistic care and deemed to be a crucial component of culturally competent care. For instance, sensitivity to and reverence for spiritual beliefs, preferences and needs are recognized as required competences (CNA, 2011).

The CNA (2011)*Position Statement on Spirituality, Health and Nursing Practice* also acknowledges the role of the parish nurse. A **parish nurse** is a registered nurse with specialized spiritual knowledge who is called to promote health, healing and wellness through ministry to the clients in their care (Webster, 2016). They serve many roles such as health educators, counsellors and advocates for spirituality (Webster, 2016). The CNA also accepts The Canadian Association for Parish Nursing Ministry (CAPNM) as a legitimate component of nursing practice. The CAPNM's (2019) vision is to promote the integration of religious devotion and health within diverse faith communities throughout Canada.

The Ethic of Care & Spirituality

"Caring itself is coexistent with suffering. In times of illness, dying and death, professional and lay caregivers feel, through compassion, the pain of the others." Author Unknown.

The ethic of care can be viewed as a means to spiritual connection because, like religion, spirituality values the relationship between people and all that exists in life (Ray, 2016; Watson, 2008). The nurse is called to care for the whole person, not just the body and mind but also to tend to the human soul (Watson, 2008). Burkhardt *et el.,* (2015) asserts that the nurse must recognize all three levels of a person, body, mind and spirit. Other theorists maintain that as nurses engage in caring in general and spiritual care practices in particular, the bonds of common humanity are strengthened (Ray, 2016; Watson, 2008; Miller-Tiedeman, 1999). The practice of compassion and mercy is also viewed by the ethic of care to be as crucial as any other duty-based response from the nurse and compassion or identifying with the suffering of other, illuminates the spiritual in all of us (Watson, 2008; Ray 2016).

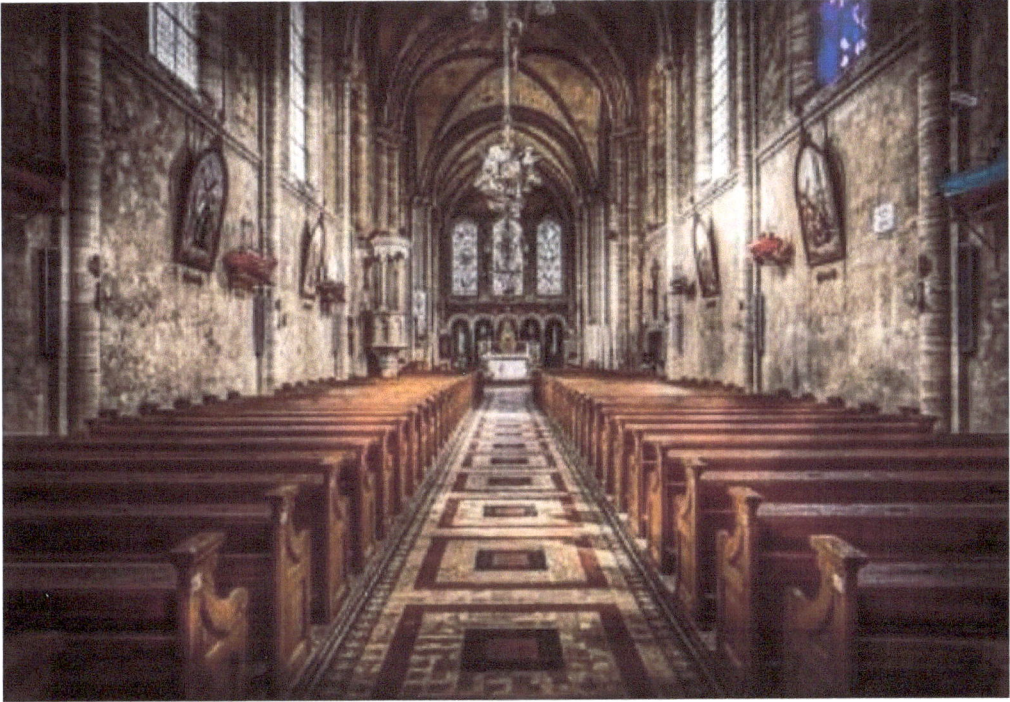

Fig. (11.3). Christian Church. Source: www.pixabay.com

DEALING WITH LOSS & DEATH: THE ROLE OF FAITH

Having faith in a religion can be helpful when circumstances drastically change or tragedy strikes and when people experience stressful times they often turn to religion or spirituality, even if they are non-believers (Levine, 2003). This is especially true when a person is suddenly confronted with loss or the prospect of death, either their own death or that of a loved one. As a former critical care nurse and Coroner I have witnessed many individuals turn to religion because the thought of life ending, or never expecting to see their family again, is unbearable. Kuhl (2003) is a Canadian palliative care physician and he points out that, facing death, and the fear and anxiety that accompanies it is a part of the experience of being human. Yet, although much has been accomplished to address the physical pain suffered by those with a terminal illness, Western medicine has been slow to understand or accept the psychological and painful distress that comes with knowing that death is near (Kuhl, 2003). The following story is about a woman, who shares her story that as her death was fast approaching she reignited with her faith in God. Box **(11:2).**

BOX 11:2 Narrative: Being Reunited with My Faith
I was in complete shock. I could barely hear the words, *"I am so sorry to have to tell you this but you are dying and there is nothing else that we can do."* The words, *"You are dying,"* seemed surreal and distant to me, as though the doctor was speaking to someone else. After all, death happened to old people, not to me, and I was completely convinced that they had gotten all of the cancer from my bowels or that the chemotherapy would somehow work. I thought that it was just a bad dream that I could wake up from, and everything would be okay, but that was not the case. I was only 38 years old, never smoked, barely drank alcohol and I took really good care of myself, yet I developed colon cancer and it was going to kill me. At first I pretended that I had never been told that I was dying but that didn't last very long. The constant tiredness and abdominal pain reminded me that the end was near, I became angry and miserable. What did I do to deserve this punishment? Days of rage and anger were soon replaced with an overwhelming sense of sadness, hopelessness and buckets of tears. I didn't know that a peson could cry that much. I was mortal after all. Even if they some how came up with a miracle treatment, I was still looking face to face into the mirror of death. We are all going to die no matter how hard we try to convince ourselves otherwise. That was when I started to spend a great deal of time thinking about God. I returned to my Babtist upbringing, the religious roots that I had so often shunned and ridiculed as irrelevant for almost my whole adult life. I started to read the Bible, and began to pray again. Suddenly I desperately needed to know that I would live beyond death, that I would be waiting in heven for my family to join me someday. In some ways I felt a bit better. I was less terrified even though I still had sad moments. I learned to pray to a God that I believed was listening and it helped.

HONOURING YOUR CLIENT'S FAITH

"Why not let people differ about their answers to the great mysteries of the Universe? Let each seek one's own way to the highest, to one's sense of supreme loyalty in life, one's ideal life, let each philosophy, each world-view bring forth its truth and beauty to a larger perspective, that people may grow in vision, statue and dedication." Algeron Black, Leader of Ethical Culture & Defender of Social Justice.

It is beyond the scope of this textbook or knowledge base of the author to even attempt to educate others about the various religious or spiritual traditions. Nurses are encouraged to examine the sacred books and literature on their own or consider asking their clients to educate them about what they believe. As stated at the onset, the key aim of this Chapter is to encourage nurses to work with their clients' religious or spiritual values and not to discriminate when they differ from their own. The good news is that nurses can succeed in this task by implementing the following six transcultural caring guidelines for spirituality into their practice. Box **(11:3)**.

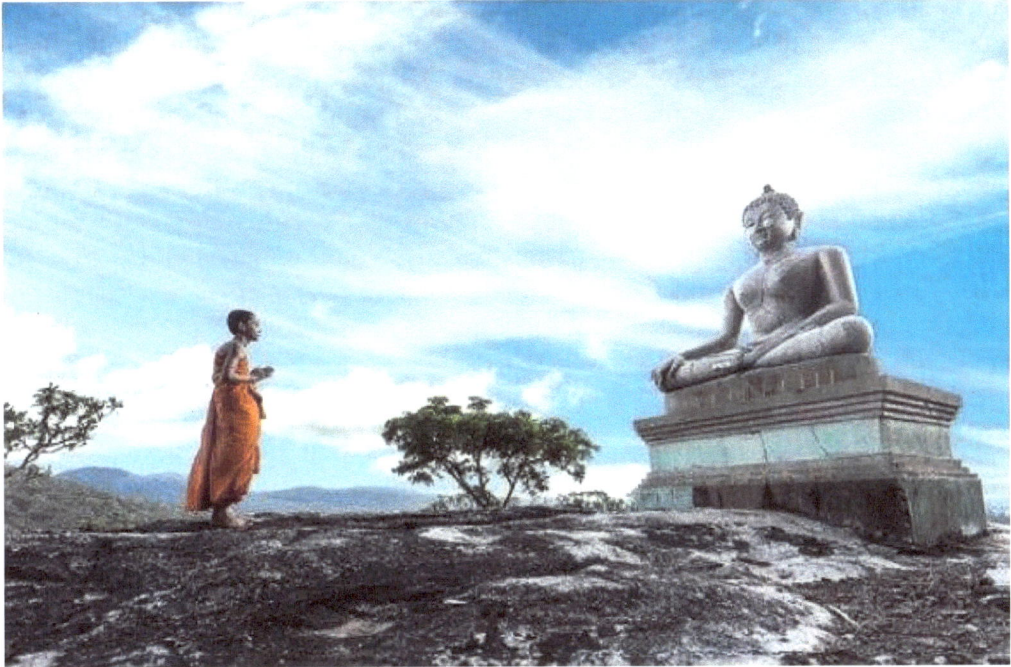

Fig. (11.4). Buddhism. Source: www.pixabay.com

BOX 11:3 Transcultural Caring Guidelines for Spirituality (as adapted from Ray, 2016)
1. Set your intention on respecting everyone, not just some people but all people, no matter what color of skin, creed or culture.
2. Be open to and respectful of, all religious/spiritual beliefs.
3. Seek to embrace and understand the meaning of moral and spiritual development in self and in others.
4. Be accountable to, and responsible for, helping others in any way that you can, regardless of their religious or spiritual values.
5. Uphold all human rights and freedoms.
6. Be involved in designing and implementing nursing care plans that facilitate choices and that improve the life of persons from all religions or spiritual premises.

WHAT TO DO WHEN YOUR CLIENT IS A NON-BELIEVER

When confronted with illness and suffering people may become confused and they may experience a spiritual struggle between faith and hope. Their spiritual beliefs may increase or decrease depending on the emotions that they are experiencing (Ray, 2016). What is a nurse to do when their client does not believe in anything or declares that they are an atheist? Atheism must be respected. It is a term that is derived from Greek with the "a" standing for "without" and the "theism" means "belief in God" (Stanford, 2010). The definition of **atheism** is essentially a denial in the existence of God or gods or any spiritual being outside of the human experience (Merriam-Webster Dictionary, n.d.). Stanford (2010) points out that originally atheism was considered to be a rejection of religion but now Western scientific, secular philosophies considers it to be a religion of its own. As a practicing nurse, whether you are a religious or spiritual person or you are not, the rule of ethical advice is that you must work with your client's faith or their lack of faith. This directive applies because you are mandated by the CNA (2017) Code of Ethics not to discriminate for any reason. It is also a relevant directive because it is the caring, compassionate approach to what really matters to the client who is the center (Ray, 2016).

As a nurse, therapist and Coroner I always worked with the client's values. If the individual who was sitting in front of me was talking about how devastated they were feeling about a recent loss, I would pose the question, *"Do you have any religious or spiritual beliefs that would help you through this difficult time?"* If they said yes, I would ask them who or what group I could contact for spiritual help. If their answer was, *"I don't believe in anything,"* I would connect them to whatever supportive network may help them through their situation (*e.g.*, family, friends, support groups and/or therapist) (Fig. **11.5**).

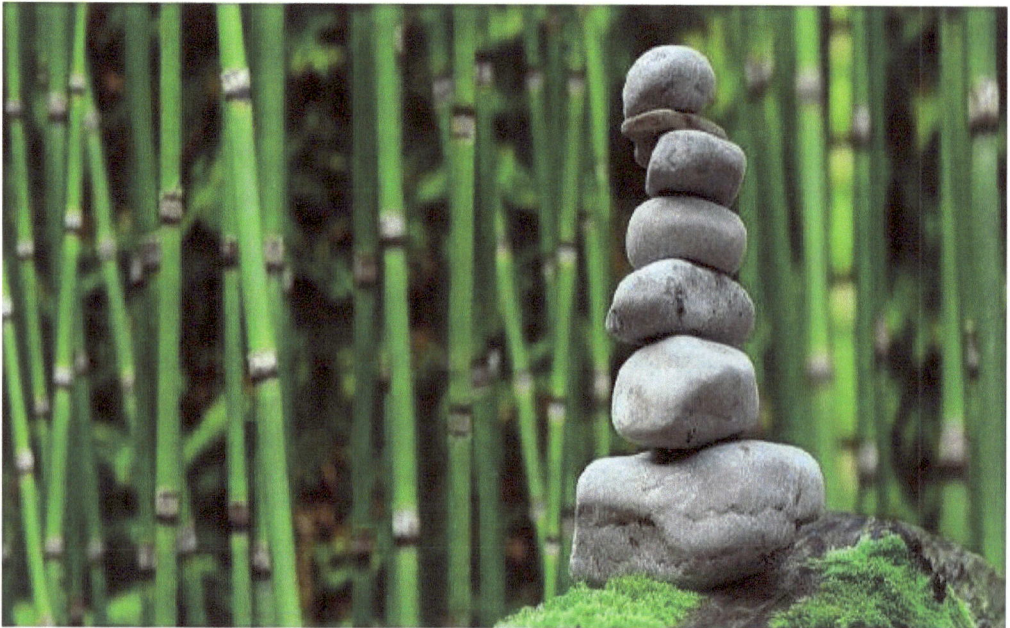

Fig. (11.5). Zen Garden. Source: www.pixabay.com

BOX 11:4 CASE IN POINT: WHEN A PRACTICING CHRISTIAN NURSE IS ASSIGNED TO CARE FOR AN ATHEIST
May is 21 years old and graduated as a registered nurse with distinction from a Canadian nursing school that was Christian based. In fact, Mary chose this particular school because it had a good academic reputation and the curriculum also aligned well with her religious beliefs. Mary was working on her first job when she experienced an existential crisis. She was assigned to care for Mrs. Brown who was dying from renal failure secondary to a long history of poorly controlled diabetes. Mary noticed that on Mrs. Brown's admission form she did not have any religious affiliation written down. Mary asked Mrs. Brown if she wanted any spiritual care. Mrs. Brown's reaction startled Mary. Her patient got very angry at her for even asking. Mrs. Brown yelled out, *"Where was God when I lost my twin daughters and where is he now? Leave me alone."* Mary obliged and left the room in a hurry. Although she felt terrible for her patient, she didn't know what she could do to help her. Mrs. Brown had no close family and she seemed so alone, yet Mary avoided her as much as she could for the rest of the shift. Mary went home after her shift ended. However, she couldn't stop thinking about Mrs. Brown. Mary was sure that is Mrs. Brown didn't believe in God she would likely go to Hell once she died. Mary said a prayer for her patient and eventually fell asleep. The next morning when Mary arrived to work she learned that Mrs. Brown had passed away during the night shift. Mary felt extremely sad and couldn't stop thinking that there must have been something else she could have done to help her patient. Mary was having difficulty sorting through her feelings. Because Mary was new to the ward and didn't know any of the other nurses that well, she kept quiet and suffered in silence.

Questions Pertaining to the Case in Point

1. Is there anything more that Mary could have done that would have helped Mrs. Brown through the process of dying?

2. What should Mary do to ensure that she is able to sort through her emotional and spiritual anger?

3. If you were a senior nurse working with Mary what kind of things could you recommend that would help her through this situation?

REFLECTING BACK

Summary of Key Points Covered in Chapter 11

* The goal of this Chapter is to encourage nurses to respect their client's religious and spiritual values and not discriminate when their views differ from their own.

* The desire to believe in God or something beyond the physical was deemed universal.

* Theology, religion and spirituality are integral parts of the search for something more. However, even though they have much in common they are not one and the same.

* What most religious and spiritual beliefs share is the notion that there is more to

life than physical existence.

* The profession of nursing has a long and enduring history of a close association with spirituality and religion and nursing has often been referred to as a religious mission or calling.

* It was argued that religion and spiritual practice are still valid for present day nursing and the CNA supports this stand.

* The CNA also recognizes parish nursing as valid.

* Religion and spirituality align well with the ethic of care and the emphasis on the relationships between people and all that exists.

* It was determined that religion and spirituality may offer comfort when a person is dealing with loss or death.

* It was beyond the scope of this book to examine the various world religions or spiritual traditions. Nurses are encouraged to examine the sacred texts on their own to become more understanding of their client's religious beliefs and practices

* Six guidelines from transcultural nursing were put forward as a way for nurses to learn to respect their clients' religious values.

* The idea that atheism is a belief that is worthy of being respected was also discussed.

SOMETHING TO PONDER

1. Do religious or spiritual values influence how a person approaches health? Yes or No? Support your point of view with evidence.

2. Does learning about different spiritual practices help you to be more effective as a nurse?

3. Consider spending some time reflecting on your own ideas about life and death and the greater meaning of things. You need to know what you believe if you are going to be effective with your clients.

4. As a nurse you may be confronted with issues that will test your faith. If this happens to you, what will you do to ensure that you will be okay?

5. Do you think that spiritual healing is a relevant part of the profession of nursing? Why or why not?

CLASSROOM GROUP EXERCISES

1. It was argued that theology, religion and spirituality have some things in common and other aspects that differ. As an open class discussion or in small groups, expand on this discussion.

ON YOUR OWN

1. The controversial subject of war and violence in the name of religion was not explored in this Chapter. How can human beings change this sad reality and what role can nurses play? Spend some time thinking and reflecting on constructive but caring ways to begin to end this trend.

2. Consider researching and writing a paper or doing a presentation on a religious or spiritual following hat differs from your own. Make sure that you read the original sacred books or documents, because sometimes secondary sources may miss key aspects that are important. After completing the project ask yourself these questions, *"What did I learn? Were any of my preconceived assumptions challenged?"*

Recommended Readings

Chopra, D. (2000). *How to know God: The soul's journey into the mystery of mysteries.* New York: Harmony Books.

His Holiness the Dalai Lama (2010). *Toward a true kingship of faiths: How the world'sreligions can come together.* New York: Doubleday Religion.

Salzberg, S. (2002). *Faith: Trusting your own deepest experience.* New York: Riverhead

Books. Stanford, P. S. (2010). *Religion: 50 ideas you really need to know about religion.* United Kingdom: Chartwell Books.

Web Resource

Web Resource: World Religions Web Resources. Index to sites covering a broad range of religious topics and religious studies. https://marymount.libguides.com/c.php?g=271944&p=1813434

CONSENT FOR PUBLICATION

Not applicable.

CONFLICT OF INTEREST

The authors confirm that this chapter contents have no conflict of interest.

ACKNOWLEDGEMENTS

Declared none.

REFERENCES

Atheism.(n.d.). In Merriam-Webster Dictionary.com. Retrieved from: https://www.merriam-webster.com/dictionary/atheism

Burkhardt, MA, Nathaniel, AK & Walton, NA (2015) *Ethics and issues in contemporary nursing* Nelson Education Limited., Toronto, Ontario.

Buscaglia, LF (1982) *Personhood: The art of being fully human.* Ballantine Books, USA.

Canadian Association for Parish Nursing Ministry (CAPNM) (2019). Mission, vision,role and guiding principles. Retrieved from: http://www.capnm.ca/

Canadian Nurses Association (CNA). (2011). The CNA Position Statement on spirituality, health and nursing practice. Ottawa: Author. Retrieved from: http://pnig.rnao.ca/ news/2011/02/25/cna-position-stateme-t-spirituality-health-and-nursing-practice

Canadian Nurses Association (CNA) (2017) *CNA Code of Ethics for Registered Nurses* Author, Ottawa.

Kuhl, D (2003) *What dying people want: Practical wisdom for the end of life.* Anchor Canada, Canada.

Levine, M (2003) *Seven lessons from Noah's ark: How to survive a flood in your own life.* Celestial Art Publishing, Toronto.

McDonald, L (2010) *Florence Nightingale at first hand.* Wilfred Laurier University Press, Canada.

Miller-Tiedeman, A (1999) *Learning, practicing, and living the new careering.* Taylor & Francis Group, USA.

Morehouse, D (2008) *Remote viewing.* Sounds True Inc., Canada.

Perlman, HH (1979) *Relationship: The heart of helping people.* The University of Chicago Press, Chicago.

Ray, M (2016) Transcultural caring dynamic in nursing and health care, 2nd ed. F. A. Davis Company, Philadelphia, PA.

Stanford, PS (2010) *Religion: 50 ideas you really need to know about religion.* Chartwell Books, United Kingdom.

Watson, J (2008) Nursing: The philosophy of caring. Revised edition University Press of Colorado, Boulder, Colorado.

Webster, AM (2016). Foundations in parish nursing: Bringing the healing love of Christ to those we serve. (Ed.) Institute for Ongoing Formation at St. Peter's Seminary, London, Ontario.

CHAPTER 12

Ethical Nursing Leadership for the 21ˢᵗ Century: The Importance of Being the Change

Abstract: Ethical leaders ensure that moral conduct is a standard expectation for people in positions of power and Chapter twelve introduces ethical leadership as the new way of leading for nurses. Many people have ingrained beliefs as to what leadership consists of. Therefore, the Chapter begins with an overview of the five most common myths of leadership. An explanation is given as to why the topic of ethical leadership has become popular in recent years. Ethical leadership has four key aims. It brings the person back into focus, it encourages organizations to invest in human potential as a valuable resource, it pursues greater social justice, and it makes protecting the environment a priority. It is argued that ethical nurse leaders are needed because the 21ˢᵗ Century presents unique challenges for the nursing profession. The association between ethical nursing leadership and the ethic of care is explained and nurses are inspired to take on the challenge of being agents for change. In the Case in Point a student nurse recounts a leadership strategy that empowered them.

Keywords: Ethical leadership, Ethical nursing leadership, Entrepreneur, Ethical fitness, Ethic of care, Moral principles, Pioneer, Social justice.

LEARNING GUIDE

After Completing this Chapter, the Reader Should be Able to

* Become aware of the five myths of leadership.

* Describe what it means to be an ethical leader.

* Understand the reasons why ethical leadership is becoming popular.

* Give reasons why ethical nursing leadership is needed.

* Explain the four key aims of ethical leadership.

* Understand the association between ethical nursing leadership theory, moral values, effective communication skills, ethical fitness and the ethic of care.

* Apply what was learned to the Case in Point: When a student nurse recounts a leadership strategy that empowered them.

* Be inspired to take on the challenge of being the change.

Ethical leaders ensure that moral conduct is a standard expectation for people in positions of power and this final Chapter of this book introduces ethical leadership as the new way of leading for nurses. The discussion begins by reviewing five common myths of leadership. An explanation is given as to why the topic of ethical leadership has become popular in recent years. The four key aims of ethical leadership are presented. Reasons are given as to why ethical nurse leaders are needed. The association between ethical nursing leadership and the ethic of care are explained and nurses are inspired to take on the challenge of being agents for change. In the Case in Point a student nurse recounts a leadership strategy that empowered them.

THE FIVE MYTHS OF LEADERSHIP

Leadership is often not what we assume it to be, yet many people have ingrained beliefs and ideas as to what leadership consists of. Some view leadership as something that is for the elite few and see a leader as a person who is larger than life (Myers, 2012). They often assume that for someone to be a leader they must possess an impressive title, but titles have very little to do with actual leadership (Maxwell, 2007). According to Maxwell (2007) authentic leadership cannot be bestowed, appointed or inherited. It must be earned. We will now review the five most common myths that are associated with leadership as identified by Maxwell (2007).

1. The Management Myth

Many people assume that management and leadership are the same but they are not. One key difference between the two is that management is most often concerned with maintaining systems and the process of running the organization, whereas leadership is more focused on investing in people (Maxwell, 2007; Langlois, 2011). Traditional autocratic managers have been known to expect those who work for them to follow their advice whether they agree with it or not. On the other hand, effective leaders ensure that they get the people who work for them to buy into the vision of the organization by including them and their ideas, in the development and implementation of organizational goals. By investing in others effective leaders easily influence others to want to follow their guidance (Maxwell, 2007).

2. The Entrepreneur Myth

An **entrepreneur** is someone who has a business idea that they turn into profit (Dictionary.com, n.d.). Often people assume that entrepreneurs are leaders because they possess ideas, see opportunities and understand how to turn all of that into a financial success. However, not everyone who is good at business and finances is able to lead other people, especially if they put making money above people. If an entrepreneur genuinely wants to lead, they need to be able to pass their excitement for a project onto others and include them in the plan for action and success (Maxwell, 2007; Langlois, 2011).

3. The Knowledge Myth

We sometimes assume that the smartest person in the room should be the leader. However, people can be extremely knowledgeable in their field of expertise and still be inept when it comes to leadership skills. For example, they may be unable to convey what they know to others in a way that will motivate them to want to get involved, especially if they treat other people in condescending ways. Being smart is not enough Maxwell, 2007).

4. The Pioneer Myth

An additional misconception about leadership is that a pioneer is a natural leader. A **pioneer** is the first or earliest in a field to come up with a unique idea (Dictionary.com, n.d.). Some pioneers lack the people skills. They may have great ideas, but they must be able to act on a vision, set achievable goals, and be able to influence others to want to follow them (Maxwell, 2007).

5. The Position Myth

One of the biggest misunderstandings about leadership is that it is based on position (Maxwell, 2007). You get a promotion, you have an important title, you are the boss and you have people working for you, so everyone assumes you are the leader. Being the boss doesn't make you an effective leader especially if you are controlling and autocratic. An effective leader must know how to influence the people who work for them by investing in them and motivating them to do their best (Myers, 2012).

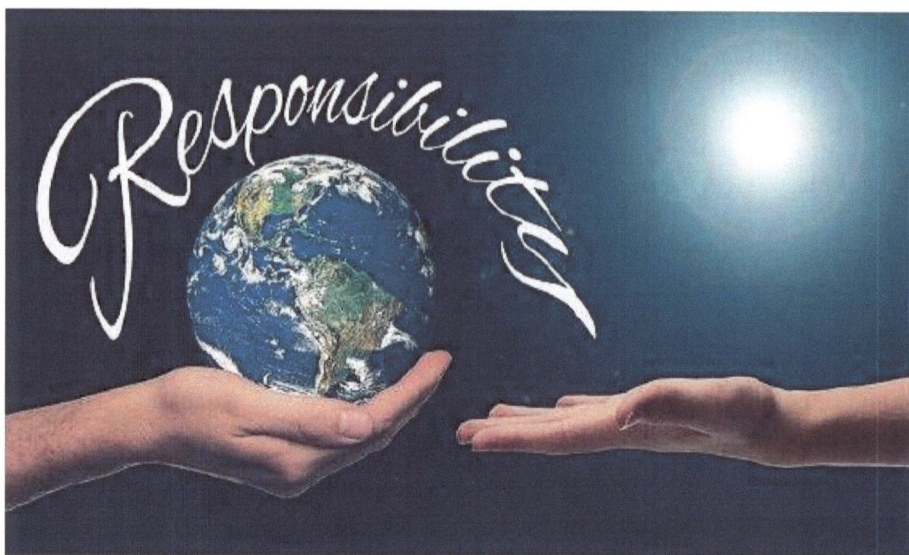

Fig. (12.1). Ethics, Leadership & Responsibility. Source: www.pixabay.com

The Definition of Ethical Leadership

"Leadership responsibility is multidimensional and cannot be described in one or two words. It is personal, interpersonal, environmental and societal." Linda Fisher Thornton, Author of the book, *7 Lenses: Learning the Principle and Practices of Ethical Leadership* (Fig. **12.1**).

While ethics is concerned with wanting to do the right thing, leaders mobilize and inspire others to work toward a common purpose, to be responsible and to pursue honorable goals, and **ethical leaders** ensure that moral conduct is a standard expectation for people in positions of power ((Kouzes & Posner, 2014; Barkhordari-Sharifabad, Ashktorab, & Atashzadeh-Shoorideh, 2017).

ETHICS & A CALL FOR VALUES-DRIVEN LEADERSHIP

"I believe that the financial crisis of 2008/9 exposed more of a lack of ethics and morality – especially by the financial sector – rather than a problem of regularity or criminality. There were of course, regulatory lessons to be learned, but at the heart, there was a collective loss of our moral compass." Paul Polman, Entrepreneur & Promoter of Equitable Business.

There are key reasons why ethical leadership has become increasingly popular in the past decade. The call for values-driven leadership in all sectors of our lives has never been louder. We live in an era when all of us, adults and youth, are bombarded on a daily basis – in the press, on the internet, or on television – with stories of ethical transgressions, short-term thinking, and moral shortcuts, surrender to group pressure, or a simple lack of attention to values (Gentile, 2015).

Furthermore, the corporate scandals associated with the financial crisis in 2008, have led to the increased interest in ethics in the workplace and generated a renewed fascination with the subject of ethical leadership (Skabinn & Herzog, 2016). The reasons for the current focus on ethics and leadership is also due in part to a recognition that modern society has been following a morally flawed standard that causes human suffering. For example, corporate economic paradigms with their ultimate quest for financial profit have circumvented the value of humans (Langlois, 2011). People are regarded as a mere resource of the enterprise and a means for corporations to achieve financial success (Langlois, 2011). The corporate aim has been to prioritize cash flow and economic transactions to the exclusion of all ethical concerns. Issues that are largely ignored include but are not limited to: the disparity between the rich and the poor, the rise in poverty, exploitation of people, unequal power in relationships, and problems associated with exclusion, intolerance and discrimination (Langlois, 2011). The realization that the former direction of a sole emphasis on corporate profit regardless of the consequences, has culminated in a new and clear goal of developing leaders who will passionately want to change that negative trajectory into something that will benefit everyone in society (Langlois, 2011). A renewed interest in ethical leadership is the direct result of this realization.

The Four Aims of Ethical Leadership

Ethical leadership has four key aims. It brings the person back into focus, it encourages organizations to invest in human potential as a valuable resource, it pursues greater social justice, and it makes protecting the environment a priority (Langlois, 2011). Profit should not be the primary focus. People are considered a value resource rather than just a commodity to be exploited or ignored. Social justice matters and too many decisions by top executives are made with a complete disregard for how those who are less fortunate in society will be impacted. Ethical leadership also challenges the conscience of the person who is a position of authority, by inviting reflection on the actions to be taken along with a commitment to an ethical perspective (Langlois, 2011). Box **(12:1)** summarizes the four aims of ethical leadership.

Why Ethical Nurse Leaders are Needed

"We have another chance to navigate, perhaps in a slightly different way than we did yesterday. We cannot go back. But we can learn." Jeffrey R. Anderson, Author of, *The Nature of Things: Navigating Everyday Life with Grace*

Box 12:1 THE FOUR AIMS OF ETHICAL LEADERSHIP (as adapted from Langlois, 2011)
1) Ethical Leadership brings the person back into focus.
2) Ethical Leadership encourages organizations to invest in human potential as a valuable resource.
3) Ethical Leadership pursues greater social justice.
4) Ethical Leadership makes protecting the environment a priority.

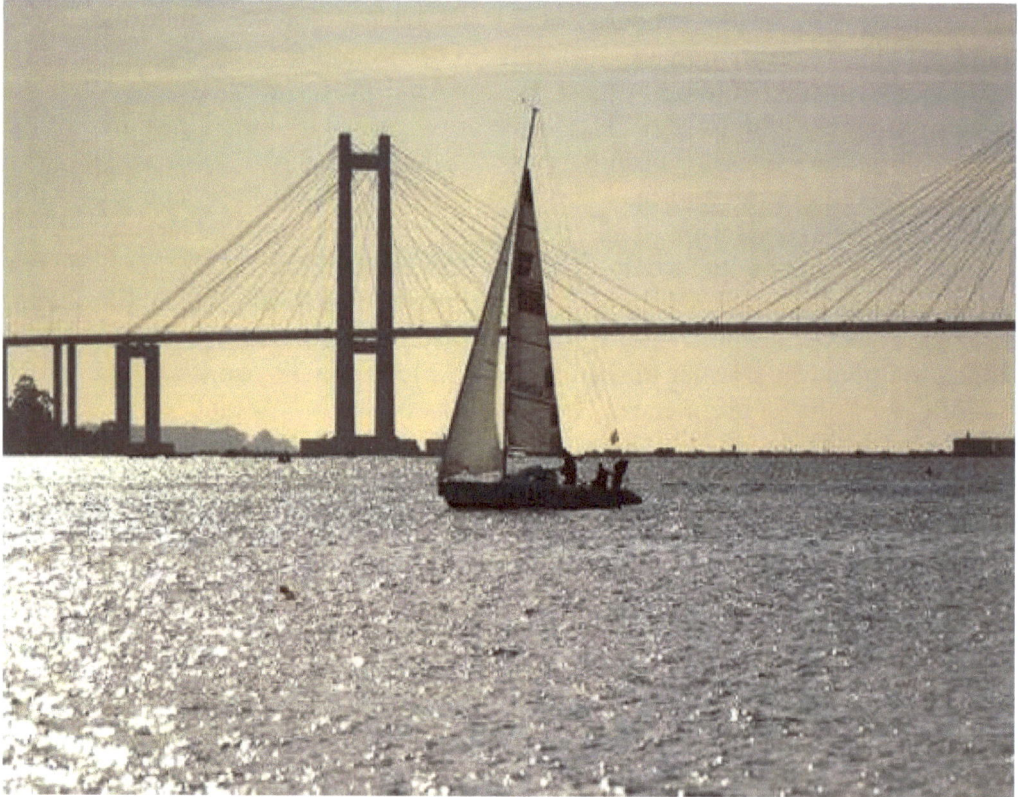

Fig. (12.2). Navigating our way. Source: www.pixabay.com

The 21st century presents unique challenges for the profession and for nursing practice. Due to advancements in technology, globalization, innovation, constant changes in health care, heavy workloads and higher societal demands, the focus of client care has become riddled with ethical dilemmas (Pangman, & Pangman, 2010; de Veer, Francke, Struijs & Willems, 2013). Subsequently, if today's nurse leaders are going to be able to successfully navigate their way in an ever-changing health care environment they need to take on the challenge of becoming ethical nurse leaders, because **ethical nurse leadership** ensures that nurses in leadership roles support other nurses to do what is morally right (Fig. **12.2**).

Nurses Feel Ill-Equipped to Deal with Ethical Challenges

Ethical nursing leadership is necessary because many nurses report that they feel ill-equipped to deal with ethically challenging situations (Makaroff, Storch, Pauly, & Newton, 2014). For instance, nurses often admit that they do not possess the skills to sort through the ethical problems in practice because ethical competencies are not taught to them in their undergraduate training (Makaroff *et al.,* 2014). A contributing factor to this problem may be related to not incorporating nursing ethics into the leadership curriculum, and since many nursing textbooks on leadership fall short in the area of ethics. For example, a review of the literature revealed that recent textbooks on nursing leadership, administration and management include very little content on ethics. Less than half of the textbooks that were reviewed had a Chapter on ethical responsibilities and many others combined ethics with law, with the focus being on law. Other nursing leadership textbooks did not include any ethical content (Makaroff *et al.,* 2014).

There are additional reasons why ethical nursing leadership is crucially needed. Although nurses are experiencing morally related stressors in their work environment, the focus on ethics has decreased over time. Nurses are also leaving the profession in alarming rates as a direct consequence of feeling unsupported by their managers to practice ethically (Makaroff *et al.,* 2014). Yet, ideally, every nurse should be given the opportunity to develop ethical leadership skills to add to their own moral compass in a way that guides the delivery of ethical, competent nursing care, and that serves as a model for other nurses to follow (Smith, 2017).

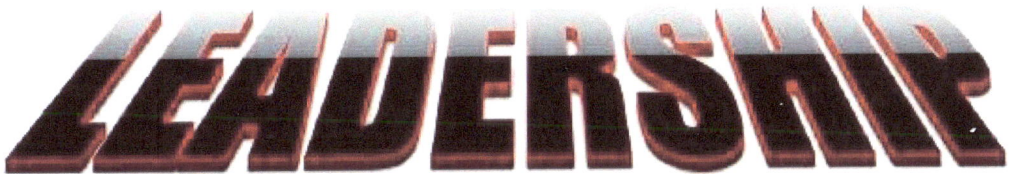

Fig. (12.3). Leadership. Source: www.pixabay.com

Box 12:2 LEADERSHIP ICE BREAKER ACTIVITY: WHO WOULD YOU BE AS A LEADER?
Sit in a large circle. Write down on a recipe card the following question, *"If you could be any leader in the world, past or present, who would you want to be and why?"* Pass the card to each person one at a time and give them a couple of minutes to answer this question.

What is Ethical Nursing Leadership?

Ethical leadership is now considered the gold standard in the business world and has made its debut into the field of nursing (Skabinn & Herzog, 2016; Barkhordari-Sharifabad *et al.,* 2017). **Ethical nursing leadership** is moral leadership and focuses on nurses in positions of power supporting other nurses to do what it is ethically right. It includes abiding by a Code of Ethics, following standards of practice and putting patients first (Skabinn & Herzog, 2016; CNA, 2017; Bjarnason & LaSala, 2011). The goal of ethical nursing leadership is to ensure that all patients are treated with care in a safe, ethical, competent, compassionate manner and with the utmost respect (CNA, 2017). Ethical nurse leaders are concerned with a commitment to fairness and trust as well as being proactive and not reactive (Bjarnason & LaSala, 2011; Kangasniemi *et al.*, 2015). They also embrace ethical values such as honesty, care, respect, accountability, courage, competency, compassion and effective communication skills (Smith, 2017).

Box 12:3 LEARNING ACTIVITY: TELL US YOUR STORY
Sit in a large circle. Now think about someone in your life who stands out as a leader, perhaps someone who had a positive or profound impact on you or your life. They do not have to be a nurse or a person who has a title. They can be anyone, either in the past or present. What makes them a leader and why? Each person should of an opportunity to tell their story. You may want to pass around a talking stick if you have one. Ensure that you only share with the group what you feel safe sharing.

Ethical Nursing Leaders make Investing in Others a Priority

"Divorced from ethics, leadership is reduced to management and politics to mere technique." James MacGregor Burns, American Historian & Political Scientist.

Ethical nurse leaders are most successful when they invest in others and they understand that investing in people is the key to an effective and safe work environment. Subsequently, they set out to form strong relationships by taking a genuine interest in everyone on their team. They make time to get to know their fellow workmates and what is going on in their lives. Maxwell (2007) would refer to this as the ability to connect with others on a human to human level. The following story illustrates what a positive effect that ethical nursing leadership can have on another nurse (Fig. **12.4**) Box **(12:4)**.

Ethical Nursing Leadership & Ethical Fitness

Ethical nurse leaders strive to achieve ethical fitness. **Ethical fitness** consists of the way in which one prepares to make good choices and to take actions that will benefit others, especially those under our watch and care (Storch, 2013). To be fit ethically can be compared to getting physically fit. It involves achieving moral fortitude through continual practice, a commitment to achieving better and more morally sound practices, and applying ethical principles to decision-making

(Kiddler, 2009 as cited in Storch, 2013; Bjarnason & LaSala, 2011). Some of the ethical principles practiced by ethical nurse leaders include but are not limited to autonomy, advocacy, beneficence, non-maleficence and respect for dignity (Bjarnason & LaSala, 2011).

Box 12:4 Narrative: When Caring Matters

I can remember when my mother died suddenly in a car accident. I was working as a new nurse on a medical ward at the time. Most of the people that I worked with on that ward had heard that my mother had died but no one said anything to me, except for my Nurse Manager. When she learned that my mother had been killed in a fatal car crash she immediately called me into her office. She told me how sorry she was for my loss and asked me how she could better support me through my time of grief. I burst into tears and she just stayed quiet and allowed me to cry. I don't remember what else my Nurse Manager said to me after that, but I do remember that she was really understanding and that I felt that she genuinely cared about me. Over the course of the next six months, this same Manager checked in with me from time to time to see how I was doing. This made me feel valued. I have never forgotten My Manager's acts of kindness at a time when I was going through so much pain and grief.

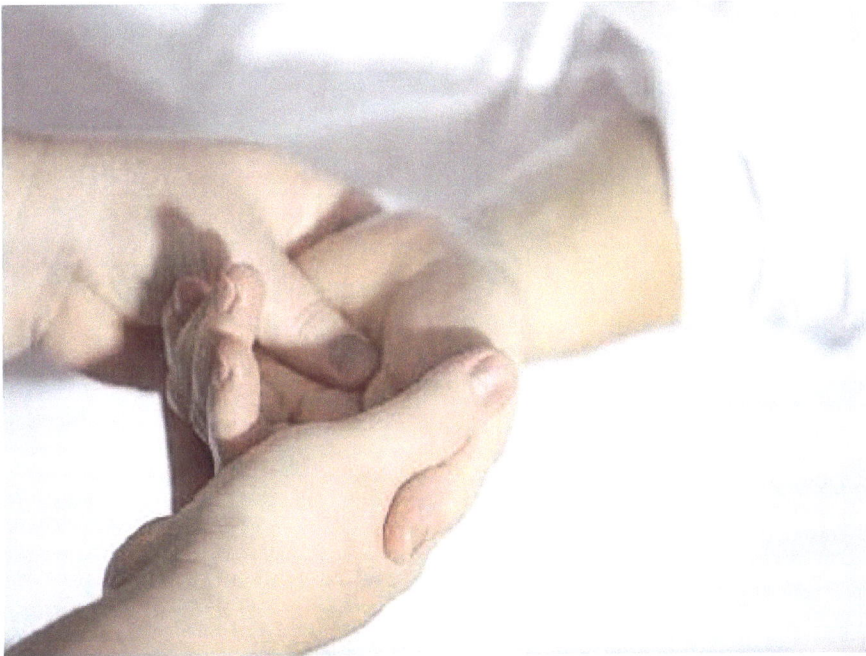

Fig. (12.4). Caring hands. Source: www.pixabay.com

In order to work toward ethical fitness a nurse must increase their capacity for self-awareness and other awareness through the process of on-going reflection and by consultation with other colleagues (Stephany, 2015). It is about nurses having conversations with other nurses about how they can best apply or incorporate ethics into their daily round and how they can evaluate what each person could do better next time (Storch, 2013).

Ethical Nursing Leadership & The Ethic of Care

"We have no means of discriminating between right and wrong if we do not take into account others' feelings, others' sufferings." His Holiness, the 14th Dalai Lama.

The ethic of care is an essential component of ethical nursing leadership. The ethic of care places significant importance on all relationships, incorporates caring, context and meaning making into decisions concerning patients and ensures that no one is intentionally hurt or harmed (Langlois, 2011; Stephany, 2012). The ethic of care and ethical nursing leadership share these key values: autonomy, beneficence, non-maleficence, advocacy, caring-concern, empathy and compassion. Both theories oppose discrimination, support social justice, emphasize human goodness and value lived experiences (Langlois, 2011; Stephany, 2012). Box **(12:5)** summarizes the key components of ethical nursing leadership and Box **(12:6)** points out the similar focus of the ethic of care and ethical nursing leadership.

Box 12:4 KEY ASPECTS OF ETHICAL NURSING LEADERSHIP
(as adapted from Skabinn & Herzog, 2016; Smith, 2017; Kiddler, 2009; Storch, 2013; CNA, 2017; Stephany, 2012)
1. Ethical nursing leadership explicitly focuses on nurses in positions of power supporting other nurses to do what is ethically right.
2. The goal of ethical nursing leadership is to ensure that all patients are treated with care in a safe, ethical, competent, compassionate manner and with the utmost respect.
3. Ethical nurse leaders embrace ethical values such as honesty, care, respect, accountability, courage, competency & compassion.
4. Ethical Nurse leaders possess effective communication skills.
5. Ethical nurse leaders strive to be ethically fit.
6. Ethical nurse leaders and the ethic of care share the same key values. They abide by the same moral principles, they promote social justice, they emphasize human goodness & value lived experiences.

Box 12:5 (as adapted from Stephany, 2012; Langlois, 2011)	
THE ETHIC OF CARE:	**ETHICAL NURSING LEADERSHIP:**
Emphasizes the interconnectedness of all of life	Human connection is important
Ethical Decision making should occur in a caring environment	Caring nurses should be involved in decision making

Relationships matter	Values relationships
Principles & Values include: autonomy, beneficence, non-maleficence, advocacy, caring-concern, empathy, compassion & unconditional positive regard	Principles & Values include advocacy, autonomy, beneficence, non-maleficence, trust, honesty, transparency, compassion, caring-concern & empathy
Context is important	Effective communication is essential
Opposes discrimination	Emphasizes respect & dignity in the workplace
Promotes social justice	Endorses and supports causes of social justice
Goal is a healthy society	Aim is to create and sustain a healthy work environment for the delivery of health care
Emphasizes human goodness	Views humans as the most valuable component of the organization
Values lived experience and listening to a patient's story	Values lived experience

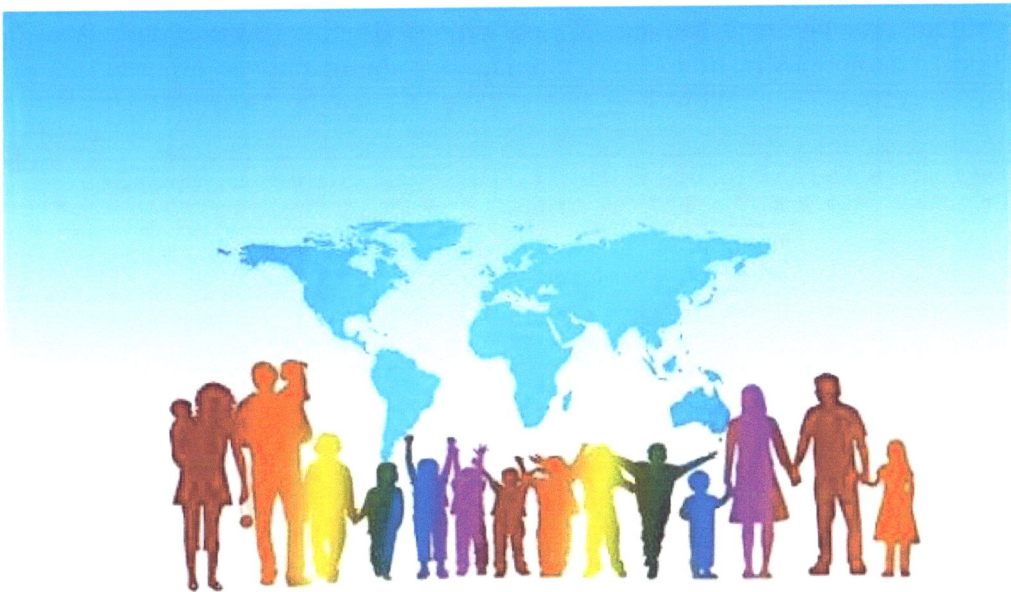

Fig. (12.5). Coming Together. Source: www.pixabay.com

NURSES TAKING THE LEAD BY BECOMING THE CHANGE

"Be the change you wish to see in the world." Mahatma Gandhi, Indian Civil Rights Activist.

This is the last Chapter of a revised edition of a book on the ethic of care as a moral compass for Canadian nursing practice. In closing, it is my hope that nurse leaders will be inspired to embrace the ethic of care as a lived virtue in order to make our world a better place for everyone (Fig. **12.5**). How do we begin this journey? Deepak Chopra (2005) asserts that all change begins when we alter our attitude. The attitude that we must adopt has been a reoccurring theme throughout this book: that understand that we are all connected and what happens to someone else affects us all. Other people's suffering is our suffering. Therefore, we must live a compassionate life and be willing to get involved (Pipe & Bortz, 2009). We can't just stand by and watch from a distance and hope that someone else will make things better. As nurses we need to be willing to take political action if necessary (CNA, 2017). We must be visionary and take on what may seem like an impossible task and do it anyways (Grossman & Valiga, 2005). Problems don't have to scare us. They can force us to look for solutions. However, if we are to succeed in problem solving we will have to work together, to connect with other like-minded individuals and challenge what always has been, with new and innovative ideas (Grossman & Valiga, 2005). We must cultivate forgiveness and gratitude and facilitate healing of past wrongs (Pipe & Bortz, 2009; Watson, 2008). The notions in Box **(12:7)** summarize some of the ways that nurses can make change happen followed by an inspirational poem by Algeron Black.

Box 12:6 NURSES TAKING THE LEAD BY BECOMING THE CHANGE (as adapted from Grossman & Valiga, 2005, CNA, 2017; Pipe & Bortz, 2009; Watson, 2008)
1. Be willing to get involved (politically if needed) in order to use single and collective voices to make a case for progressive change for people who have no voice.
2. Be visionary by being willing to suggest what might seem impossible (*e.g.*, like working to end all poverty and hunger).
3. Aim to transform problems into solutions.
4. Be able to resolve conflict.
5. Focus on cooperation rather than competition.
6. Be able to form relationships with all stakeholders and connect with others of like mindedness to challenge old, bureaucratic organizational structures and old ways of doing things.
7. Be willing to develop meaningful rituals for cultivating forgiveness, gratitude and healing interactions.

This Is a Call to the Living

This is a call to the living,
To those who refuse to make peace with evil,
With the suffering and the waste of the world.
This is a call to the human, not the perfect,
To those who know their own prejudices,
Who have no intention of becoming prisoners of their own limitations.

This is a call to those who remember the dreams of their youth,
Who know what it means to share food and shelter,
The care of children and those who are troubled,
To reach beyond barriers of the past
Bringing people to communion.
This is a call to the never ending spirit,
Of the common man, his essential decency and integrity,
His unending capacity to suffer and endure,
To face death and destruction and to rise again,
And build from the ruins of life.
This is the greatest call of all,
The call to a faith in people.

Algeron Black, Leader of Ethical Culture & Defender of Social Justice

Box 12:7 CASE IN POINT: GETTING A SECOND CHANCE
My name is Sonya and I want you to hear my story of how an instructor helped me to succeed. It was my fifth semester in nursing school. I had just failed my mental health clinical rotation and I felt devastated. Lucky for me I was allowed a second chance, but I was petrified that I would fail again. One more failure and I was out of the program. For my repeat clinical experience, I was assigned a different nursing instructor, Mr. Narang. I met with Mr. Narang before the start of the semester. At our first meeting I tried my best to be up front concerning what I perceived were my main reasons for being unsuccessful. I told Mr. Narang that I was a very poor communicator and that people with mental illness just scared me. That was why I hid and tried my best not to spend time with mental health patients. I expressed that in my opinion, my previous instructor had failed me for all the right reasons. Mr. Narang just listened as I rambled on and on. After I had finished talking, he finally spoke. He told me that he had read thorough my file and noted that I was an exceptional nursing student in many ways. He pointed out that I was academically strong and that more than one previous instructor had commented in my evaluation summary that I was especially compassionate and caring with very ill, frail and elderly patients. This seemed like news to me, although I did feel especially compassionate to some of the patients that I had cared for in the past. Mr. Narang went on to explain that my caring skills for these patients could be transposed to patients suffering from mental illness. He then handed me an article with a title, *The Experience of Living with Chronic Mental Illness: A Photovoice Study*. Mr. Narang asked me to read the article carefully so I could better understand the experiences of mental health patients and stigma, especially their experience of being judged by health care providers. Mr. Narang went on to explain, *"People who suffer from mental illness are just people first. You don't have to be afraid of them. You are more at risk of being assaulted in a domestic dispute than by a mental health patient. Furthermore, I will do everything that I can, as your instructor to support you to gain the confidence and courage that you need to realize this fact, but the rest is up to you."* The next thing that he said rang loudly in my ears, *"You are in the driver's seat. It is up to you to ensure that you do what it takes to pass. I cannot make it happen without your commitment to succeed."* I knew then that I was under pressure and that made me feel frightened, but somehow I was less scared than I had been. Mr. Narang also suggested that I take advantage of free and confidential counselling sessions at Student Services to work on any issues that I was experiencing. I agreed that this was a very good idea. He also asked that I write down daily and weekly goals, and to bring them to clinical so that we could work on them together.

Cont.....

I left that meeting feeling a little less defeated than I had felt going into it. It felt good to have an instructor that was willing to help me to succeed. Nevertheless, I was still afraid of failing again and my anxiety over doing it right interfered with my confidence. I was trying so hard to get it all perfect that I handed in my first assignment late.

Mr. Narang was not at all impressed. He met with me and was very clear that this was not the right attitude and that perhaps I was determined to sabotage my own success as a self-fulfilling prophesy. I explained to him that I wanted to get it perfect. He gave me some very good advice. *"Sonya, you are better off turning in a slightly sub-standard assignment on time so you don't forfeit the whole grade and you will get feedback on how to do it better next time. Secondly, it is okay to ask for help."* I heeded Mr. Narang's advice and made sure I handed in all subsequent assignments on time.

I did try harder in clinical this second time around, not just for my teacher but for me. I attended counselling and I even went to drop-in sessions in Open Communications Lab to do extra role playing to increase my confidence. But I must confess, I was still anxious in the clinical setting. But instead of hiding away, I would seek out my instructor and ask for his advice on how to best to approach specific situations that scared me. Mr. Narang would sometimes do a short role play with me and then make me go and interact with the patients. Afterwards we would debrief to examine what I did well and explore what I could do differently next time. I felt supported and my confidence in my ability to effectively communicate with mental health patients steadily improved with time. I am happy to report that by the end of my clinical rotation I had passed and I was ecstatic. But more importantly, I was no longer afraid of people with mental illness and I had renewed confidence in my abilities as a nurse. I am not sure if I would have been successful if it weren't for Mr. Narang. I think that because he believed that I could do it, that helped me to believe in my own ability to succeed.

Question Pertaining to the Case in Point:

1. What specific actions by Mr. Narang demonstrated ethical nursing leadership and why?

REFLECTING BACK

Summary of Key Points Covered in Chapter 12

* There are five known myths concerning leadership: the management myth, the entrepreneur myth, the knowledge myth, the pioneer myth and the position myth.

* Ethical leadership ensures that moral conduct is a standard expectation for people in positions of power.

* There are key reasons why ethical leadership has become increasingly popular in the past decade. The call for values-driven leadership in all sectors of our lives has never been louder. We live in an era filled with stories of ethical transgressions, short-term thinking, moral shortcuts, group pressures and a simple lack of attention to values.

* Ethical leadership has four key aims. It brings the person back into focus, it encourages organizations to invest in human potential, it pursues greater social

justice, and makes protecting the environment a priority.

* Ethical nursing leadership is needed because even though the delivery of patient care has become increasingly complex, many nurses report that they feel ill-equipped to deal with these ethically challenging situations.

* Ethical nursing leadership focuses on nurses in positions of power supporting other nurses to do what it is ethically right.

* Ethical nurse leaders possess moral values, effective communication skills & ethical fitness.

* The ethic of care is closely aligned with the practice of ethical nursing leadership because they share key values, they emphasize human goodness, value lived experiences and promote social justice

SOMETHING TO PONDER

1. Can you recall a situation in practice that was handled poorly by a nurse leader? What if anything could have improved the outcome for all involved?

2. Describe an ethical issue that occurred in a clinical setting. Did you feel adequately supported by your nurse manager to do the right thing, yes or no? Please explain.

3. Is there a situation that was ethically challenging that was handled well by a nurse leader? What did they specifically do that stood out for you as an example of an effective leadership strategy?

Recommended Readings

Langlois, L. (2011). *The anatomy of ethical leadership: To lead our organizations in a conscientious and authentic manner.* Edmonton, Alberta: Athabasca University Press.

Maxwell, J. C. (2007). *The 21 irrefutable laws of leadership: Follow them and people will follow you.* Dallas, Texas, USA: Thomas Nelson.

Myers, B. (2012). *Take the lead: Motivate, inspire, and bring out the best in yourself and everyone around you.* USA: Simon & Schuster, Inc.

Web Resources

Web Resource: Ethical Systems and Leadership http://www.ethicalsystems.org/content/leadership

Web Resource: Five Traits of an Ethical Leader: The Conversation
http://theconversation.com/five-traits-of-an-ethical-leader-51181

CONSENT FOR PUBLICATION

Not applicable.

CONFLICT OF INTEREST

The authors confirm that this chapter contents have no conflict of interest.

ACKNOWLEDGEMENTS

Declared none.

REFERENCES

Barkhordari-Sharifabad, M, Ashktorab, T & Atashzadeh-Shoorideh, F (2017) Obstacles and problems of ethical leadership from the perspective of nursing leaders: a qualitative content analysis. *J Med Ethics Hist Med,* 10, 1.
[PMID: 28523116]

Bjarmason, D & LaSala, A (2011) Moral leadership in nursing. *J Radiol Nurs,* 30, 18-24.
[http://dx.doi.org/10.1016/j.jradnu.2011.01.002]

Canadian Nurses Association (CNA) (2017) *CNA Code of Ethics for Registered Nurses* Author, Ottawa.

Chopra, D (2005) *Peace is the way.*Three Rivers Press, USA.

de Veer, A J E, Francke, A L, Struijs, A & Willems, D L (2013) Determinants of moral distress in daily nursing practice: A cross sectional correlational questionnaire survey. *International Journal of Nursing Studies,* 50, 100 – 108.
[http://dx.doi.org/10.1016/j.i.jnurstu2012.08.017]

Entrepreneur. (n.d.). In Dictionary.com. Retrieved from: www.dictionary.com/browse/entrepreneur

Gentile, MC (2015) Learning about ethical leadership through giving voice to values curriculum. *New Dir Stud Leadersh,* 2015, 35-47.
[http://dx.doi.org/10.1002/yd.20133] [PMID: 26894902]

Grossman, SC & Valiga, TM (2005) The new leadership challenge: The future of nursing, 2nd ed. F. A. Davis Company, Philadelphia.

Kangasniemi, M, Pakkanen, P & Korhonen, A (2015) Professional ethics in nursing: an integrative review. *J Adv Nurs,* 71, 1744-57.
[http://dx.doi.org/10.1111/jan.12619] [PMID: 25598048]

Kiddler, RM (2009) *How good people make tough choices: Resolving the dilemmas of ethical living.*Harper, New York.

Kouzes, JM & Posner, BZ (2014) *The student leadership challenge: Five practices for becoming an exemplary leader.*Wiley & Sons, New Jersey.

Langlois, L (2011) *The anatomy of ethical leadership: To lead our organizations in a conscientious and authentic manner.*Athabasca University Press, Edmonton, Alberta.

Makaroff, KS, Storch, J, Pauly, B & Newton, L (2014) Searching for ethical leadership in nursing. *Nurs Ethics,* 21, 642-58.

[http://dx.doi.org/10.1177/0969733013513213] [PMID: 24418739]

Maxwell, JC (2007) *The 21 irrefutable laws of leadership: Follow them and people will follow you.*Thomas Nelson, Dallas, Texas, USA.

Myers, B (2012) *Take the lead: Motivate, inspire, and bring out the best in yourself and everyone around you.*Simon & Schuster, Inc., USA.

Pangman, VC & Pangman, C (2010) *Nursing leadership from a Canadian perspective.*Lippincott Williams & Wilkins, Philadelphia, USA.

Pioneer. (n.d.). In Dictionary.com. Retrieved from: www.dictionary.com/browse.pioneer

Pipe, TB & Bortz, JJ (2009) Mindful leadership in healing practice: Nurturing self to serve others. *Int J Hum Caring,* 13, 35-40.
[http://dx.doi.org/10.20467/1091-5710.13.2.34]

Schwartz, AJ (2015) Inspiring and equipping students to be ethical leaders. New *Directions for Student Leadership,* (146), 5 – 14. *Doi,* 10
[http://dx.doi.org/10.1002/yd.20131] [PMID: 26894900]

Skabinn, R & Herzog, L (2016) Internalized identity in ethical leadership. *J Bus Ethics,* 133, 249-60.
[http://dx.doi.org/10.1007/s10551-014-2369-3]

Smith, M A (2017) The ethics/advocacy connection: What are the ethical leadership qualities of nurses and how do these traits contribute to competent, safe care? *Nursing Management,* 48, 18 – 23.
[http://dx.doi.org/10.1097/01.NUMA.0000521571.43055.38]

Stephany, K (2012) *The ethic of care: A moral compass for Canadian nursing practice.*Bentham Science Publishing Ltd., United Arab Emirates.
[http://dx.doi.org/10.2174/97816080530491120101]

Stephany, K (2015) *Cultivating empathy: Inspiring health professionals to communicate more effectively.*Bentham Science Publishing Ltd., United Arab Emirates.

Storch, JL (2013) Nursing ethics: The moral terrain.*Toward a moral horizon: Nursing ethics for leadership and practice* Pearson, Toronto 1-19.

Watson, J (2008) Nursing: The philosophy of caring. Revised edition University Press of Colorado, Boulder, Colorado.

GLOSSARY

Acceptance is the act of taking people as they are and where they are.

Accountability is concerned with responsible action and being answerable to someone outside yourself for what you do.

Act Deontology views each act as unique and separate. The decision to label a situation as right or wrong must be made by consulting our conscience or intuition and our choices must be also be made without the application of rules.

Act Utilitarianism applies the pleasure criteria to each specific action. An individual judges the moral status of each action by its consequences.

Active Listening is intentionally being fully present and listening to what is being said while also giving your full attention to the person who is speaking.

Advance Care Planning consists of an ongoing process of reflection communication and documentation regarding a person's values and wishes for future health and personal care if they become incapable of consenting to or refusing treatment.

Advocacy entails being the voice for or acting on behalf of the client or a cause.

Affirmative Action consists of an active effort to improve the employment or education of members of known minority groups.

Alternating Rhythms of Care consists of the notion of flexibility and spontaneity in helping relationships.

Applied Nursing Ethics is a sub-category of ethics and is more involved with the practice of nursing and less concerned with just applying philosophical rules for decision-making.

Atheism is a denial in the existence of God or gods or any spiritual being outside of the human experience.

Attitude consists of our opinion on an object person or matter.

Autonomy is having the freedom to make personal choices about issues that affect one's life without interference from others.

Belief consists of having confidence in the existence of something that is not necessarily susceptible to actual verification that it exists.

Beneficence is the obligation for do what is beneficial for the client.

Boundary Violations consist of intentional or unintentional actions between two people that go against well accepted social expectations.

Bullying is a drastic form of incivility that constitutes workplace violence. It consists of repeated unreasonable and purposeful cruel actions of either individuals or groups, that is directed toward a person or group of employees. The goal of bullying is to intimidate and belittle.

Calling can be described as a way in which our work allows us to demonstrate passion dignity, integrity and greater service to the greater good for all.

Canadian Nurses is a statement of the ethical values of nurses and of nurse's commitments to
Association (CNA) *Code* persons with health-care needs and person receiving care.
of Ethics for Registered
Nurses

Caring as Technology refers to caring in relationship to technology and such things as virtual reality
machines that support life and robots.

Caring-Concern is about being concerned about the person's present set of circumstances but also
about everything else that is going on in their life.

Caritas refers to the belief that caring and love are the most important forces in all of
life.

Categorical Imperatives in philosophy consist of commands that direct what a person ought to do that are
associated with morality and moral maxims.

Case Law refers to precedent decisions made in previous cases.

Civil Law is a body of laws that deal with disputes between individuals and does not deal
with criminal cases.

Civility consists of behaviour that is tantamount with respectful gracious, polite and
courteous conduct.

Cognitive Behavioural is a therapeutic strategy that teaches clients to change negative self-talk and a
Therapy (CBT) negative world view into something positive.

Common Law (sometimes called case law) is a system based on rules principles, and doctrine
based on common sense. Laws of conduct are not formally written down. A
judge makes decisions made from past legal cases.

Communities of consist of a group of people who share a common concern or interest in a topic
Practice and who come together to achieve individual and mutual goals.

Compassion is concerned with identifying with another's suffering.

Confidentiality is concerned with keeping medical information about a client private.

Conflict of Interest occurs when any aspect of nursing care clashes with a nurse's own moral beliefs
but in keeping with professional practice.

Conscientious occurs when a nurse informs their employer about a conflict of conscience and
Objection the need to refrain from providing care because of a practice or procedure
conflicts with the nurse's moral beliefs.

Consequentialism (also known as **utilitarianism**) is an ethical theory considers an action useful or
valuable if the result of that action is good. For example an action is considered
right by whether it has good consequences.

Contract is a legal agreement between two or more people that can be enforced by law.

Courage consists of working to improve something for the good of others and includes
purposeful perseverance through opposition.

Criminal Law is derived from statutory law and regulates the arrest charging, and trying of
suspected offenders. It includes decisions that are made regarding the
punishment of individuals convicted in the courts of committing a criminal act

Criminally Negligent refers to a person who in doing anything or omitting to do anything that is his duty to do shows wanton or reckless disregard for the lives or safety of other persons.

Cultural Awareness consists of the action of wanting to know what values beliefs and behaviours are important to people who are from cultures other than our own.

Cultural Competence is a skill that helps nurses to deal with cultural issues in practice in positive and helpful ways and includes cultural awareness cultural sensitivity and cultural safety.

Cultural Humility consists of a dynamic process of caregiver self-reflection whose goal is to uncover personal and systemic biases and to genuinely replace them with respectful behaviours that enhance dignity.

Cultural Safety promotes respectful engagement and strives to address the power imbalances inherent in the health care system. It also strives to cultivate an environment that is free of racism and discrimination.

Cultural Sensitivity goes beyond cultural awareness and understanding and seeks to incorporate a client's cultural beliefs directly into nursing practice.

Culture consists of the beliefs values, behaviours, customs and way of living of any group of individuals and is not limited to ethnicity.

Democracy is defined as a form of government where a constitution guarantees basic personal and political rights fair and free elections, and independent courts of law.

Demonstrating Patience contributes to the caring relationship through the process of tolerance and encouraging personal growth.

Deontology is an ethical theory that asserts that the rightness or wrongness of an act is dependent on the very nature or morality of the act and not on its outcome or consequences.

Distributive Justice as an aspect of utilitarianism is concerned with the notion of fairness and requires that the privileges of people in given situations be distributed proportionately and equally.

Diversity reflects variations in belief systems and ways of living.

Electroconvulsive is a treatment modality in psychiatry induces a self-limiting seizure in a
Therapy (ECT) controlled fashion under general anesthesia and results in changes in mood.

Emotional Intelligence is the ability to think about the consequences of your choices before acting.

Empathetic Listening is listening with the deliberate intention of wanting to understand what the other person is really experiencing.

Empathy is the action of trying to understand or experience all the feelings of another person either good or bad.

Empowerment is the process of assisting and encouraging another person to find the strength to pursue their goals.

Engrossment is the process of receiving the other person's experience into oneself.

entrepreneur is someone who has a business idea that they can turn into profit.

Esthetics is a branch of philosophy that is focused on the study of beauty.

Ethic of Care is a special proponent of applied nursing ethics. It emphasizes the interconnectedness of all of life places significant emphasis on relationships, context and lived experiences, and incorporates caring and meaning making into decisions concerning clients.

Ethic of Justice is related to distributive justice. It proposes that ethical decisions should be made by making use of universal principles and rules and that decision making be impartial.

Ethical Dilemma exists when there are two or more morally defensible courses of action that could be taken but only one can be played out in practice.

Ethical Problem is a basic statement of the key moral issues as they currently appear and sets the stage for further inquiry.

Ethical Leadership is based on an ethical foundation of trust honesty, transparency, compassion, empathy and an emphasis on obtaining positive results.

Ethical Nursing Leaders embody ethical values rights, duties, and responsibilities into their personal character and role model these values for others.

Ethical Nursing Leadership is explicitly focused on nurses in positions of power supporting other nurses to do what is morally right.

Ethics is the study of moral conduct or the right and noble action of groups and how we all should ideally act.

Ethics Committees or panels exist for the purpose of providing education advice, guidance and support in relation to ethical issues.

Ethnicity refers to a group of people who share a common and distinctive culture religion and language, often from a specific country or part of the world.

Feminism is concerned with subjectivity of experience and the ways that politics and the establishment shape experience. It also aims to end discrimination against women and all other minorities.

Fidelity is the act of keeping promises and being loyal.

Fiduciary Relationship is a special confidence in a professional who in good conscience, is obligated to act in good faith and in the interests of the person(s) in their care.

Fitness to Practice consists of ensuring that a nurse is physically mentally and emotionally able to practice safely and competently.

Gender Non-Conforming is a term that refers to persons who do not conform to cultural or social expectations of what is usually associated with their gender.

Generosity in nursing consists of the imparting of non-material substance. It is the giving of care through our actions.

Genuineness consists of honesty and being authentic and real in our interactions and communication with others.

Health is a state of complete physical mental, and social wellbeing and not merely the absence of disease or infirmity.

Health Promotion teaches people to envelope healthier lifestyles and emphasizes the importance of client empowerment.

Heterosexism refers to the stereotypical bias that assumes that the most preferred and only accepted form of sexual practice is heterosexuality.

Hope is the belief that beneficial outcomes can be realized. It is not blind optimism but consists of unwavering confidence that anything is possible if we only believe.

Humanism is a psychological theory that emphasizes the human capacity for goodness creativity, and freedom.

Humility consists of being able to admit when you are wrong as well as taking responsibility for when you do not know.

Hypothetical are associated with philosophy and consist of statements of what a person ought
Imperatives to do given the existence of a certain desire or goal.

Incivility consists of activity that is intentionally rude intimidating and hostile toward others.

Indigenous is used as an inclusive and international term to describe individuals and collectives who consider themselves as being related to and/or having historical continuity with "First Peoples," whose civilizations in many parts of the world predate those of subsequent invading or colonizing populations.

Informed Consent is consent that is given with a full understanding of available treatment options and the likely effects of those treatments if their effects are known.

Injustice equals unlawfulness and/or unfairness.

Integrity consists of integrating honest ways consistently into one's everyday actions.

Justice as an ethical principle is based on the notion of fairness and theories of justice focus on how we treat individual and groups within society. Justice as a moral virtue includes lawfulness (universal justice) and fairness (particular justice).

Law is concerned with the rules and regulations formed by government.

Logic is a branch of philosophy that is involved with research.

Maxim is the principle behind an action and in Kantianism a moral maxim is consistently expressed in the form of a universal command.

Mental Competence measures the capacity for informed choosing and whether an individual is capable of rational self-determination. Is the person mature enough to choose? Are their reasoning powers intact? Are they capable to choosing their own medical treatment? Individuals may be cognitively proficient relative to some tasks but not to others.

Metaphysics is a sub-category of philosophy and focuses on perception and knowledge and the surreal or the ultimate reality of all things.

Mindful Listening refers to actively listening to what is being said and to the overall theme of what is shared. It is concerned with holding time still and listening from the heart.

Moral Agency is the ability of a nurse to be able to act on their moral beliefs.

Moral Agency Violation occurs when the nurse is unable to act on what they believe to be morally right.

Moral Courage is the ability to adhere for the fundamental law of integrity ethics and perseverance even in the face of rejection or opposition.

Moral Disengagement consists of distancing oneself from relational aspects of nursing practice and resorting to merely performing tasks.

Moral Distress occurs when there is only one ethically right avenue of action that can be taken but institutional or other constraints prevent that right action from happening.

Moral Outrage is experienced when someone in the health care setting performs an act the nurse believes to be immoral but the nurse feels somewhat disempowered likely because of being on the fringes of the moral situation rather than directly involved in it.

Moral Principles are a set of ethical values that are used to guide decision making.

Moral Residue consists of feelings of guilt or remorse because you are unable to act on your personal moral beliefs.

Moral Silence occurs when the ability to voice your moral convictions is stifled.

Morality or **Morals** are concerned with the good or bad thoughts and actions of individuals and have been traditionally associated with religious views.

Morally inclusive practice celebrates what people have in common as well as their differences and involves the action of whole heartedly embracing diversity.

Morbidity refers to the types of health challenges in a particular group.

Mortality consists of the relative frequency of deaths in a specific population.

Mosaic is a pattern created by small pieces of material that when viewed together form an artful picture that is beautiful to behold.

Narratives are real situations and encourage an inductive process in which one can examine the notions of morality that are embedded in the story.

Non-Binary is a gender term that refers to those who are not exclusively masculine or feminine.

Non-Maleficence is derived from the concept of beneficence and is the duty to prevent harm whether intentional or unintentional.

Nurse Follower is someone who either works with or for, a nurse leader.

Nursing Leadership is a much broader concept than nursing management and includes the personality skills of the nurse leader such as the ability to influence others.

Nursing Management has been traditionally concerned with hierarchy position and authority and nurse managers are most often associated with a formally designated role of power.

Nursing Competence is essential and implies that nurses draw from evidence-based data that they are life-long learners and that they maintain competency in their field of expertise.

Ontology is the study of the basic nature of human beings.

Parish Nurse is a registered nurse with specialized spiritual knowledge who are called to promote health healing and wellness through ministry to the clients in their care.

Paternalism occurs when doctors make decisions for clients without their consent because they believe that they know what is best for their clients.

Phenomenology is a psychological theory that accentuates each person's uniqueness and focusses on lived experience.

Philosophy as a discipline studies the fundamental nature of knowledge and is dedicated to the pursuit of truth.

Pioneer is first or earliest in a field who comes up with a unique idea.

Politics is a sub-category of philosophy and is concerned with social organization and the dynamics of power.

Practice Standards guide nursing practice and the scope of nursing is legally legislated.

Precedent is an aspect of a previous legal case where a judge writes out the reasons for a decision in a specific legal matter.

Presencing involves being a safe non-judgmental place for someone and in its purest form it occurs in complete silence.

Principlism proposes that clinical decisions in medical practice be evaluated, not by philosophical theory, but by four moral principles autonomy, beneficence, non-maleficence and justice.

Professional is an educated skilled and knowledgeable individual who offers a particular service to the community and professions exist for the purpose of meeting the needs of society.

Professional Boundary is a limit that is set and determines how far a relationship can go and when it is in appropriate for the relationship to proceed.

Professional Standard is the minimal expected level of performance expected of nurses in their practice.

Race refers to a group of individuals that are connected by ancestral origin and certain biological differences such as skin pigmentation.

Racialized Ethnicity refers to the problems faced by people who are automatically associated with an ethnic background and are assumed to follow the characteristics of that ethnic group.

Reflection involves paraphrasing what you think the client may have said to ensure that you have truly understood their intended message.

Reflective Journaling involves writing about your experiences while they occur or afterwards.

Relationship-Based Care is central to the creation of a healing environment and consists of purposeful acts of compassion offered by health care professionals to the persons that they are assigned to care for and about.

Religion is the worship of a greater power or a being outside of the individual person. It involves the following of sacred texts or a book of laws and rules and emphasizes prayer service, and earning your place in the afterlife.

Resiliency is the ability to gain strength from adversity.

Respect for Self-Worth inspires nurses to embrace the intrinsic value of every person even when they have acted in less than desirable ways.

Rule Deontology embraces the notion of universality in addition to making moral judgments and argues that moral rules are universal.

Rule Utilitarianism asserts that the moral status of general rules of conduct are evaluated by judging the possible consequences if everyone is expected to behave according to the same moral rules in order to maximize happiness and decrease unhappiness.

Safety Plan is a written prioritized list of coping strategies and resources for reducing suicide risk.

Self-Awareness is the act of looking at oneself as the observer in order to gain a clearer understanding of the motives behind our actions.

Social Determinants of Health consist of the situations that people are born into live in, work in, and age in. They are shaped by the distribution of money and resources at the global, national and local levels of government.

Self-Disclosure occurs when a nurse shared some personal information about themselves that they believe may help the client.

Self-Regulation allows nursing members to set requirements for entrance into the profession devise educational requirements, set standards of practice, investigate complaints and instigate disciplinary action when indicated.

Sexual Orientation can be used to refer to sexual identity sexual behavior or both.

Social Justice focuses on the relative position of one social group in relation to others in society as well as on the root causes of disparities and what can be done to eliminate them.

Social Injustice is a relative concept about the claimed unfairness or injustice of a society.

Spirituality focusses on the energy within the individual and the connection with an animating life force that permeates every aspect of life.

Statutory Laws are laws that politicians make such as acts or statutes.

Stereotyping is expecting all people from a particular group to respond in a certain way based on perceived ideas.

Synergism refers to the energy in nature that ensures that everything is related to everything else.

Systemic Racism is also called structural or institutional racism and consists of actions, practices and policies that either maintain, perpetrate or reinforce unfair inequalities among ethnic or racial groups.

The Canadian Constitution establishes the fundamental rules and principles of how the country of Canada is ordered how its laws are made and the extent of the power of its government and its courts.

The Charter of Rights and Freedoms articulates the basic legal and democratic rights of Canadians. The rights as set out by the Charter cannot be infringed upon by government unless justifiable and any government action or law that breaches a person's constitutional rights is itself illegal and invalid.

The Supreme Court of Canada is the highest court in Canada as well as the final court of appeals within the Canadian justice system.

Theology is the study of the transcendent and supernatural often referred to as God, and includes the study of all religions and topics relevant to spirituality.

Tort is a legal term that refers to an alleged wrongdoing or harm done to another.

Transgender can be defined as identifying with a gender that differs from the one which corresponds to the person's sex at birth.

Trauma-Informed Care (TIC) is strength based and is founded on the premise of sincere responsiveness to the full impact of trauma.

Trauma-Responsiveness is acting with understanding when confronted with somewhat reactive behaviours associated with past trauma.

Trauma Sensitive is understanding that trauma is prevalent in our society and that it has negative impacts on individual health and relationships.

Two Spirit or 2-Spirit refers to Indigenous persons who identify as trans gender diverse or gender-non-conforming.

Utilitarianism also referred to as **consequentialism**, is a moral theory that asserts that any action is judged as good or bad relative to the consequences or outcome resulting from that action. What is deemed good is anything that brings us pleasure and/or freedom from pain.

Unconditional Positive is the act of offering an atmosphere that demonstrates that you truly do care and **Regard** that there are no obstacles or conditions to your capacity to help your client or client.

Values are standards that are esteemed desired important or have merit or worth.

Values Clarification as a progressive process where persons seek to understand what values are important to them and how important they are.

Veracity is the duty to tell the truth.

Victim Blaming tends to hold people burdened by social conditions as accountable for their own situations and responsible for needed solutions rather than identifying social injustice as a primary contributing factor.

Virtue is concerned with the pursuit of moral excellence.

Virtue Ethics is commonly taken to represent a fundamentally different approach to ethics. Rather than focus on right or wrong action or justified or unjustified principles, virtue ethics is said to focus on moral character.

Warmth is positive lively, outgoing and genuine interest in another person's experience that is physically felt by the person on the receiving end of the experience.

Whistle-Blowing is a form of advocacy that is more drastic than merely calling attention to an ethical issue and it must be used as a last resort.

SUBJECT INDEX